Springer Japan KK

K. Hayashi · H. Ishikawa (Eds.)

Computational Biomechanics

With 204 Figures

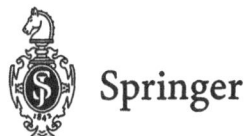 Springer

Kozaburo Hayashi, Ph.D.
Department of Mechanical Engineering, Faculty of Engineering Science,
Osaka University, 1-3 Machikaneyama-cho, Toyonaka, Osaka, 560 Japan

Hiromasa Ishikawa, Ph.D.
Department of Mechanical Engineering II, Faculty of Engineering, Hokkaido
University, N13 W8 Kita-ku, Sapporo, 060 Japan

ISBN 978-4-431-66953-1   ISBN 978-4-431-66951-7 (eBook)
DOI 10.1007/978-4-431-66951-7

Printed on acid-free paper

© Springer Japan 1996

Originally published by Springer-Verlag Tokyo in 1996.

Typesetting: Best-set Typesetter Ltd., Hong Kong

Preface

It is widely recognized that numerical analysis is a useful tool common to the fields of engineering, applied mathematics and mechanics, and medical science. Computer simulation and modeling have contributed much to the understanding of a wide variety of biomedical phenomena. In particular the use of numerical techniques is essential for solving problems involving extremely complex geometry and physical properties that arise in a wide range of biomechanics. The increased speed and expanded storage capacity of modern computers, together with newly advanced numerical and programming techniques, have greatly improved the potential for studying complicated biomedical processes.

Computer modeling techniques and their applications in the field of biomechanics have shown remarkable development in Japan in the past few years. This book focuses on these advances and shows how computer modeling and simulation are being utilized to aid and assist researchers, scientists, and clinicians in their understanding of biomedical systems from the biomechanical point of view.

The papers included in this book fall within three main areas of interest: orthopedic, orthodontic, and skeletal mechanics; circulatory mechanics; and biological and living systems. This book contains highly original papers that have been carefully selected from the studies financially supported by a 3-year Grant-in-Aid for Scientific Research on Priority Areas (Biomechanics, Nos. 04237101~04237104) from the Ministry of Education, Science and Culture, Japan, with Kozaburo Hayashi as the principal investigator. It is evident from the papers presented in this book that we can learn a great deal from the activities of researchers working on related problems in different fields of computational biomechanics. We would therefore encourage readers not only to read the papers that relate directly to their specific research interests, but also to examine the papers that at first sight might appear to be outside their field of study.

This publication was supported financially in part by a Grant-in-Aid for Publication of Scientific Research Result (No. 78023). Finally, we wish to thank the editorial and production staff of Springer-Verlag for their care and cooperation in producing this book.

Kozaburo Hayashi
Hiromasa Ishikawa

Contents

Orthopedic, Orthodontic, and Skeletal Mechanics

Circulatory Mechanics

Biological and Living Systems

List of Contributors

Orthopedic, Orthodontic, and Skeletal Mechanics

Model and Simulation of Bone Remodeling Considering Residual Stress

MASAO TANAKA[1] and TAIJI ADACHI[2]

Summary. In bone remodeling, some bone material is resorbed and new bone material is then synthesized. In this context, the new bone material may have its own natural state which is different from that of the old bone materials in its neighbors, and this nonuniform distribution of the natural state is suggested to cause the stress/strain that remains even when all external loads are removed. Our preliminary observations have also suggested the existence of residual stress/strain in the bone structure, and the model of bone remodeling is expected to take these into account. This chapter describes a mathematical model of the bone remodeling that considers residual stress from the statical indeterminacy of the bone structure. The basic idea is discussed by using a lumped parameter system and is then extended to distributed parameter systems of the conventional continuum. The idea is also combined with the lattice continuum, that is, a continuum consisting of the rigidly interconnected elastic members as the microstructure, and this is used as a mechanical model of cancellous bone with trabecular architecture. The fundamental characteristics of the model are examined through remodeling simulations of the diaphysis bone under axial load by using a cylindrical model. The proposed model for the conventional continuum and the lattice continuum is applied to remodeling simulations of leporine tibiofibula bone and bovine vertebral bone. The capability of the remodeling simulation is demonstrated by the morphology of the bone structure as well as residual stress in comparison with experimental observations.

Key words: Bone mechanics—Mechanical bone remodeling—Residual stress—Uniform stress hypothesis—Remodeling simulation

---

[1] Department of Mechanical Engineering, Faculty of Engineering Science, Osaka University, 1-3 Machikaneyama-cho, Toyonaka, Osaka, 560 Japan
[2] Department of Mechanical Engineering, Faculty of Engineering, Kobe University, 1-1 Rokkodai, Nada-ku, Kobe, Hyogo, 657 Japan

1 Introduction

Bone remodeling is a process that occurs in response to mechanical stimuli, and the bone is altered in its internal and external structure in adapting to the mechanical environment. The mechanical approach to bone remodeling is aimed at understanding the fundamental mechanism of the adaptation of living bone, clinical engineering applications such as the design and operational planning of surgical devices including implants or prostheses, mechanical engineering applications to the optimal biomimetic design of materials and systems, and so on.

A mathematical model of the bone remodeling process is the basis for these ends, and classical engineering model studies have a long history, from the nineteenth century [1–4]. In the past several decades, studies have moved from a qualitative description of the process to the quantitative one [5,6], and current studies have proceeded to mechanical models based on modern mechanics and mathematical physics [7–18]. Computer simulation encourages the detailed mathematical model and has become a standard tool in this field. The basic concept of the model of bone remodeling is described as the remodeling rate equation, that is, the constitutive equation connecting the response of the tissue resorption and deposition or its resultant with mechanical stimuli [19]. It is also described as the characteristics of the remodeling equilibrium attained as the result of the mechanical adaptation by remodeling. Both concepts must work in a complementary fashion and not conflict with each other.

In soft tissue mechanics, the residual stress or strain is understood as an important factor in stress/strain regulation at the normal state, that is, at the remodeling equilibrium, and its role is discussed from the point of view of uniformity of the stress or strain [20–22]. The authors have reported the preliminary observation of the residual stress at the zero-load state in bone structure [23,24], and have discussed the nonuniform natural state in bone tissue in accordance with uniform stress distribution at the loaded state. In bone remodeling, some bone material is resorbed and new bone material is then synthesized, and the newly synthesized bone material may have an individual natural state which is different from that of the remaining bone tissue. This suggests the nonuniform natural state does not conflict with the preliminary observation.

In this chapter, we describe a mathematical model of bone remodeling that considers residual stress and several bone remodeling simulations. First, the basic idea of the model is discussed, regarding the way in which the natural state becomes nonuniform and the residual stress remains, by using a lumped parameter system. The idea is applied to distributed parameter systems, and diaphyseal bone remodeling is described for the centric and eccentric axial load to demonstrate the fundamental characteristics of the model. Remodeling simulation is described for the leporine tibiofibula bone, and residual stress at remodeling equilibrium is compared with experimental observation. The idea is also extended to the lattice continuum, that is, a model of cancellous bone with trabecular architecture; remodeling of the bovine coccygeal vertebral body is simulated and the residual stress is examined by comparing with experimental data.

2 Basic Idea of Bone Remodeling Considering Residual Stress

We discuss here how residual stress can be taken into account for mechanical remodeling by considering the statical indeterminacy of bone structure. The basic concept of our model is described by referring to the preliminary suggestion by Seguchi [25], and the rate equations are then discussed for the parameters describing remodeling and the natural state [26].

2.1 Residual Stress Caused by Remodeling

Let us consider two linear elastic members i (= 1 and 2) with different Young's moduli E_i and cross-sectional areas A_i, which are interconnected in a statically indeterminate manner (Fig. 1a). For simplicity of the explanation, no initial stress or strain is assumed for these members, and the conventional linear elastic constitutive relation

$$\sigma_i = E_i \varepsilon_i \tag{1}$$

holds for the stress σ_i and strain $\varepsilon_i = \varepsilon$ of each member i. When the structure is exposed to the external load P, both members deform elastically to the strain ε_p, as shown in Fig. 1b and Fig. 2a, and stress σ_{pi} satisfies the equilibrium condition

$$\sigma_{p1} A_1 + \sigma_{p2} A_2 = P \tag{2}$$

When bone remodeling is activated under this mechanical condition, the stress of these two members may be regulated toward some desired condition.

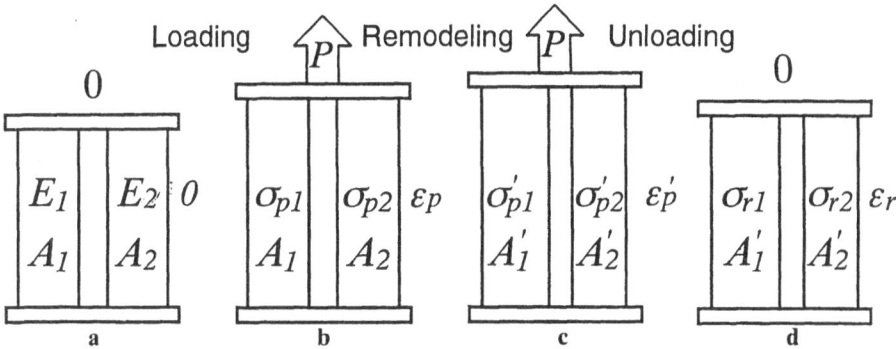

FIG. 1a–d. Statically indeterminate two-bar structure of a lumped parameter system. **a** Initial. **b** Loaded. **c** After remodeling. **d** Unloading. E, Young's modulus; A, cross-sectional area; σ, stress; ε, strain

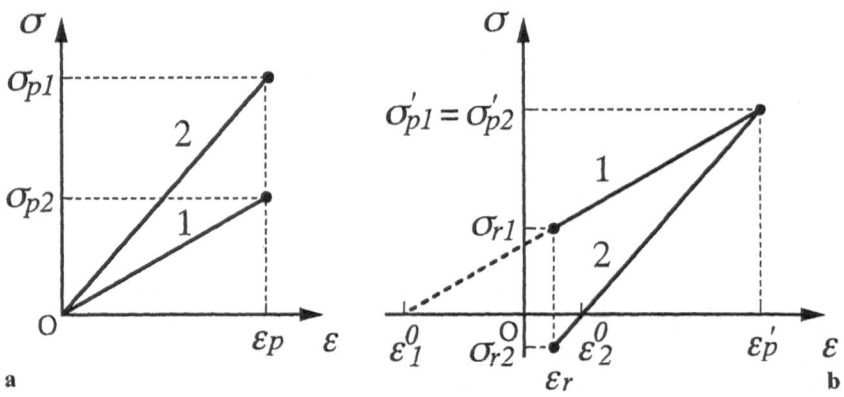

FIG. 2a,b. Change in stress–strain relationship from remodeling. **a** Loading. **b** Unloading

As the criteria to be regulated by the remodeling, different mechanical parameters have been recruited by different mathematical models of remodeling simulation. Stress, strain, and strain energy are typical examples in the context of the continuum mechanics, and a certain value or range is used to characterize the remodeling equilibrium. From the standpoint of a mechanical optimality of bone structure, the uniform stress state is assumed as the remodeling equilibrium in this study; that is, the stress state as the result of the remodeling is characterized as

$$\sigma'_{p1} = \sigma'_{p2} \tag{3}$$

under the external load P, as shown in Fig. 1c and Fig. 2b. The cross-sectional areas or the natural lengths of the members are the possible parameters of remodeling in this two-bar system, and the constitutive relation is apparently altered as

$$\sigma_i = E_i\left(\varepsilon_i - \varepsilon_i^0\right) \tag{4}$$

where ε_i^0 is the initial strain that represents the change of the natural state. This also means that residual stresses σ_{ri} and residual strain ε_r remain even when the external load P is removed, as shown in Fig. 1d and Fig. 2b, and they satisfy the self-equilibrium condition

$$\sigma_{r1} A'_1 + \sigma_{r2} A'_2 = 0 \tag{5}$$

where A'_i is the cross-sectional area as the result of remodeling. Figure 2 illustrates this change of the constitutive relation schematically. This is the summary of Seguchi's preliminary suggestion.

The uniform stress state characterized by Eq. 3 only states the relative relationship between members and is not sufficient to specify the desired stress value to be attained as the result of remodeling. That is, this model has the capability to accommodate the residual stress in the remodeling, but it is not closed yet as a mathematical model of remodeling. Thus, some constitutive relations are needed to determine the remodeling parameters resulting in the remodeling equilibrium condition of Eq. 3.

2.2 Remodeling Rate Equation

The remodeling rate equation is the most fundamental relation in characterizing the mechanical regulation process in bone remodeling. For the uniform stress state at remodeling equilibrium, nonuniformity of the stress distribution is the primal driving force in the rate equation. That is, the stress difference between members

$$\Delta\sigma_i(t) = \sigma_i(t) - \sigma_j(t) \qquad (i \neq j) \tag{6}$$

works as that for the two-bar system of Fig. 1 where t denotes the time. The effective value of the driving force is sometimes determined by taking the lazy zone into account [9], and we also define the effective stress difference $\Delta\sigma_i^e(t)$ as

$$\Delta\sigma_i^e(t) = \text{sng}\{\Delta\sigma_i(t)\} \max\{|\Delta\sigma_i(t)| - \Delta\sigma^s, 0\} \tag{7}$$

for an individual member by using a positive threshold $\Delta\sigma^s$.

As the elementary remodeling rate equation, the rate of cross-sectional area change per unit area is assumed to be proportional to the effective stress difference $\Delta\sigma_i^e(t)$ as

$$\frac{1}{A_i}\frac{dA_i}{dt} = K_i \Delta\sigma_i^e(t) \tag{8}$$

where the parameter K_i is the positive constant of remodeling rate. As the result of the cross-sectional change of each member, the effective stress difference decreases in time and the stress distribution over the two bars tends to the uniform state. Thus, the value of stress at remodeling equilibrium is determined uniquely depending on the ratio of the remodeling rate constants K_1 and K_2 [26].

2.3 Rate Equation of Initial Strain

We discuss here how the natural state could be altered by remodeling and what constitutive relation might be expected for the natural state. When the cross-sectional area increases by remodeling under a certain external loading condition P, the new bone tissue cannot refer to the natural state of the old tissue at the strain ε_i; thus, the new tissue has a different natural state from that of the old tissue, assuming the typical case in which the new tissue is formed with no initial stress or strain. As the result of remodeling, an individual member consists of old and new tissues and its natural state is determined by superposing both tissue materials. This change in the natural state is expressed as an initial strain ε_i^0 in the constitutive relation in Eq. 4, and its rate is derived as

$$\frac{d\varepsilon_i^0}{dt} = \frac{1}{A_i}\frac{dA_i}{dt}\left(\varepsilon_i - \varepsilon_i^0\right)$$

(9)

This process is schematically illustrated in Fig. 3.

3 Diaphyseal Remodeling Simulation

The basic idea of remodeling considering residual stress in the previous section is now examined for the fundamental case of the diaphyseal remodeling under centric axial load. The model is then extended to the one-dimensional distributed parameter system of time and space, and is examined again with diaphyseal remodeling under centric and eccentric axial load.

3.1 Under Centric Axial Load: A Lumped Parameter System

Diaphyseal remodeling under repeated centric axial load is studied by simulation with the lumped parameter model, and the characteristics of the rate type model of Eqs. 8 and 9 are examined. The diaphysis of a long bone is idealized as an axisymmetrical two-layered hollow cylinder (Fig. 4a). The inner layer of $i = 1$ stands for the cancellous bone and the outer layer of $i = 2$ for the cortical bone, and Young's moduli of layers $i = 1,2$ are denoted by E_i. When a centric load acts on this cylinder, the stress distributes uniformly in the circumferential direction, so that this model reduces to the lumped parameter system model in Fig. 1. The thickness $W_i(t)$ of layer i plays the role of the remodeling parameter A_i in Eq. 8,

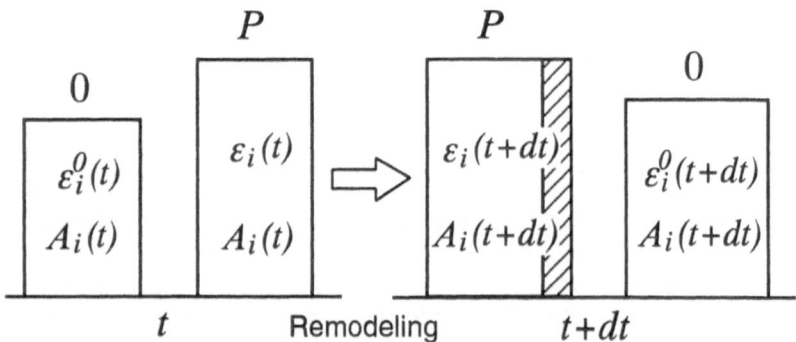

FIG. 3. Change in natural state from change of cross-sectional area. t, time

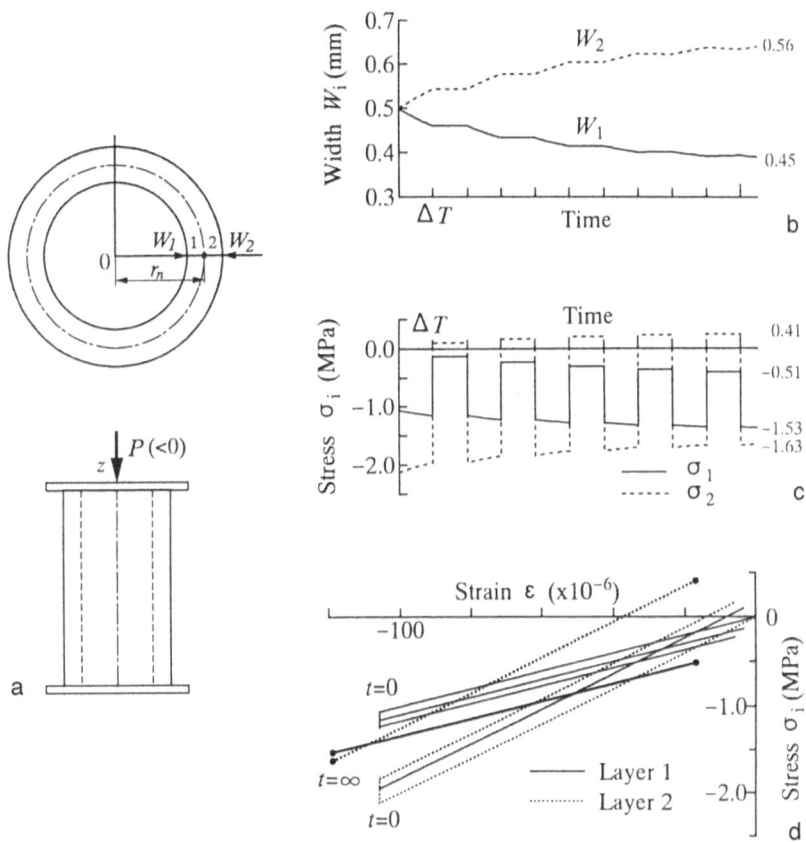

FIG. 4a–d. Diaphyseal remodeling: a lumped parameter system. **a** Diaphyseal model under centric axial load. **b** Thickness history. **c** Stress history. **d** Change in stress–strain relation (**a** adapted, from [24] with permission)

and the rate of thickness change per unit thickness of layer i is then expressed as

$$\frac{1}{W_i}\frac{dW_i}{dt} = K_i \Delta \sigma_i^e(t) \tag{10}$$

For a case study, the natural state is assumed to be uniform with no initial strain or stress at the initial state, and the remodeling simulation is studied under a symbolic repetitive load between zero and P with the period of $2\Delta T$. The simulation parameters used are as follows. The initial thicknesses are $W_1(0) = W_2(0) = 0.5\,\mathrm{mm}$, the radius of the boundary between two layers is $r_n = 2.5\,\mathrm{mm}$, Young's moduli are $E_1 = 10\,\mathrm{GPa}$ and $E_2 = 20\,\mathrm{GPa}$, the remodeling rate constants are $K_1 = K_2 = 0.1/(\mathrm{MPa}\cdot\Delta T)$, and the threshold of the lazy zone is $\Delta\sigma^s = 0.1$ MPa. The value of remodeling constant K_i is determined such that the thickness change becomes 1% for the first unit time period of ΔT.

Figure 4b shows the time history of the thickness W_i calculated by the remodeling simulation. At time $t = 0$, the applied load of $P = -25$ N results in the stress $\sigma_{p1} = -1.06$ MPa and $\sigma_{p2} = -2.12$ MPa in each layer (Fig. 4c), and remodeling is initiated by this stress difference between layers. As the result of remodeling under the external load of P, the thickness W_2 is increased and the stress σ_{p2} is decreased. In contrast, the thickness W_1 is decreased and the stress α_{p1} is elevated. The stress difference between layers becomes smaller with time (Fig. 4c). When the external load is returned to zero at $t = \Delta t$, the residual stress σ_{ri} and residual strain ε_r remain in each layer i.

With the progress of time and repetitive remodeling in the periods with external load P, the difference in residual stresses between layers gradually increases, and remodeling is also initiated during the period with zero load. As a result of successive remodeling in both loaded and unloaded states, the process approaches the steady state, and the apparent stress–strain relationship of each layer changes with time (Fig. 4d). Thus, the process by which the tissue changes its apparent constitutive relationship can be recognized as the mechanical adaptation process of the tissue through remodeling permitting the residual stress.

3.2 Under Centric Axial Load:
A Distributed Parameter System in Time

The basic idea in a lumped parameter system is extended to the distributed parameter system. To make the discussion clear, the diaphyseal model is reduced to a single-layered cylinder with both ends attached to the rigid plates (Fig. 5a). Let us consider a centric axial load the magnitude of which is time dependent. The axial stress in the z-direction still remains uniform along the circumferential θ-direction for the cylinder with uniform thickness, and remodeling equilibrium seems to be maintained in the context of spatial distribution of the stress. However, the uniformity of the stress distribution is not maintained in the time coordinate, and this nonuniformity may also drive the remodeling.

The uniformity of the stress in time is represented as the memory or inertia effect, that is, the past stress history is accumulated in terms of the convolution as

$$\sigma^m(t) = \int_0^\infty \sigma(t-s)g(s)ds \tag{11}$$

where the function g represents the effect of fading memory. Thus, the rate of remodeling is, for example, described as

$$\frac{1}{W}\frac{\partial W}{\partial t} = C_t \frac{|\sigma| - |\sigma^m|}{|\sigma^m|} \tag{12}$$

for the cylinder thickness, where the parameter C_t is the positive remodeling rate constant.

Consider the diaphyseal cylinder of radius $r_n = 2.5$ mm with the unit wall thickness $W = 1.0$ mm initially. Young's modulus is assumed to be $E = 15$ GPa. It is also assumed that the bone cylinder is at remodeling equilibrium with the uniform stress of $\bar{\sigma}$ under the centric compressive load $P = -15$ N, and with no initial strain $\varepsilon^0 = 0$. The rate constant is set to be $C_t = 0.16$/day. When the centic compressive load is increased from $P = -15$ N to $P = -30$ N, the stress difference between the instantaneous stress $\sigma(0)$ and the memory stress $\sigma^m(0)$ becomes positive, and remodeling is activated to increase the bone wall thickness. As the wall thickness W increases by remodeling with the memory function of $g(t) = C\exp(-Ct)$, $C = 0.1$, the stress $\sigma(t)$ is regulated to decrease and the stress difference becomes smaller (Fig. 5c). A new equilibrium is then attained in about 20 days. In this adaptation process, cross-sectional area increases from 15.71 mm² to 24.20 mm² (Fig. 5b).

3.3 Under Eccentric Axial Load: A Distributed Parameter System in Space

When the axial load acting on the diaphyseal cylinder becomes eccentric, the stress in the z-direction distributes along the circumferential θ-direction. This nonuniformity of the stress in space is considered to drive remodeling as well. The nonuniformity is evaluated in terms of the spatial derivative of the distribution of the stress, and the remodeling rate of the wall thickness W is related to the second derivative with respect to space coordinate θ as

$$\frac{1}{W}\frac{\partial W}{\partial t} = -C_s \frac{\partial^2 |\sigma|}{\partial \theta^2} \tag{13}$$

where C_s is the positive remodeling rate constant.

The position of the axial load acting is denoted by $(r_e, 0)$ in cylindrical coordinates system (r, θ) for the single-layered diaphyseal cylinder with unit thickness (Fig. 6a). This is a case of remodeling simulation in accordance with the shift of the load acting position from the centric position of $r_e = 0$ to the eccentric position of $r_e = 0.5$ mm at time $t = 0$. This brings the stress distribution in the circumferential direction of θ as shown by the solid line in Fig. 6c, and remodeling is initiated. The stress is regulated by the thickness change, and the uniform stress state in space is attained at time $t = \infty$ (broken line in Fig. 6c), where the remodeling rate constant is assumed to be $C_s = 0.63$ mm²/(MPa·day). As a result, the wall thickness distributes nonuniformly (Fig. 6b), showing an increase in wall thickness at the load acting side and a decrease at the opposite side. Although the total cross-sectional area remains almost the same as the initial condition, the centroid of the cross section is altered to become the position of eccentric axial load.

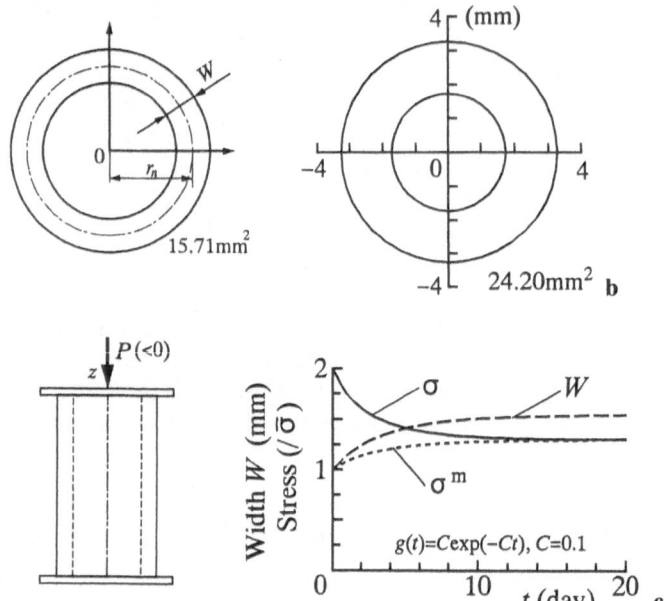

FIG. 5a–c. Diaphyseal remodeling under centric axial load. **a** Diaphyseal model at initial conditions. **b** At remodeling equilibrium. **c** Stress history (**a, b, c** adapted, from [24] with permission)

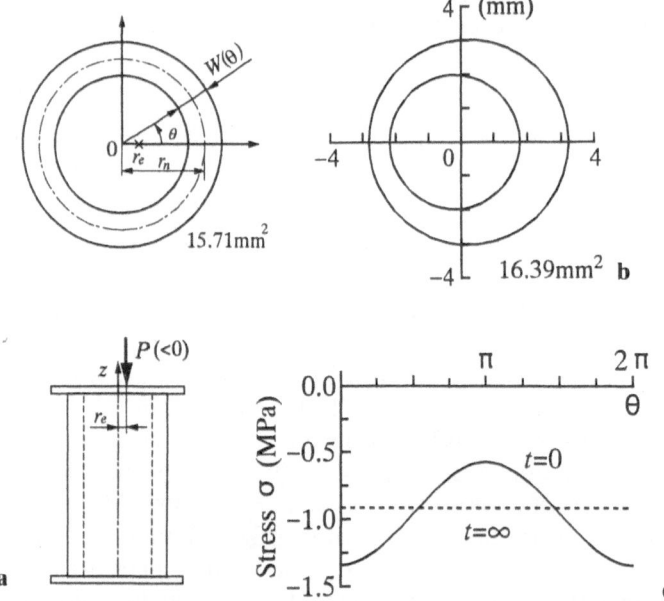

FIG. 6a–c. Diaphyseal remodeling under eccentric axial load. **a** Diaphyseal model at initial conditions. **b** At remodeling equilibrium. **c** Stress distribution (**a, b, c** adapted, from [24] with permission)

4 Remodeling Simulation of Tibiofibula Bone

The leporine fibula is interconnected to the midshaft of the tibia making a tibiofibula bone with statical indeterminacy. The remodeling equilibrium of the tibiofibula bone is simulated by using the proposed model and is examined through the residual stress release experiment by comparing with experimental observations.

4.1 Model of the Tibiofibula Bone

The tibia is modeled as a hollow cylinder with thickness $W(0) = 1.0$ mm at $r_n = 2.5$ mm, and the fibula as a circular solid column of radius $r_f = 1.0$ mm at $r_m = 6.0$ mm (Fig. 7a), making a statically indeterminate structure. Young's modulus of the bone material is $E_t = E_f = 15$ GPa for both tibia and fibula. The initial state is considered to be at the remodeling equilibrium under the force of $P = -15$ N at $r_e = 1.0$ mm, that is, the geometrical center of the tibia and fibula. The uniform natural state is assumed to be the initial state.

In this case study, the remodeling, toward the stress uniformity in both time and space, is considered for the shift of the loading point from $r_e = 1.0$ mm to $r_e = 0.0$ mm at time $t = 0$. To make the problem simple and clear, the fibula

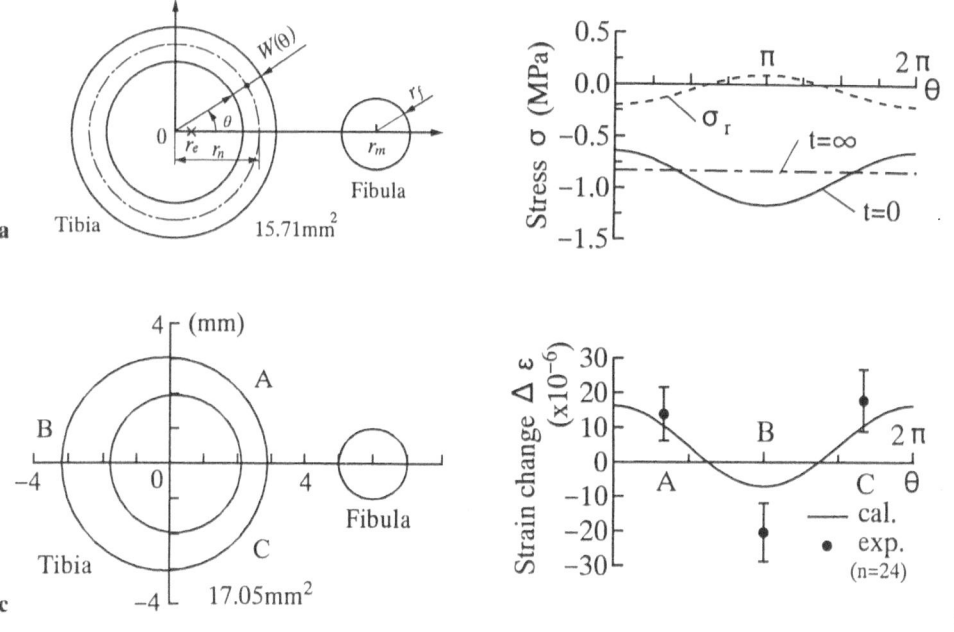

FIG. 7a–d. Leporine tibiofibula remodeling simulation. **a** Tibiofibula model. **b** Stress distribution in tibia. **c** Cross-sectional change. **d** Strain change caused by cutting fibula (**b, c, d** adpated, from [24] with permission)

is assumed to be of conventional elastic material and only carries a part of the load; that is, mechanical remodeling is considered only for the tibia. The remodeling rate equation of the thickness change of the tibia is expressed as

$$\frac{1}{W}\frac{\partial W}{\partial t} = C_t \frac{|\sigma| - |\sigma^m|}{|\sigma^m|} - C_s \frac{\partial^2 |\sigma|}{\partial \theta^2} \tag{14}$$

by superposing the rates in Eqs. 12 and 13, and the rate parameters used are identical to those in Sections 3.2 and 3.3. It is noted again that the rate equation of the natural state in Eq. 9 is always accompanied by the rate equation of the remodeling parameters.

4.2 Remodeling Equilibrium and Fibula-Cutting Experiment

The initial stress distribution in the tibia under load P is shown by the solid lines in Fig. 7b. Although the position of the loading point r_e is the same as that in the case of Section 3.2, the axial stress distribution is not uniform in the tibia because of the fibula, and the magnitude of stress in the tibia becomes maximum at the site of $\theta = \pi$. As the result of remodeling, the stress is regulated toward uniformity (Fig. 7b, dash-and-dotted line). The bone wall thickness decreases at the lateral site of the tibia facing the fibula, and the thickness increases at the medial site. The cross-sectional shape changes to that shown in Fig. 7c at remodeling equilibrium ($t = \infty$). This remodeling results in the residual stress σ_r in the tibia (broken line, Fig. 7b), and the tensile residual stress is 0.15 MPa in the fibula.

We have reported the strain change in the tibia observed by cutting the fibula of a Japanese white rabbit. To examine the remodeling equilibrium obtained by the simulation, the numerical fibula-cutting experiment is conducted here. The external load is removed from the remodeling equilibrium and that is used as the reference for the strain change in the fibula-cutting study. When the fibula is cut numerically, the residual stress in the tibiofibula bone is partially released. That is, the positive strain change is observed at the lateral site of $\theta = 0$, and the negative strain change is observed at the medial site of $\theta = \pi$ (Fig. 7d). In this figure, circumferential positions labeled A, B, and C correspond to the gauge sites employed in the experiment of the previous study [23], and the experimentally observed strain changes in microstrains are $\Delta\varepsilon_A = 13.9 \pm 7.7$, $\Delta\varepsilon_B = -20.3 \pm 8.4$, and $\Delta\varepsilon_C = 17.8 \pm 8.9$ (mean $\pm$ SD) as shown by solid marks in the figure. It is confirmed that the strain change by numerical study shows reasonable correlation with that of experimental observations.

5 Lattice Continuum Model of Bone Remodeling

Cancellous bone has trabecular architecture, and it is closely related to the mechanical remodeling of cancellous bone. Therefore, the mechanical responses of bone must be studied at two hierarchical levels of structure [27]. The external load condition acting on the bone structure determines the macroscopic stress and strain of the bone tissue as a continuum, and these govern the mechanical condition at the microstructure of the trabecular architecture. This is critical in mechanical bone remodeling of the trabeculae, in which resorption and deposition of the bone material are found. In this section we discuss the model of remodeling of the cancellous bone with trabecular architecture, that is, the extension of the model in the previous section to the lattice continuum.

5.1 Lattice Continuum of Cancellous Bone

The lattice continuum is a continuum made of rigidly interconnected elastic rod/ beams as the microstructure, and is used as a model of cancellous bone tissue with trabecular architecture [28]. Consider a two-dimensional lattice with unit thickness (Fig. 8) in which the coordinate axes x_i are chosen to be parallel to the principal axes of the microlattice structure. We denote the lattice interval as L_i, the member width as A_i, and Young's modulus of the member material as E_i.

The couple stress theory [29] is a tool to handle the continuum with the microstructure, and the constitutive relation of the lattice continuum is expressed in tensor components as

$$\sigma_{ii} = \overline{E}_i \gamma_{ii}, \quad \sigma_{ij} = 2\overline{G}\gamma_{ij}, \quad m_i = 4\overline{G}\,\overline{L}_i^2\kappa_i \quad (i,j = 1,2; \ i \neq j)$$

$$\overline{E}_i = E_i S_i, \quad \overline{G} = \frac{E_i E_j S_i^3 S_j^3 L_i^2 L_j^2}{E_i S_i^3 L_j^4 + E_j S_j^3 L_i^4}, \quad \overline{L}_i = \frac{L_i}{4}\sqrt{\frac{1}{3}\left(1 + \frac{E_i S_i^3 L_j^4}{E_j S_j^3 L_i^4}\right)} \tag{15}$$

where σ_{ij} and m_i are the symmetrical parts of stress T_{ij} and the deviatoric part of couple stress μ_i, and γ_{ij} and κ_i stand for the strain and curvature [28]. The summation convention is not assumed in this chapter. Apparent material constants $\overline{E}_i$, $\overline{G}$, and $\overline{L}_i$ as the continuum depend on the geometrical parameter of the microstruc-

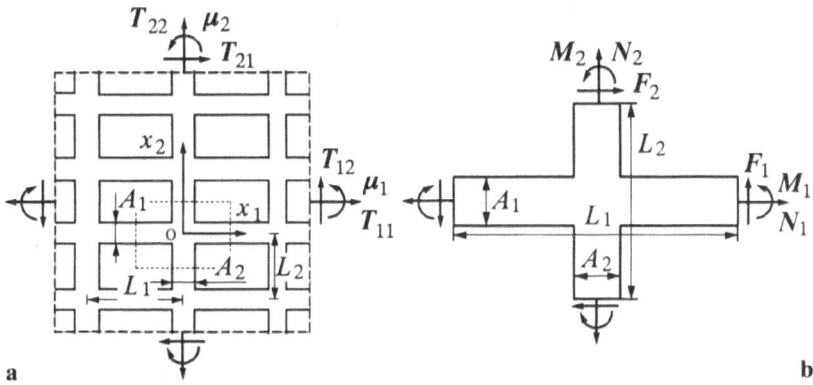

FIG. 8a,b. Lattice continuum model of bone with microstructure. **a** Macroscopic stresses. **b** Unit lattice

ture, that is, the member width ratio $S_i(= A_i/L_j)$ and the lattice interval L_i, as well as Young's modulus E_i of the lattice material itself.

The effective stress of the microstructural members is determined from the normal force N_i, the shear force F_i, and the bending moment M_i acting on the unit lattice (Fig. 8b); that is, the equilibrium of the unit lattice is written as

$$N_i = T_{ii}L_j = T_{ii}^e A_i, \quad F_i = T_{ij}L_j = T_{ij}^e A_i, \quad M_i = \mu_i L_j = \mu_i^e A_i \qquad (16)$$

and the effective stress and couple stress, $T_{\alpha\beta}^e$ and μ_α^e, are defined as

$$T_{i\alpha}^e = \frac{T_{i\alpha}L_j}{A_i} = \frac{T_{i\alpha}}{S_i}, \quad \mu_i^e = \frac{\mu_i L_j}{A_i} = \frac{\mu_i}{S_i}. \quad (i,j,\alpha = 1, 2; \ i \neq j) \qquad (17)$$

This gives us the link between the macroscopic stress T_{ij} at the continuum and the microscopic stress T_{ij}^e at the unit lattice element, that is, the effective stress at the trabeculae.

5.2 Remodeling Rate Equations

The sequence of lattice members, making a ladder structure in its transverse direction in the lattic continuum, is a recursion of the two-bar system of Fig. 1a, and the remodeling rate equation of the lumped parameter system of Section 2.2 is extended for the width A_i of the lattice member referring to the nonuniformity of the axial stress T_{ii}^e. The nonuniformity of the stress in two-dimensional space is evaluated in terms of the second derivatives as in Section 3.3, and the remodeling rate equation is written as

$$\frac{1}{A_i}\frac{\partial A_i}{\partial t} = -R_i \nabla^2 \left| T_{ii}^e \right| \qquad (18)$$

where Laplacian ∇^2 describes the difference in the neighbors, and R_i is the positive remodeling rate constant [30,31].

As to the change of the member width A_i by remodeling, the natural state is altered for the same reason as discussed in the lumped parameter system. That is, the normal component of the initial strain γ_{ii}^0 changes because of the change in the natural state of the lattice member, and is written as

$$\frac{\partial \gamma_{ii}^0}{\partial t} = \frac{1}{A_i}\frac{\partial A_i}{\partial t}\left(\gamma_{ii} - \gamma_{ii}^0\right) \qquad (19)$$

Thus, the normal strain γ_{ii} in the constitutive equation (Eq. 15) is replace by $(\gamma_{ii} - \gamma_{ii}^0)$. As a result of remodeling, the member width A_i and the initial strain γ_{ii}^0 have the nonuniform distribution in the bone tissue. Because the volume fraction of V_f of the tissue is defined as

$$V_f = S_1 + S_2 - S_1 S_2 = \frac{A_1}{L_2} + \frac{A_2}{L_1} - \frac{A_1 A_2}{L_1 L_2} \tag{20}$$

the distribution of the member width corresponds to the distribution of the volume fraction. The distribution of the natural state means the residual stress distribution in the bone tissue. It is only noted that the nonuniformity of the effective shear stress is the driving force of the mechanical remodeling, yielding the change of the lattice orientation of the microstructure when the similar rate equation model is recruited [32], while the nonuniformity in the effective normal stress is primal in relation to the tissue volume fraction.

6 Remodeling Simulation of Vertebral Body

The remodeling simulation based on the lattice model is now demonstrated for a vertebra body under repetitive bending with compression.

6.1 Simulation Model

A bovine coccygeal vertebra body is simplified as a solid cylinder of cancellous bone covered with cortical bone, and the coronal section is modeled as the plane strain problem in the radial axis r and the cephalocaudal, that is, longitudinal, axis z. It is observed that the orientation of the trabecular architecture approximately coincides with the radial and the cephalocaudal directions in the coronal section [33], and the orientations of the lattice structure are assumed to align along the r- and z-axes. The member width ratios S_z and S_r distribute in the z-r plane.

By referring to the measured values, the dimensions for the vertebra body model are determined so that the radius of the boundary between cancellous and cortical bones is r_1 = 8.0 mm, the radius of the outer surface of cortical is r_2 = 10.0 mm, the cephalocaudal length is $2 L$ = 40.0 mm, and the thickness of the end-plate is δ = 2.0 mm. Young's modulus of the member material itself is determined as E_i = 4.32 GPa by substituting the apparent Young's modulus $\bar{E}_z$ = 1.21 GPa in the cephalocaudal direction obtained in the compression test and the average area ratio S_z = 0.28 in that direction into Eq. 15. The lattice interval is L_i = 0.5 mm, and the remodeling rate parameter is R_i = 10 mm²/(MPa·day).

Assuming symmetry with respect to the r-axis, the cranial half of $z \geq 0$ is used for the remodeling simulation, and is discretized by using finite elements (Fig. 9a). The finite elements are in the form of quadrilateral crossed-triangles, and 9 × 8 elements are used for the cancellous bone inside, 9 × 1 for the cortical bone at the both radial ends, and 1 × 10 for the end-plate.

The compressive load of $\widetilde{P}$ = –3.2 N and the repetitive bending moment between $\widetilde{M}$ = 4.2 N·mm and – $\widetilde{M}$ are applied on the end-plate surface of the two-dimensional model. This is equivalent to a compressive load of P = –50 N and repetitive bending moment of M = 50 N·mm for the whole vertebra body. It is also assumed for the initial condition that the member width ratio is $S_r = S_z$ = 0.1 for the cancellous and $S_r = S_z$ = 1.0 for the cortical bone, and that initial strains are

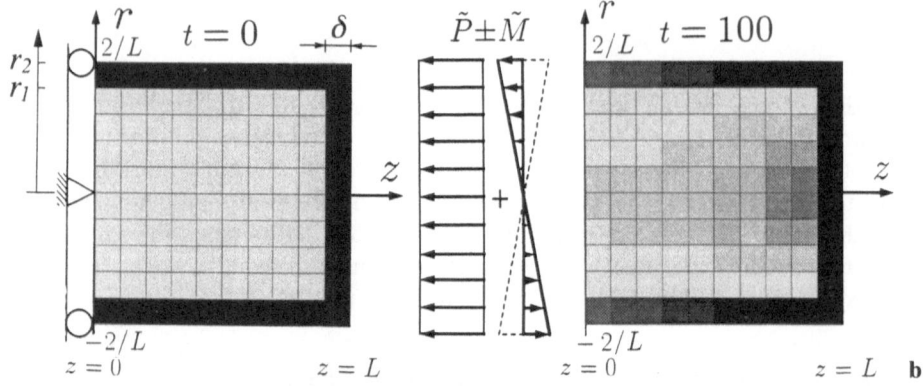

FIG. 9a,b. Bovine vertebral remodeling simulation. **a** S_z ($t = 0$) and boundary condition. **b** S_z ($t = 100$)

$\gamma^0_{zz} = \gamma^0_{rr} = 0$. The elements corresponding to the end-plate are assumed to be cortical throughout the simulation.

6.2 Stress Regulation and Residual Stress

The effective stress distribution along the z-axis is shown in Fig. 10, in which the stress is averaged over $\tilde{P} + \tilde{M}$ and $\tilde{P} - \tilde{M}$ as $\bar{T}^e_{zz}$. At $t = 0$, the effective stress distribution is significant, as is shown by the broken line in Fig. 10. The member width ratio S_z increases at the cancellous region with relatively large effective stress (see Fig. 9b), and the effective stress is regulated to become almost uniform at $t = 100$ (dash-and-dotted line, Fig. 10) as the result of the remodeling under repetitive bending. As is found in Fig. 9b, a triangular high-density region is

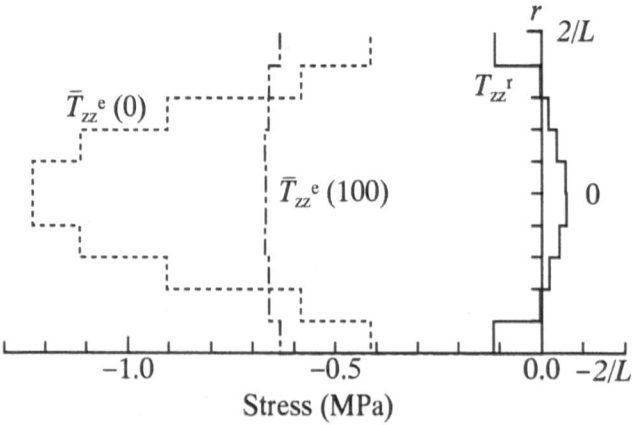

FIG. 10. Effective stress and residual stress

formed near the surface facing the intervertebral disk, which is also found in the coronal section of the vertebra body, and its apparent volume fraction is almost 0.3, similar to that of 0.28 of the real bovine coccygeal vertebral body.

At the time $t = 100$, the initial strain is no longer uniform, so that the residual stress remains in the vertebra (as shown by a solid line in Fig. 10), when all the external forces are removed. To examine the residual stress caused by the remodeling simulation, the cortical cylinder at the radial surface is isolated numerically and the strain at the cortical surface is calculated referring to the zero-load state. Experimental observations with a strain gauge, by removing the end-plate and the cancellous bone, gave $\Delta \varepsilon^{exp} = 34.0 \pm 22.1$ microstrains ($n = 9$) [24]. The calculated strain was $\Delta \varepsilon^{cal} = 38$ microstrains on the cortical surface at $z = 0$, showing reasonable agreement with the experimental values.

7 Conclusions

This chapter describes a mathematical model of bone remodeling considering residual stress. A basic idea of how the residual stress remains in the bone was considered by taking the statical indeterminacy of the bone structure, and the change of the natural state from remodeling was described in terms of the initial strain. The rate equation of the initial strain was related to the rate equation of the morphological remodeling parameter of the bone structure, and the framework of the mathematical model was established by using a lumped parameter system. This idea was extended to the distributed parameter systems of the conventional continuum and of the lattice continuum with microstructure that is considered as a mechanical model of the cancellous bone with trabecular architecture.

The model for the conventional continuum was applied to the remodeling simulation of the leporine tibiofibula bone, and the results were confirmed with the simulated morphology of the cross section and the residual stress release experiment by cutting the fibula from the remodeling equilibrium. The model for the lattice continuum was examined with the remodeling simulation of the bovine coccygeal vertebral body. The simulated distribution of the volume fraction of cancellous bone showed good correlation with that of real vertebra, and the numerical residual stress release analysis also compared well with the experimental results. The capability of the simulation model discussed here is confirmed through these studies. The model for the lattice continuum is under extension to include three-dimensional cases and considering arbitrary lattice angles; these will be reported in the near future.

Acknowledgment. This work was supported in part by the Grant-in-Aid for Scientific Research on Priority Areas [Biomechanics] (Nos. 04237101 and 06213225) and for Encouragement of Young Scientists (No. 06855015) from the Ministry of Education, Science, Sports and Culture, Japan.

References

1. Wolff J (1986) The law of bone remodeling (trans by Maquet P, Furlong R). Springer, Berlin
2. Currey JD (1984) The mechanical adaptations of bones. Princeton University Press, Princeton, NJ
3. Martin RB, Burr DB (1989) Structure, function, and adaptation of compact bone. Raven, New York
4. Cowin SC (1989) Bone mechanics. CRC Press, Boca Raton
5. Frost HM (1964) Mathematical elements of lamellar bone remodeling. Thomas, Springfield
6. Kummer BKE (1972) Biomechanics of bone: mechanical properties, functional structure, functional adaptation. In: Fung YC, Perrone N, Anliker M (eds) Biomechanics: its foundations and objectives. Prentice-Hall, Engle Wood Cliffs, NJ, pp 237–271
7. Cowin SC, Hegedus DH (1976) Bone remodeling: I. Theory of adaptive elasticity. J Elasticity 6(3):313–326
8. Hart RT, Davy DT, Heiple KG (1984) A computational method for stress analysis of adaptive elastic materials with a view toward applications in strain-induced bone remodeling. Trans ASME J Biomech Eng 106:342–350
9. Huiskes R, Weinans H, Grootenboer HJ, Dalstra M, Fudala B, Slooff TF (1987) Adaptive bone-remodeling theory applied to prosthetic-design analysis. J Biomech 20(11/12):1135–1150
10. Carter DR, Fyhrie DP, Whalen RT (1987) Trabecular bone density and loading history: regulation of connective tissue biology by mechanical energy. J Biomech 20(8):785–794
11. Carter DR, Orr TE, Fyhrie DP (1989) Relationships between loading history and femoral cancellous bone architecture. J Biomech 22(3):231–244
12. Fyhrie DP, Carter DR (1990) Femoral head apparent density distribution predicted from bone stresses. J Biomech 23(1):1–10
13. Beaupre GS, Orr TE, Carter DR (1990) An approach for time-dependent bone modeling and remodeling-application: a preliminary remodeling simulation. J Orthop Res 8:662–670
14. Weinans H, Huiskes R, Grootenboer HJ (1992) The behavior of adaptive bone-remodeling simulation models. J Biomech 25(12):1425–1441
15. Cowin SC, Sadegh AM, Luo GM (1992) An evolutionary Wolff's law for trabecular architecture. Trans ASME J Biomech Eng 114:129–136
16. Van Rietbergen B, Huiskes R, Weinans H, Sumner DR Turner TM, Galante JO (1993) The mechanism of bone remodeling and resorption around press-fitted THA stems. J Biomech 26(4/5):369–382
17. Sadegh AM, Luo GM, Cowin SC (1993) Bone ingrowth: an application of the boundary element method to bone remodeling at the implant interface. J Biomech 26(2):167–182
18. Weinans H, Huiskes R, Grootenboer HJ (1994) Effects of fit and bonding characteristics of femoral stems on adaptive bone remodeling. Trans ASME J Biomech Eng 116:393–400
19. Cowin SC (1993) Bone stress adaptation models. Trans ASME J Biomech Eng 115:528–533
20. Fung YC (1984) Biodynamics: circulation. Springer, Berlin, p 64

21. Takamizawa K, Hayashi K (1987) Strain energy density function and uniform strain hypothesis for arterial mechanics. J Biomech 20(1):7–17

22. Liu SQ, Fung YC (1989) Relationship between hypertension, hypertrophy, and opening angle of zero-stress state of arteries following aortic construction. Trans ASME J Biomech Eng 111:325–335

23. Tanaka M, Adachi T, Seguchi Y, Morimoto Y (1992) Residual stress of biological tissues and model of adaptation by remodeling. In: Fujiwara H, Abe T, Tanaka K (eds) Residual stress: III. Science and technology, vol 1. Elsevier, New York, pp 134–139

24. Tanaka M, Adachi T, Tomita Y (1993) Bone remodeling considering residual stress: preliminary experimental observation and theoretical model development. In: Held DK, Brebbia CA, Ciskowski RD, Power H (eds) Computational biomedicine. Computational Mechanics, Southampton, pp 239–246

25. Seguchi Y (1989) Preliminary study on adaptation by remodeling. In: Woo SL-Y, Seguchi Y (eds) Tissue Engineering-1989, BED-14. American Society of Mechanical Engineers, New York, pp 75–78

26. Tanaka M, Adachi T (1992) Preliminary study on mechanical bone remodeling permitting residual stress. Trans Jpn Soc Mech Eng 58(551):1022–1029

27. Cowin SC, Moss-Salentijn L, Moss ML (1991) Candidates for the mechanosensory system in bone. Trans ASME J Biomech Eng 113(2):191–197

28. Adachi T, Tomita Y, Tanaka M (1994) Cosserat continuum model of bone structure and simulation. In: Proceedings, 37th Japanese Congress on Materials Research, Society of Materials Science, pp 215–221

29. Koiter WT (1964) Couple-stress in the theory of elasticity. Proc K Ned Akad Wet Ser B Palaeontol Geol Phys Chem Anthropol 67:17–44

30. Tanaka M, Adachi T, Tomita Y (1994) Regulation model of microstructural stress in trabecular bone remodeling. In: Abstracts of second world congress on biomechanics, 10–15 July 1994. Amsterdam, p 240

31. Adachi T, Tomita Y, Tanaka M (1994) Mechanical bone remodeling considering residual stress: a lattice continuum model. In: Askew MJ (ed) 1994 Advances in bioengineering, BED-28. American Society of Mechanical Engineers, New York, pp 255–256

32. Adachi T, Tanaka M, Tomita Y (1995) Skew lattice continuum model of trabecular bone remodeling (in Japanese). Jpn Soc Mech Eng 95(3):110–111

33. Adachi T, Tomita Y, Matsui O, Tanaka M (1995) Measurement of quantitative characteristics of vertebral trabecular architecture: distribution of trabecular density and orientation. Journal of Japanese Society for Clinical Biomechanics and Related Research, 16:173–176

Functional Adaptation of Mandibular Bone

Norio Inou[1], Yuzuru Iioka[2], Hiroshi Fujiwara[3], and Koutarou Maki[4]

Summary. This study examined the human mandible from the biomechanical point of view. This chapter covers two subjects: mechanical events that occur in the human mandible during biting, and the basic behavior of the functional adaptation of bone. To estimate mechanical response in the mandible, we proposed an individual modeling method based on X-ray computed tomography (CT) data of the individual that consists of four parts. First, we extracted contour images of the mandibular shape from the X-ray CT data. Second, we made a surface model covered with polygons. Third, we provided an approximate model modified from a standard type of model. Finally, we obtained an individual finite-element model by transforming the approximate model so that it fitted the shape of the surface model. Using the model, we analyzed the stress distribution of the mandible during biting. The stress distributes in the whole area of the mandible, although there are some regions that are highly stressed. The stress distribution was compared with the bone density distribution, and a strong correlation was found. This correlation tells us that the human mandibular bone also has functional adaptation. Based on the analytical results, we discussed the mechanical rationality of the human mandible and the basic behavior of functional adaptation. To examine mechanical rationality, we determined bone robustness by calculating the ratio of stress value to bone strength for every element. The result shows that the human mandible takes a rational structure because the ratio is almost uniform throughout the mandible. To examine the basic behavior of functional adaptation, we proposed a model of functional adaptation and showed that the proposed model self-organizes a proper mechanical structure. We also showed that mechanisms of mandibular deformity can be explained successfully by the proposed model.

[1] Department of Mechanical and Environmental Informatics, Tokyo Institute of Technology, O-okayama, Meguro-ku, Tokyo, 152 Japan
[2] Seiko Corporation, Akanehama, Narashino, Chiba, 275 Japan
[3] Ricoh Corporation, Ohta-ku, Tokyo, 143 Japan
[4] Department of Orthodontics, Showa University, Ohta-ku, Tokyo, 145 Japan

Key words: Mandibular bone—Stress analysis—Individual modeling—Functional adaptation—Mandibular deformity

1 Introduction

Mandibular bones are essential organs for the mastication of foods. They can be regarded as mechanical parts that receive outer forces from teeth and the masticatory muscles. We expect that the mandibular bones have mechanical rationality because they endure large forces during biting. It is often said that bones appear to be well- designed from the point of view of structural engineering. The "maximum-minimum law" claimed by Roux [1] is a famous concept to explain the mechanical rationality of bone. Roux's law states that a bone provides a maximum of strength with a minimum of constructive material. According to his interpretation, stress distribution in the bone will be almost uniform under a set of loading conditions. The finite-element method (FEM) is a useful tool to examine the problem. However, there are few reports on this theme although there are many studies on stress analyses. The main reason is the difficulty of making a model. For validation, an accurate model is required because the fidelity of the model directly affects the mechanical profile.

Roux also proposed an idea of functional adaptation that means "adaptation of an organ to its function by practicing the latter." He assumed that functional adaptation achieves the maximum-minimum design of a bone. Based on Roux's law, Pauwels explained the functional adaptation as a kind of feedback mechanism [2]. The basic mechanism is as follows: when a stress at a part of bone is not present for a long time, the part is weakened by decrease in bone density. Conversely, when a part of bone is highly stressed, the part is strengthened by an increase in bone density. As a result of the continuous process, the whole bone forms a proper structure relative to outer circumstances. We expect this phenomenon also to operate in the human mandible.

In this chapter, we discuss two subjects from an engineering point of view, focusing on the human mandible. One is estimation of mechanical events in the human mandible during biting and examination of the rationality of the bone. If the bone is rational, we will find the proof in the mechanical analysis. Figure 1 shows our scheme for examining the mechanical characteristics of the human mandible. Mechanical events are calculated by finite-element analysis based on X-ray computed tomography (CT) data around the human mandible. For the stress analysis, we developed an individual modeling method. Bone density is also important information because it is related to mechanical strength. It is possible to extract the information from the same X-ray CT data. We can discuss the mechanical rationality of the human mandible by comparing stress distribution and bone density distribution.

We also examine the basic behavior of functional adaptation. We propose a mathematical model and simulate the behavior of a mechanical system on

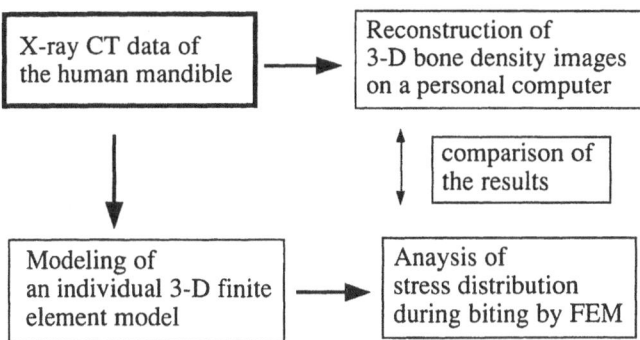

FIG. 1. Scheme for examining mechanical rationality of a mandibular bone. *CT*, computed tomography; *3-D*, three-dimensional; *FEM*, finite-element model

a computer. We further try to explain mechanisms of deformation of a nonsymmetrical mandible by the proposed model.

2 Methods

Making an individual three-dimensional finite-element model is very important to obtain precise stress distribution because the mandibular shape and way of biting are different for each person. We must perform an individual mechanical simulation to obtain reliable computational results. First, this chapter describes the simulation method based on X-ray CT data.

Figure 2 shows our simulation system. The X-ray CT data taken by a CT scanner were used in several ways. We used the data to reconstruct a three-dimensional bone density distribution and generate a finite-element model of an individual mandible on a personal computer. From the same CT data, we estimated muscular forces by measuring muscular areas using a three-dimensional image instrument (Voxel Flinger, Reality Imaging, San Francisco, CA, USA). For measuring reaction forces exerted on the teeth, we used a pressure sheet made with polyethylene terephthalate that changes color where the forces are exerted. We estimated the biting forces from the degree of color development on a personal computer. Providing these data, we computed stress analysis during biting using a workstation.

There are some reports on making an individual finite-element model of a bone based on X-ray CT data [3–5]. Hart et al. [3] have developed such a method to generate a three-dimensional finite-element model of the human mandible. The method is powerful because it directly generates a model from X-ray CT data. There is, however, some room for improvement as generated elements do not reflect the mandibular shape at some portions because they are consistently divided by a regular rule. Keyak and coresearchers [4,5] developed another

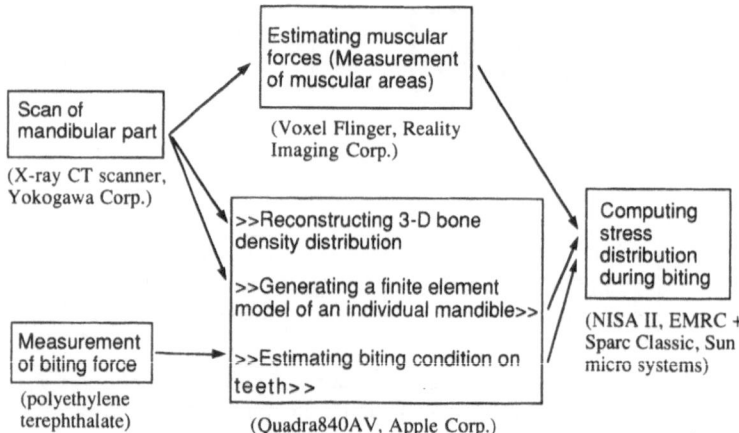

FIG. 2. Utilization of X-ray CT data for the individual mechanical simulation

individual modeling method that expresses a bony shape with small cubic elements. It will be a leading method in the future as the algorithm of the modeling method is simple and fits current computer graphics such as the volume-rendering technique. However, it is difficult to execute stress analysis with this model because it has numerous elements. If we desire an exact mandibular model, we must provide a model that includes more than 100000 elements. It requires a lot of time for such a stress analysis, even using the latest supercomputer.

We focused on generating an effective finite-element model that can be executed on a personal computer (Fig. 3). The basic idea is a geometrical transformation that consists of four parts. First, we made a three-dimensional mandibular image of contours from X-ray CT data as pictured. Each contour was extracted by the CT image. We obtained an external shape image of the mandible by stacking the contours at the same intervals. Second, we made a surface model from the shape image. The surface model is, as it were, a polygonal image that is covered with small triangles. Third, we provided an approximate model of the objective person. The approximate model was modified from a standard model that has 1596 elements and 2380 nodes. We modified the standard type of model by adjusting characteristic lengths of the mandible using the contour image. Finally, we matched the approximate model to the surface model, moving all nodes of the model by iterative transformation, and obtained the individual finite-element model.

As the corpus mandibulae (front part of mandible) has a kind of shell structure, thickness of cortical bone was also considered. Figure 4 shows the method that reflects bone thickness. We moved inside nodes located in the nearest position to the surface nodes so that these nodes coincided with a borderline of the inner cortical bone using a cross-sectional image reconstructed from the same X-ray

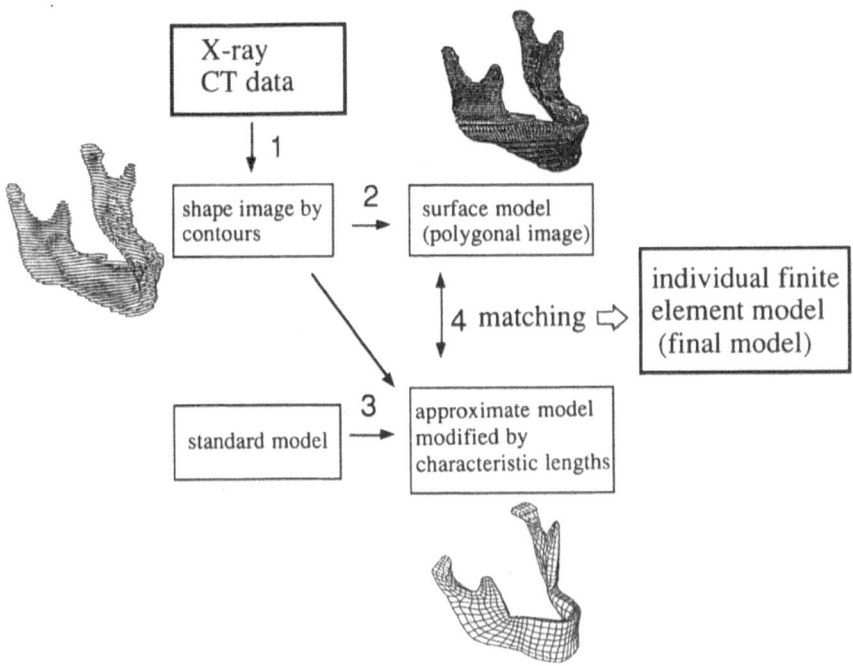

FIG. 3. Proposed modeling method of the human mandible based on X-ray CT data (adapted, from [15] with permission)

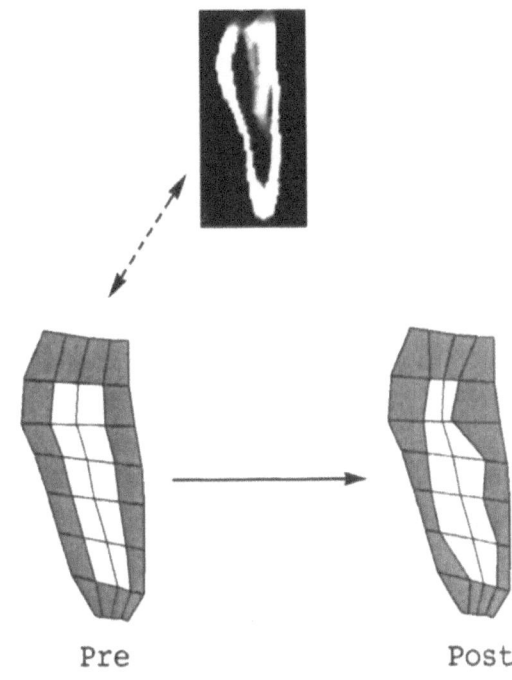

FIG. 4. Geometrical transformation considering thickness of cortical bone

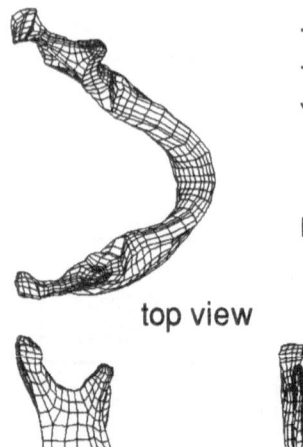

Total elements   1596
Total nodes   2380
Young's modlus
    outside elements: 1.0x10⁴ MPa
    inside elements: 1.0x10² MPa
Poisson's ratio   0.3

Fig. 5. Final model of the individual human mandible

top view

side view   front view

CT data. The representative elasticity of inside elements was selected as 1/100 compared with the outside elements. Figure 5 is the final three-dimensional finite-element model of the individual mandible.

To execute stress analysis, we must determine values of muscular forces and boundary conditions. Many kinds of masticatory muscles control the mandibular bone. For stress analysis, we assumed the following muscles: temporalis, masseter, pterygoideus medialis, and pterygoideus lateralis. As we cannot directly measure these muscular forces during biting, we assumed that muscular forces are proportional to the muscular areas. The muscular areas and the directions were measured with the Voxel Flinger, which generates an arbitral cross-sectional image of the mandible. For estimation of masticatory data, other researchers' data [6,7] were also used. The biting forces on the teeth and the locations were determined by a pressure sheet as described previously. We asked the experimental subject to bite the sheet in a bilateral manner and estimated the biting forces and the locations from the colored spots. We assumed that biting forces act on teeth in the vertical direction.

For the boundary condition of the model, we set up a supporting system (Fig. 6). Both condyles can turn in any direction like pivots, and one side of the condyle can also move freely along one direction. The moments around the condyles produced by the muscular forces and the biting forces should be balanced. Using the equations in Fig. 6, we adjusted muscular forces by proportional allotment to keep the moment balance. To execute stress analysis successfully, we need to set another boundary condition to prevent rotation of the model as a rigid body. We set a restrictive condition at the front part of the model (Fig. 6) so that the model

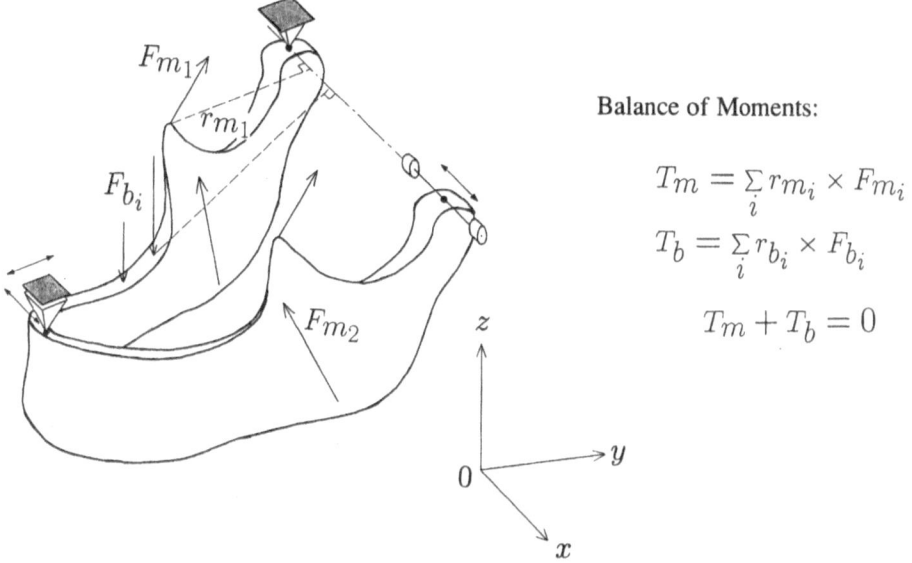

Balance of Moments:

$$T_m = \sum_i r_{m_i} \times F_{m_i}$$

$$T_b = \sum_i r_{b_i} \times F_{b_i}$$

$$T_m + T_b = 0$$

FIG. 6. Supporting system for stress analysis

TABLE 1. Masticatory muscular directions.

Muscle	Right			Left		
	i	j	k	i	j	k
M	−0.15	−3.25	9.46	2.40	−2.83	9.28
Ta	−3.33	0.00	9.43	5.14	0.00	8.57
Tm	−3.01	4.28	8.52	4.85	3.36	8.08
Tp	−3.01	4.28	8.52	4.19	5.81	6.98
Pm	5.54	−0.67	8.30	−4.32	−1.25	8.93
Pl	7.15	−6.92	−1.03	−7.87	−5.75	−2.23

Ta, anterior temporalis; Tm, median temporalis; Tp, posterior temporalis; M, masseter; Pm, pterygoideus medialis; Pl, pterygoideus lateralis. i, j, and k denote the vectors of x-, y-, and z-directions, respectively, as in Fig. 6.

TABLE 2. Ratio of muscular forces.

Muscle	Right	Left
M	187	172
T	124	99
Pm	115	115
Pl	86	100

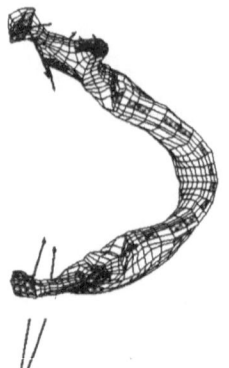

FIG. 7. Mechanical conditions of the model. *Shaded areas* denote places where muscular forces are exerted

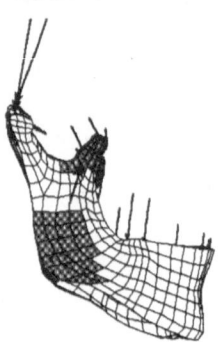
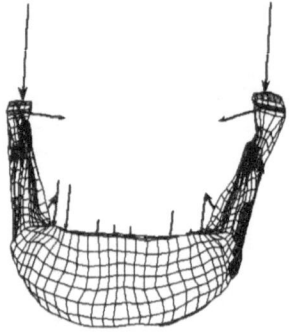

moves freely in the horizontal plane but is fixed in the vertical direction. As the moments are already balanced, this fixation does not produce any inconvenient mechanical effect on the model.

Through these modeling steps, we obtained the mechanical conditions of the model as shown in Tables 1 and 2. Figure 7 illustrates the biting conditions. Because each masticatory muscle is attached to the mandibular bone in a certain area, we distributed the forces to certain nodal points, referring to anatomical knowledge. The hatched areas in the figure indicate the distributed regions of muscular forces.

3 Results

The stress analysis was executed by a general-purpose structural program, NISA II (EMRC, Troy, MI, USA). Figures 8 and 9 are the computational results with equivalent stress. The former result (Fig. 8) was obtained by the model without considering thickness of the bone; the latter result (Fig. 9) was from the model when considering bone thickness. Comparing these results, we can see that the latter result shows more homogeneous stress distribution. The stress is distributed throughout the entire structure though there are several highly stressed portions. As the model accounting for bone thickness is more precise, we can say that the latter result presents more realistic stress distribution.

It is possible to reconstruct a bone density image using the same X-ray CT data. The X-ray CT was taken with a calibration phantom made of hydroxyapatite

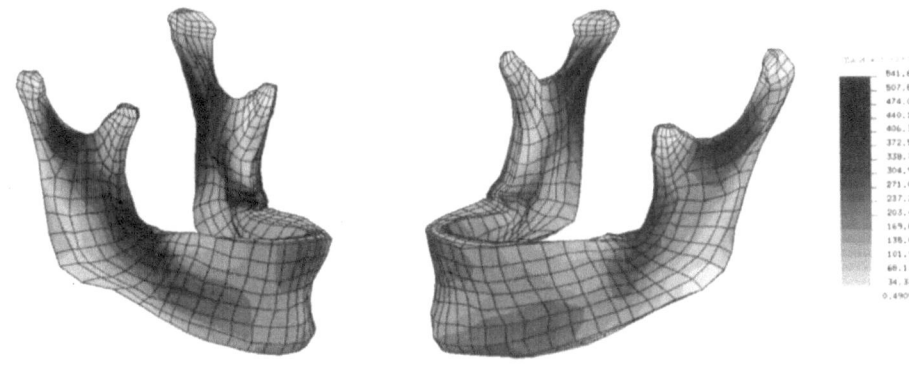

FIG. 8. Computational results with equivalent stress. Thickness transformation was not considered

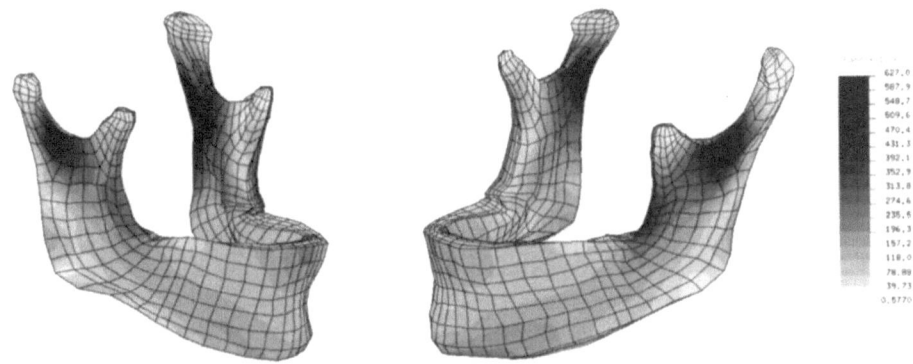

FIG. 9. Computational results with equivalent stress. Thickness transformation was considered

$[Ca_{10}(PO_4)_6OH_2]$, which is a main component of bone. As the phantom consists of several rods containing different densities of hydroxyapatite, we can make a quantitative estimation of the bone mineral content [8]. From the calibration phantom, we ensured that the CT number was approximately proportional to bone density at that position. Figure 10 shows high bone density image in the same mandible. In this case, the pattern of bone density distribution is almost the same for both sides even though the mandibular shape is rather nonsymmetrical.

We can see a pattern in the stress distribution similar to that in Fig. 9. This similarity tells us that the human mandible takes a rational structure because the portions with high bone density are stronger than other portions. At the same time, this similarity suggests to us that the mandibular bone has the function of increasing bone density so that stressed portions acquire large material strength. We discuss these subjects in some detail in the next section.

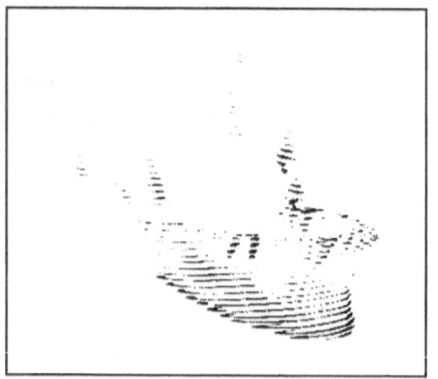 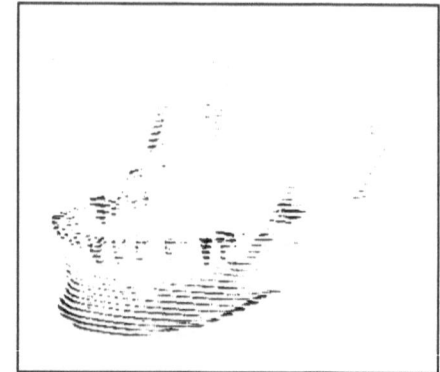

FIG. 10. Bone density distribution

4 Discussion

In this section, we discuss the human mandibular bone from several aspects. First, we evaluate robustness of bone as a mechanical structure. Second, we propose a mathematical model of functional adaption and examine the basic performance. And finally, we investigate the mechanisms of the deformation process of the human mandible using the proposed model.

4.1 Evaluation of Robustness

Fully stressed design is a optimization method that makes stress produced in the structure almost equal for a set of loading conditions. From this standpoint, we can say that the human mandible is rather well designed although there is some room to be considered. In the analysis, we assigned two values to the Young's modulus in the model. However, human mandibular bone takes various values of Young's modulus. If we estimate Young's modulus, the model will approach the actual situation much more closely.

It is said that the square of bone density is proportional to strength of bone, and the cube is proportional to Young's modulus [9,10]. We estimated Young's modulus for every finite element using an experimental equation reported by Carter and Hayes [9]. Figure 11 shows Young's modulus distribution; the maximum value was limited to 16 GPa because some CT data had large numbers. After estimating Young's modulus, we executed the stress analysis. Figure 12 shows the computational result with equivalent stress. The stress distribution looks more homogenous compared with the result when two values of Young's modulus were used (see Fig. 9).

Now, we discuss robustness of bone as a mechanical structure. If a part of the bone is hard and not highly stressed, that part is safe from damage, but wasteful. Conversely, if a part of the bone is weak and highly stressed, that portion would

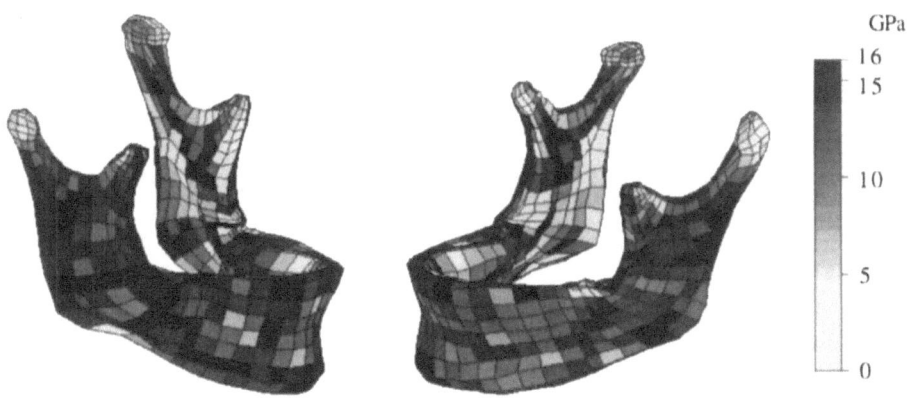

Fig. 11. Estimated Young's modulus distribution

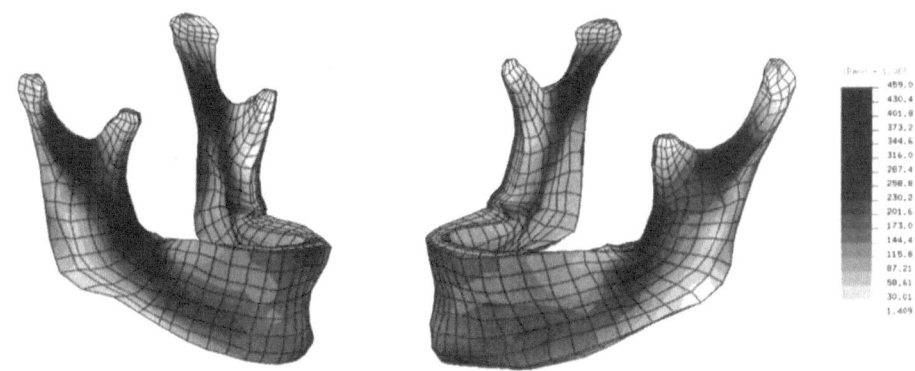

Fig. 12. Computed stress distribution considering Young's modulus distribution

be likely to fail. So the most effective state is that in which each part of the bone receives a suitable stress value for its strength.

To evaluate the robustness, we introduce the following criterion:

$$\eta = \sigma/\sigma_B \tag{1}$$

where σ is the stress value, and σ_B is the strength of the bone.

Because η is a kind of safety coefficient (but an inverse number), the condition to free the body from failure is $\eta < 1$. We can say that when η takes a small value for all elements and the distribution of η is almost homogeneous, the body is robust. In this study, we calculated $\sigma/(\text{CT number})^2$ as we did not know the actual strength of bone σ_B on the human mandible. Figure 13 shows the distribution of η. The vertical scale indicates an arbitrary value that is proportional to η. The distribution of η is almost homogeneous in the entire mandible. From this result, we understand that the mandibular bone has a robust structure.

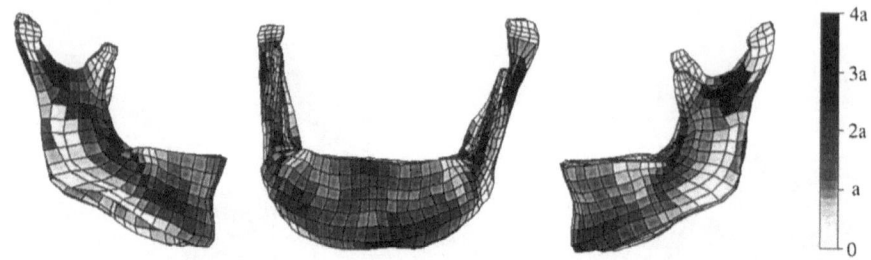

FIG. 13. Distribution of $\sigma/(\text{CT number})^2$, an inverse safety factor. Arbitrary units

4.2 Simulation of Functional Adaptation

As we have described, functional adaptation seems to play an important role in making stress distribution homogenous in the whole structure. In this section, we examine the performance of functional adaptation with a simple mathematical model [11].

The model of functional adaptation consists of many elements that connect mechanically with one another. Each element senses its mechanical condition and changes its material property appropriately. We focused on examining the performance of the model. First, we explain the simulation method, and second, we show the basic performance of the model.

The simulation is executed by the following iterative process:

Step 1. Give an initial structure composed of elements.
Step 2. Set loading forces and fixed conditions on the structure.
Step 3. Calculate stresses in the elements.
Step 4. Evaluate the stresses.
Step 5. Change material property for each element.
Step 6. Return to step 2.

The foregoing algorithm is basically the same as the growing-reforming procedure [12], which reforms the shape of a structure by partial modification. In our model, Young's modulus of each element is changed. Each element independently changes Young's modulus by the following equation:

$$E^{(t+1)} = E^{(t)}\left\{1 + \alpha\left(\sigma - \sigma_c\right)/\sigma_c\right\} \qquad (2)$$

where E is Young's modulus, t is the number of iteration steps, σ is equivalent stress, σ_c is target stress value, and α is a constant value, about 0.1.

The equation acts so that the difference between the stress of each element and the target stress at each place gradually decreases. We expect that a condition to satisfy the relation $\sigma/\sigma_c = 1$ for most elements is formed by iterative calculations. It is natural to assume that target stress value corresponds to the material strength. Consequently, σ/σ_c is essentrally equal to η, which was introduced previously.

It should be noted that target stress depends on Young's modulus. Roughly speaking, the more material density increases, the more apparent elastic modulus gains. At the same time, material strength increases with the increase of Young's modulus. However, it is very difficult to describe the relationships analytically. Here, we simply set the following linear relationship:

$$E = \left(E_0/\sigma_{c0}\right)\sigma_c \tag{3}$$

where E_0 is a reference value of Young's modulus and σ_{c0} is a value of material strength at E_0.

We provided a two-dimensional problem acting on top of a cantilever beam (Fig. 14). The initial Young's modulus was set as E_0. About 100 iterative calculations were executed using Eqs. 2 and 3. Figure 15 shows the simulation results, which correspond to the distribution of Young's modulus, equivalent stress, and σ/σ_c, respectively. The distribution of Young's modulus takes a pattern similar to that of stress distribution, which means that the beam takes an effective structure to support the loading force. The mechanical states are stably converged because σ/σ_c is almost equal to 1 except at the front part of the beam. This simulation method is easy to apply to a three-dimensional problem; we applied it to the human mandible to investigate the mechanism of the deformation process in human mandibular growth.

4.3 Application to the Human Mandible

In our previous paper [13], we reported on mechanical response during biting with two types of mandibular models: one symmetrical and the other nonsymmetrical. Both models were based on individual CT data. Figure 16 shows the nonsymmetrical type of model and the biting conditions. These masticatory data were estimated from the individual.

Using the nonsymmetrical model and the conditions, we examined the change of Young's modulus by functional adaptation. As the initial condition of Young's modulus, two values were given to the model so that the model takes a shell structure; that is, we set the elasticity of inside elements as 1/100 compared with

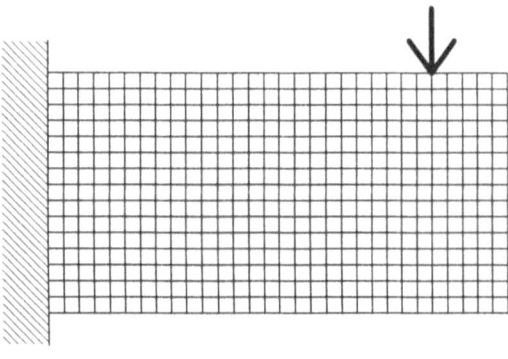

FIG. 14. Mechanical conditions for simulating remodeling process. *Arrow*; application load

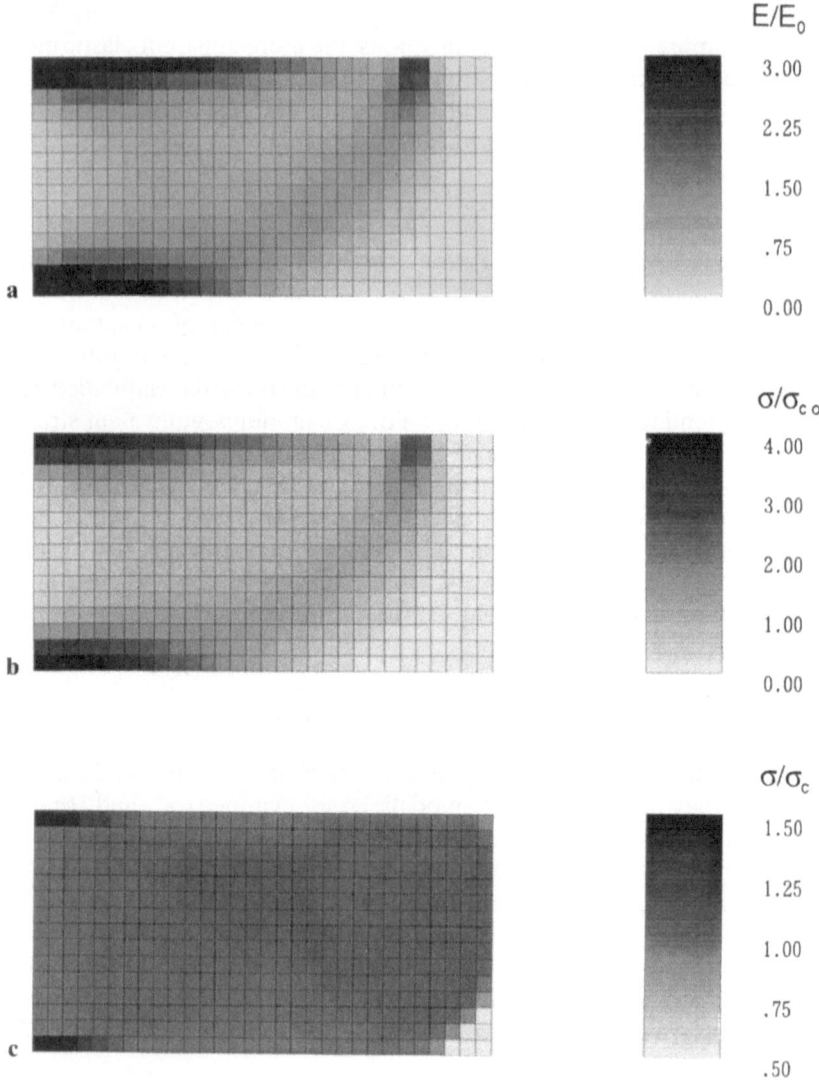

FIG. 15. Computational results. **a** Young's modulus distribution. **b** Stress distribution. **c** Distribution of σ/σ_c

outside elements. The Young's modulus of outside elements ($=1.0 \times 10^4$ MPa) was set as E_0. The simulation was executed in the same way as described in the previous section. Figure 17 shows the simulation results of the Young's modulus distribution (E/E_0); Young's modulus distributes both sides almost equally even though the manner of biting is considerably biased. As the stress distribution takes a similar pattern, we can say that functional adaptation works to make stress homogeneous in the human mandibular bone.

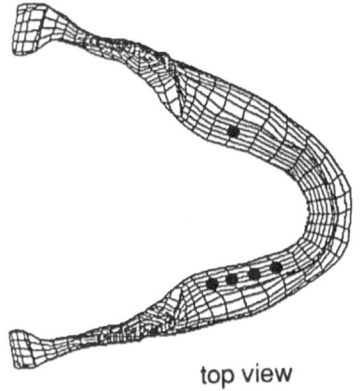

top view

Fig. 16. Nonsymmetrical mandiblular model and biting conditions (adapted, from [16] with permission)

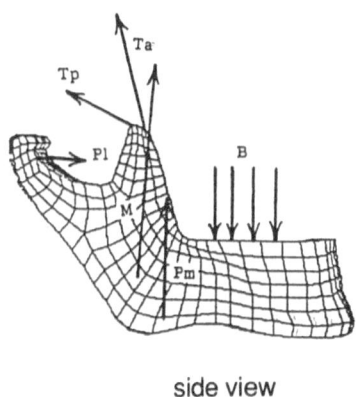

side view

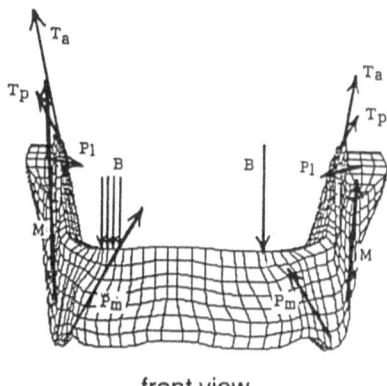

front view

It is unlikely that the nonsymmetrical shape of mandibular bone is determined inherently although the basic form is determined by genes. There must be mechanical factors to deform the mandible. We assumed that the mandible was symmetrical in shape originally, but grew at a different rate for each side under biased biting conditions maybe caused by biting habits or lost or decayed teeth. To examine the supposition, we simulated the change of Young's modulus by functional adaptation with the symmetrical model that we used in our previous paper. For the mechanical conditions, a similar biased biting for the nonsymmetrical case was provided. Figure 18 shows the simulation results of Young's modulus distribution. In this case, Young's modulus chiefly increased at the working side because a large stress was set up at this side.

Examining these simulation results, we found that the mechanisms of the deformation process of the nonsymmetrical mandibular bone can be explained as follows. In Fig. 19, all figures are drawn from a top view. Figure 19a shows the first stage of the mandibular shape of an individual. We assume that the person is relatively young in terms of growth. The mandibular shape is symmetrical, but biting is biased at one side (denoted with small circles). In this situation, the stress

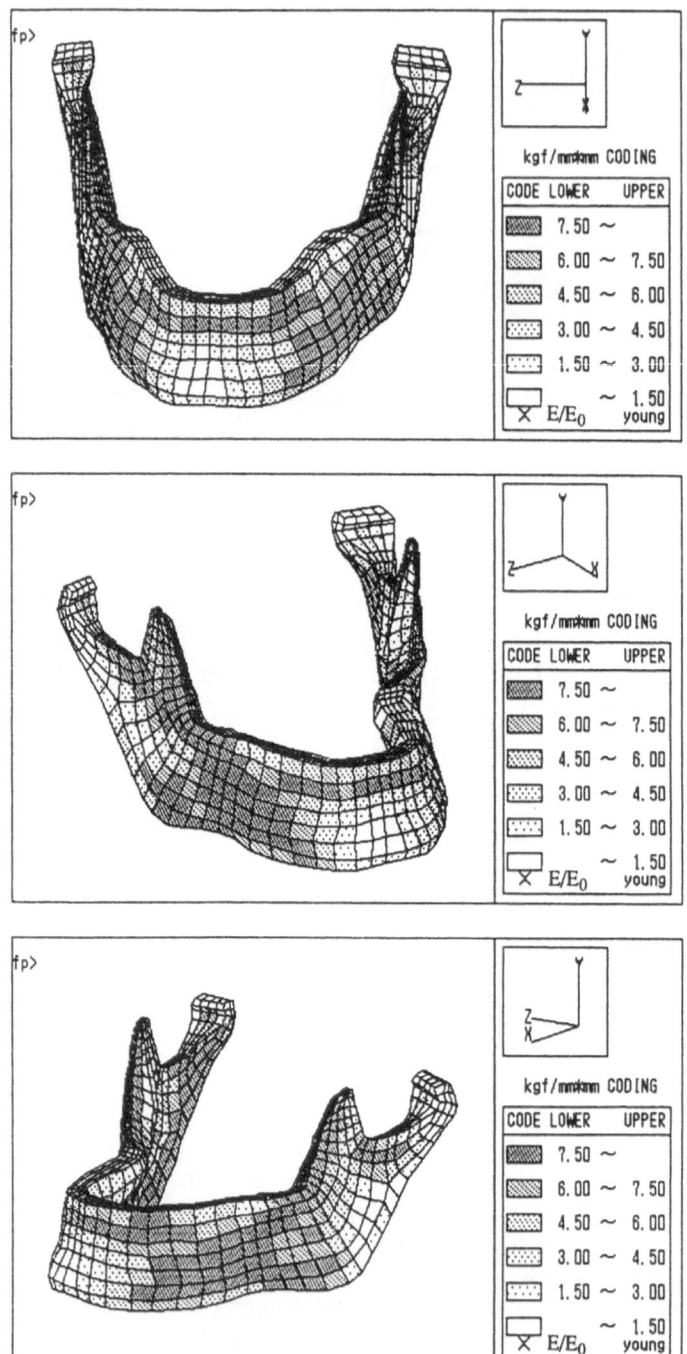

FIG. 17. Simulation results of Young's modulus distribution in case of nonsymmetrical type

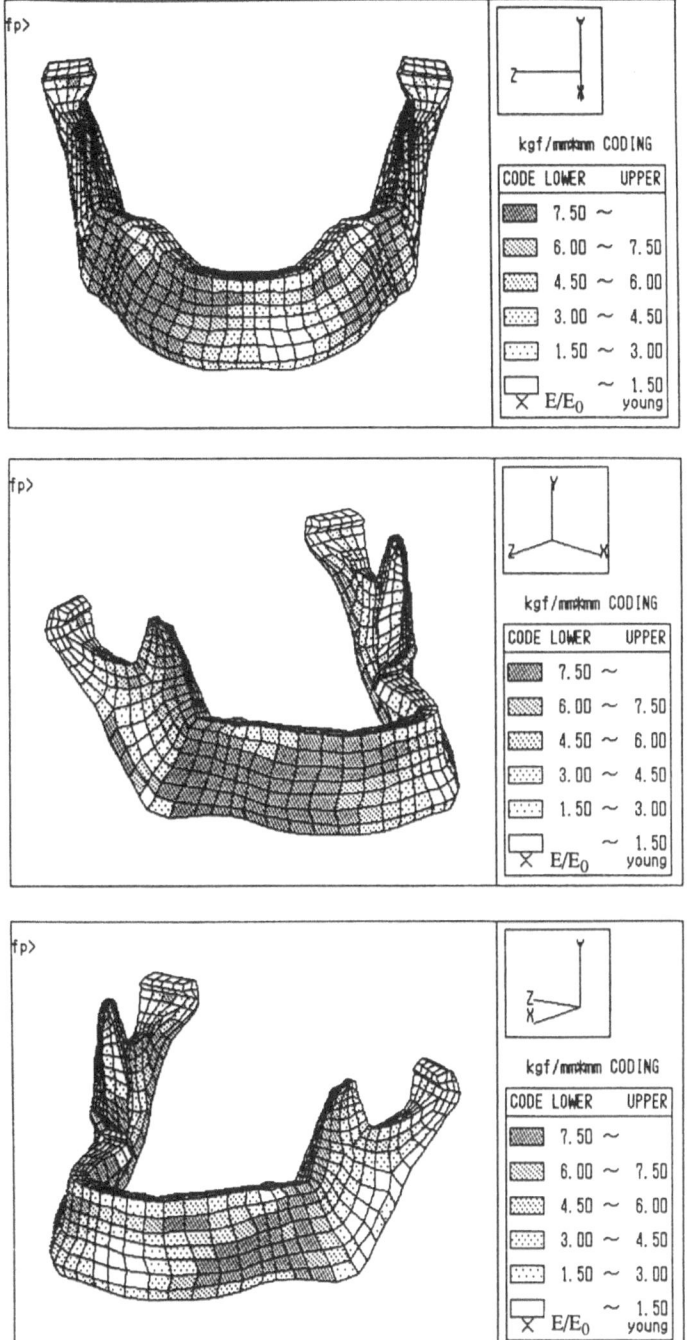

Fɪɢ. 18. Simulation results of Young's modulus distribution in case of symmetrical type

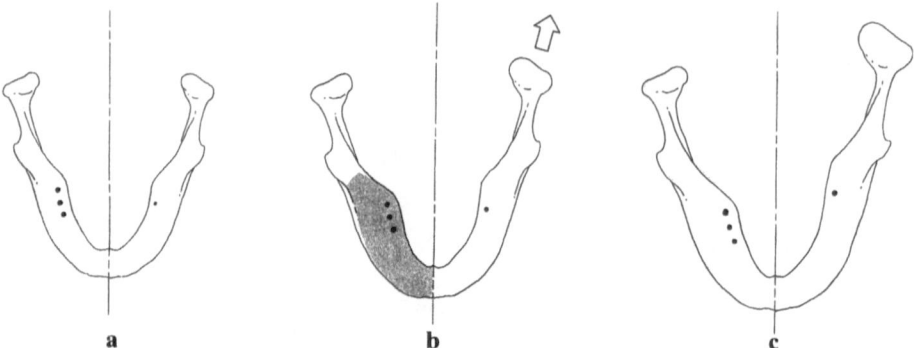

FIG. 19a–c. Hypothetical mechanism of growth process. *Small circles* denote biting forces. **a** First stage: the mandible keeps symmetrical shape and there is no differnece in the bone density distribution between the two sides. Biting forces are mainly acting on the left side. **b** Second stage: bone density increases at the left side (*shaded area*) because of the biased stress. At the same time, the mandible is growing at a different rate on each side. *Arrow*, direction of mandibular growth. **c** Final stage: mandibular shape becomes nonsymmetrical and bone density is homogenized

is high at the working side. At the highly stressed portion, bone density will increase by functional adaptation. Figure 19b shows the second stage; density became higher at the working side (denoted with the hatched area). At the same time, we must consider mandibular growth at this stage.

We sometimes observe that bones do not grow well when they are excesswively stressed. It is expected that highly stressed portions on the working side will have a slower rate of growth although the cross-sectional area of the bone may increase to support the stress. According to Enlow [14], the growth of the human mandible clearly occurs around the condyles. In the symmetrical mandible, the biased biting condition surely gives different mechanical effects to condyles on different sides of the mandible. That is, a condyle at the working side is highly stressed, but on the other (balancing) side the condyle is less stressed. Although we do not yet know the mechanisms of mandibular growth, it is also likely that the mandibular bone grows well at the balancing side where the stress is not so set up. If the rate of growth is affected by the degree of stress, the mandible will gradually deform with the growth. Figure 19b also shows the way deformity occurs (note arrow). The deformed growth will change the bone density again.

Figure 19c shows the final stage of the mandible; the bone densities have become almost equal on both sides even though the shape is nonsymmetrical. We have some evidence of this phenomenon from our investigations. We observed bone density distributions for many persons with nonsymmetrical mandibles, and found a tendency for a clear difference in bone density distribution between the two sides for young persons; it is difficult, however, to recognize the difference for older persons. We can also confirm the homogenized process with the proposed model of functional adaptation. The simulation result (see Fig. 17) essentially presents the final stage.

5 Conclusions

An individual simulation method of the human mandible based on X-ray CT data was proposed. Using the model, a stress analysis was executed and a correlation between stress distribution and bone density distribution was found. A method for evaluating robustness of bone was proposed and applied to the human mandible. These examinations showed that the mandible has mechanical rationality and functional adaptation. The model proposed to examine functional adaptation is useful for knowing the tendency of bone density to change and to explain mandibular deformity.

Acknowledgment. The authors appreciate the help of Mr. T. Uesugi and M. Koseki, who assisted in performing computer simulations and drawing illustrations. This study was supported by a Japanese Grant-in-Aid for Scientific Research on Priority Areas from the Ministry of Education, "Biomechanics" (No. 04237102).

References

1. Roux W (1985) Gesammelte Abhandlungen über Entwicklungsmechanik der Organismen, vol 1. Engelmann, Leipzig, pp 662–722
2. Kummer B (1972) Biomechanics of bone. In: Fung YC, Perrone N, Anliker M (eds) Biomechanics. Prentice-Hall, Englewood Cliffs, NJ, pp 237–271
3. Hart RT, Hennebel VV, Thongpreda N, Van Buskirk WC, Anderson RC (1992) Modeling the biomechanics of the mandible—a three-dimensional finite element study. J Biomech 25:287–295
4. Keyak, JH Meager JM, Skinner HB, Mote CD (1990) Automated three-dimensional finite element modelling of bone: a new method. J Biomed Eng 12:389–396
5. Keyak JH, Fourkas MG, Meager JM, Skinner HB (1993) Validation of an automated method of three-dimensional finite element modelling of bone. J Biomed Eng 15:505–509
6. Hatcher DC, Faulkner MG, Hay A (1986) Development of mechanical and mathematic models to study temporomandibular joint loading. J Prosthet Dent 55:377–384
7. Faulkner MG, Hatcher DC, Hay A (1987) A three-dimensional investigation of temporomandibular joint loading. J Biomech 20:997–1002
8. Maki K (1988) A study about the x-ray CT cephalmetrics providing functions as the standard for three-dimensional reconstruction and bone mineral measurement. J Orthop Soc 47:380–390
9. Carter DR, Hayes WC (1976) Bone compressive strength: the influence of density and strain rate. Science 194:1174–1176

10. Currey J (1984) The mechanical adaptation of bone. Princeton University Press, Princeton, NJ, pp 133–134
11. Inou N, Fujiwara H, Umetani Y (1993) A computational method generating three-dimensional structure based on the adaptive function of bone. Trans Soc Instrum Control Eng 29(10):1221–1226
12. Umetani Y, Hirai S (1978) Shape optimization for beams subject to displacement restrictions on the basis of the growing-reforming procedure. Bull Jpn Soc Mech Eng 21:1113–1119
13. Inou N, Fujiwara H, Maki K (1994) Biomechanical study of the human mandible on mechanical response of its shape and structure. In: Hirawasa Y, Sledge CB, Woo SL-Y (eds) Clinical biomechanics and related research. Springer-Verlag, Heidelberg Berlin New York Tokyo, pp 44–55
14. Enlow DH (1975) Handbook of facial growth. Saunders, Philadelphia
15. Inou N, Kobayashi H, Maki K (1994) A modeling method for an individual human mandible based on X-ray CT data. Trans Jpn Soc Mech Eng 60:2078–2083
16. Inou N, Fujiwara H, Maki K, (1992) 3-D FE stress analysis of mandible during biting. Trans Jpn Soc Mech Eng 58:1042–1047

Contact Mechanics in the Artificial Knee Joint

HIROMASA ISHIKAWA and HIROYUKI FUJIKI[1]

Summary. Ultrahigh molecular weight polyethylene (UHMWPE) is the material generally used for the articular plate contact surface in artificial knee joints. However, the wear of this material becomes a serious problem during the extended life of the joint. To understand the wear mechanism of the plate during walking and to improve its wear life, the cyclic contact behavior of the plate was analyzed using the constitutive equation for cyclic plasticity, because the UHMWPE is an inelastic material and the plate is subjected to cyclic contact deformation during walking. In this analysis, the two-dimensional plane strain model was employed and the contact behavior of femoral and tibial components was simulated by translating the contact stress distribution, which was calculated from elastoplastic indentation analysis of two components. The posterior cruciate ligament (PCL) retention-type artificial knee joint as the basic analytical model and two other modified contact surface models were analyzed to investigate the effect of the shape of the contact surface on the wear behavior of the plate. As a result, it is clarified that the effect of the stress history, to which the UHMWPE has been subjected, on the wear mechanism of the UHMWPE is significant, that the wear of the plate should occur from both the surface and the subsurface of the plate, and that the wear behavior of the plate is closely related to the shape of the contact surface. The optimal design of the contact surface of the plate is considered using this analysis.

Key words: Artificial knee joint—Ultrahigh molecular weight polyethylene—Tribology—Constitutive equation—Finite-element method

1 Introduction

Total arthroplasty is an operation to recover the function of a joint when the function is finally lost by trauma or disease. The operation has recently been performed mainly in the hip and knee joints and has brought remarkable benefit

[1] Department of Mechanical Engineering II, Hokkaido University, N13 W8 Kita-ku, Sapporo, Hokkaido, 060 Japan

in terms of recovery of the functions of motion and support and of release from pain. The performance of the artificial joint has been improved by optimization of the design of its shape and structure, the application of new materials, improvement of the method of surgery, and so on. The problem of wear particles of the artificial joint, however, remains serious; these affect the surrounding tissues and produce loosening of the joint [1]. This point means that the life of the current artificial knee joint is limited to about 10 years and a longer-lasting artificial knee joint has been anticipated.

Since Charnley developed an epochal artificial hip joint using a femoral head made of stainless steel and an acetabular cup made of ultrahigh molecular weight polyethylene (UHMWPE) in 1962, the combination of these materials has been employed for the bearing surfaces in various artificial joints. Various combinations of materials have been tested: for example, Co-Cr-Mo alloy (vitallium), alumina ceramic [2], pure titanium and titanium alloy [3] as the bearing material of the harder component, and carbon fiber-reinforced polyethylene [4], the composite of UHMWPE and ceramics [5], and polyvinylalcohol (PVA) hydrogel [6,7] as that of the softer component. But there is currently no superior alternative exceeding the performance of plain UHMWPE in combination with anticorrosion metal or ceramic, and plain UHMWPE is generally used for the considerations of low friction and wear resistance. The combination of harder and softer materials is employed to produce elastohydrodynamic lubrication (EHL) which improves the performance of friction and wear. Examples of fluid film measurement for the anatomical type of artificial knee joint during walking are shown in Fig. 1 [7]. The extend of fluid film formation was evaluated by the degree of separation where 1 is full separation and 0 is contact. The values were mostly around 0 except for a part of the swing phase under an extremely light load condition in Fig. 1, which indicates that significant contact occurs during walking. In the case of the anatomical-type artificial knee joint, therefore, perfect EHL does not occur because of the shape of the contact surface and the condition of the load; direct contact between the femoral and the tibial components then occurs and the UHMWPE articular plate wears off.

Many investigations have aimed to improve the life of the joint using plain UHMWPE; for example, evaluation of UHMWPE using a wear test machine [8–10] or a so-called knee simulator [3,11], and evaluation of damage in retrieved knee prostheses [12,13]. Nevertheless, there are a few investigations that make the wear mechanism of the UHMWPE clear and improve the performance of the joint aided by a mechanical method. In one of these studies, Bartel et al. analyzed the elastic contact behavior of UHMWPE [14] and a quasi-elastoplastic [15] in artificial hip and knee joints. They analyzed the contact behavior as a simple indentation problem and determined the maximum principal stress at the surface of the polyethylene for knee replacement in extension and in flexion (Fig. 2) [15]. In Fig. 2, the elliptical contours show the edge of the contact area, and the meshes shown in the first quadrant are the finite-element method (FEM) meshes on the surface of the UHMWPE articular plate. The maximum principal stresses are shown at each node near the edge of contact area and mediolateral center line of

FIG. 1. Fluid film formation in knee prosthesis with polyethylene tibial component during walking. (from [7] with permission) *S-10000*, Silicone oil lubricant (values are kinetic viscosity mm²/s at 25°C); R_p, electric resistance in parallel to rubbing specimen

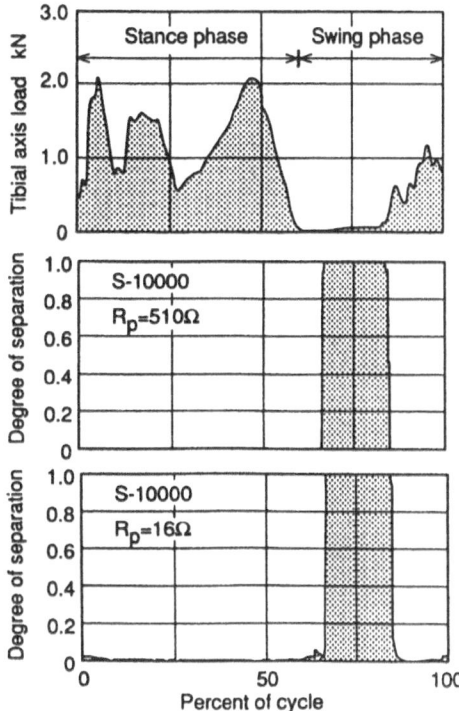

the contact area because the stresses were calculated at each node. In any plane parallel to the anteroposterior direction, the minimum (most compressive) value occurred on the mediolateral center line of the contact area and the maximum (most tensile) value occurred at the anterior or posterior edge of contact. Points on the surface of the tibial component will then be subjected to cyclic stresses that vary between tension and compression because during articulation the contact area moves with respect to the tibial component. Therefore, it is necessary to analyze the inelastic contact behavior of UHMWPE as a cyclic loading problem because UHMWPE is an inelastic material.

In this study, numerical analysis of the cyclic contact behavior of the UHMWPE articular plate in an artificial knee joint during walking was performed to better understand the wear mechanism of the plate and the effect of the stress state of the plate on wear behavior. In this analysis, the anatomical-type artificial knee joint was employed for the analytical model, and contact of the femoral and tibial components was replaced with the two-dimensional plane strain model in the sagittal plane. The contact behavior of the two components was simulated by translating the contact stress distribution, which was calculated from elastoplastic indentation analysis of the two components at each point of the walking cycle, on the UHMWPE articular plate. The contact stress distribution was not the Hertzian distribution, which has been often employed in rolling-sliding analysis, because some assumptions of Hertz are not satisfied under this

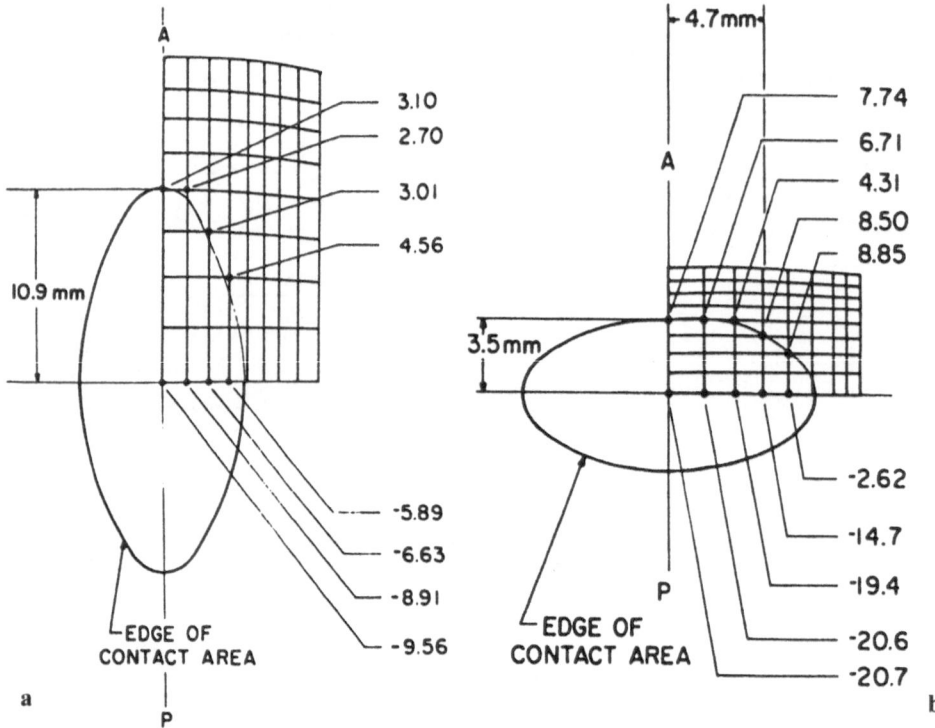

Fɪɢ. 2a,b. Values for the maximum principal stress (MPa) at the surface of polyethylene for knee replacement (from [15] with permission) **a** In extension. **b** In flexion. *A*, Anterior; *P*, posterior

situation, as pointed out by Bartel et al. [14]. The constitutive model for cyclic plasticity proposed by one of the authors [16] was employed and implemented in a plane strain FEM to simulate the behavior of the cyclic deformation of the UHMWPE articular plate because the plate is subjected to cyclic contact deformation during walking.

In the case of polymers there are three principal types of wear: abrasive wear, fatigue wear, and adhesive wear [17]. Mechanical analysis for the adhesive and abrasive wear requires microscale analysis on the contact surface. Detailed discussion about adhesive and abrasive wear could not be performed because only macroscale analysis was carried out in this study. However, in the wear test of UHMWPE, especially as regards wear from its surface, Fisher et al. [10] showed that the variation of sliding velocity in a range of 35–240 mm/s had little effect on the coefficient of friction and the amount of wear. For example, Fig. 3 shows the average wear factors for the six test conditions showing the different sliding velocities and counterface roughness [10]. This graph shows clearly that the dominant parameter affecting the wear factor in the test conditions was the

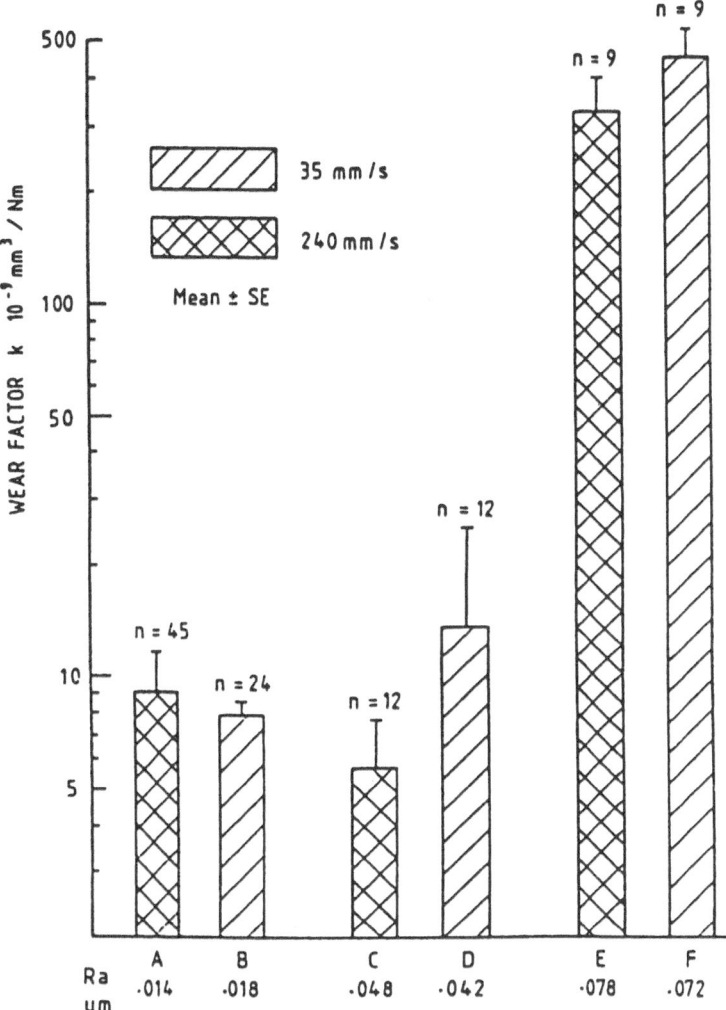

FIG. 3. Average error factors for the six test conditions show the different sliding velocities and counterface roughnesses. Error bars show +1 standard error (SE) on the mean (from [10] with permission). *Diagonal shading*, 35 mm/s; *cross-hatching*, 240 mm/s

counterface roughness but that the sliding velocity has a much smaller effect on the wear factor.

On the other hand, Blunn et al. [9] showed that the wear from rolling contact without sliding was considerably less than the wear caused by sliding because of the lack of shear stress over the surface. These findings mean that the adhesive and abrasive wear from the surface is dependent on the shear stress over the surface, but the amount of the wear and the coefficient of friction are not dependent on sliding velocity over a certain limit that exists between 0 and 35 mm/s, while the amount of wear is reduced corresponding to the decrease of sliding velocity below the limit. Consequently, in this analysis, it was considered that the amount of the wear from the surface, that is, adhesive and abrasive wear, is dependent on the contact stress without consideration of the variation of sliding velocity if sliding occurs, because the amount of the adhesive and abrasive wear is dependent on the shear stress and the shear stress is directly proportional to the contact stress. Thus, contact stress was employed as one of the parameters of evaluation of wear. As a result, it was made clear that the wear of the plate should occur from both the surface and the subsurface of the plate and that the wear behavior of the plate should be closely related to the shape of the contact surface.

2 Materials and Methods

2.1 Material Properties of UHMWPE

To evaluate the deformation behavior of UHMWPE, pure tension and compression tests and a strain recovery test were conducted at 310 K (37°C), assuming in vivo conditions. A typical uniaxial stress specimen used in this work has a gauge length of 24 mm and the radius of a solid cylinder of 10 mm, respectively. The specimens were made of UHMWPE machined from the molding of a large sheet (Chirulen, Hoechst, Frankfurt, Germany). An electric-controlled axial testing machine (5565, Instron, Canton, MA, USA), together with a computer (Compaq, Prolinea 4/50, Houston, TX, USA), was used for computerized testing and data acquisition. Strains were measured using an extensometer (A1351-1003, Instron) and the axial force was measured using a load cell incorporated in the machine. The pure compression test was conducted under three strain rates of 1.0, 0.1, and 0.01%/s, and the pure tension test was conducted under a strain rate of 0.1%/s. After these pure compression and tension tests, the strain recovery test was performed. After unloading completely to zero at the same strain rate as in the loading process, the strain recovery was measured keeping the load zero for 18 h.

Figure 4 shows the stress–strain curve during the pure compressive and tensile loading where the values of stresses and strains are shown as absolute values. The stress–strain relationships in compression and tension tests at a strain rate of 0.1%/s are almost the same, and stress increases with increase in the strain rate. Therefore, strain rate dependency in the deformation of UHMWPE is clearly observed. Figure 5 shows the relation between time and strain during strain recovery. Immediately after unloading, a large amount of strain recovery occurred in a short time and gradually stabilized. After 18 h, strain had a stabilized value of −1.3%, while the value of strain just after the unloading process was −3.4%, which is shown by the "×" mark on the x-axis in Fig. 5. Consequently, it is made clear that UHMWPE is a kind of viscoelastoplastic material.

FIG. 4. Stress–strain curve of pure compression test at three strain rates of 1.0, 0.1, and 0.01%/s, and pure tension test at a strain rate of 0.1%/s

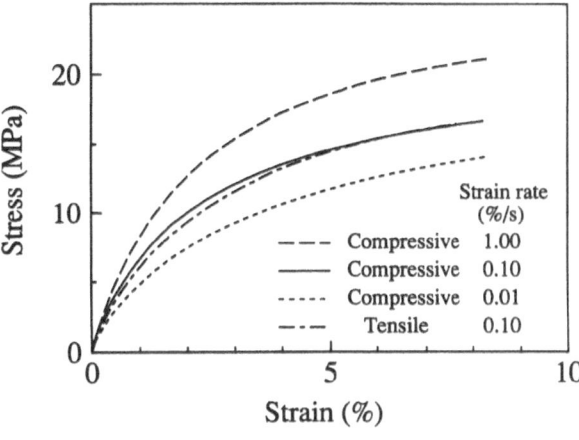

FIG. 5. Relation of time and strain in the strain recovery test after the unloading process of the pure compression test at a strain rate of 0.1%/s

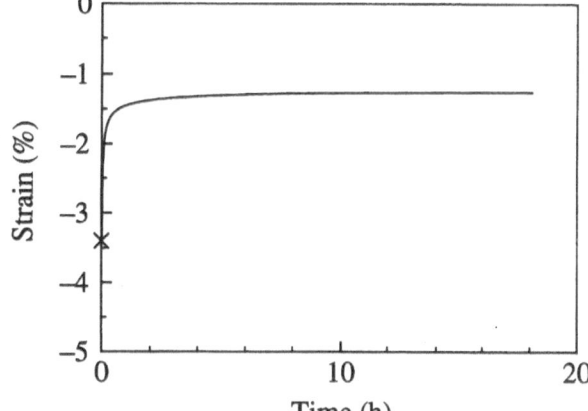

2.2 Constitutive Model for Cyclic Plasticity

Not only in the field of biomechanics, but also in several fields of mechanics, an elastic analysis had been performed as a rough approximation method instead of an inelastic analysis. The elastic analysis, however, already has been shown to be insufficient to discuss the detailed behavior of nonlinear deformation of the material, and accurate inelastic analysis has been required. Moreover, the UHMWPE articular plate in an artificial knee joint is subjected to cyclic loading. Therefore, the constitutive equation for cyclic deformation may be applied to solve this kind of contact problem. The UHMWPE is actually a viscoelastoplastic material, and the viscorecovery deformation occurs after the unloading process, as we mentioned. There is, however, no constitutive model that can completely describe this kind of behavior of the material under a multiaxial stress state. In this analysis, therefore, the UHMWPE was assumed to be an elastoplastic material as a first approximation to better understand the essential feature of wear with the aid of contact mechanics.

A brief summary of the mathematical structure of the proposed model, which combines the von Mises stress hardening form with the kinematic hardening, is reproduced from Ishikawa and Sasaki [16]. The following yield function (Eq. 1) is chosen for a cyclically stable material at temperature T:

$$f = \frac{1}{2}C_{ijkl}\left(\sigma_{ij} - \alpha_{ij}\right)\left(\sigma_{kl} - \alpha_{kl}\right) - \frac{1}{3}R^2\left(\kappa, \, T\right) = 0 \tag{1}$$

where C_{ijkl} is the plastic deformation-induced anisotropy coefficient tensor of the 4th rank, σ_{ij} and α_{ij} are stress and back stress on the current center of the yield surface, R is the flow stress, and κ is the hardening or softening parameter. Associated with Eq. 1, the modified Lévy–Mises equations of cyclic plasticity are obtained from the normality of the plastic strain increment to the yield surface:

$$d\varepsilon_{ij}^p = \frac{3d\bar{\varepsilon}^p}{2\bar{\sigma}}C_{ijkl}\left(\sigma_{kl} - \alpha_{kl}\right) \tag{2}$$

where $d\varepsilon_{ij}^p$ and $d\bar{\varepsilon}^p$ are the plastic strain increment and the equivalent plastic strain increment, respectively, and $\bar{\sigma}$ is the equivalent stress, where $\bar{\sigma} = \sqrt{(3/2)C_{ijkl}(\sigma_{ij} - \alpha_{ij})(\sigma_{kl} - \alpha_{kl})}$ and $d\bar{\varepsilon}^p = \sqrt{(2/3)C_{ijkl}^{-1}d\varepsilon_{ij}^p d\varepsilon_{kl}^p}$. Using the Ziegler type of assumption as the evolution equation of the center of the yield surface, then the motion of the center is given by

$$d\alpha_{ij} = \frac{3}{2\bar{\sigma}^2}\left\{C_{klmn}\left(\sigma_{mn} - \alpha_{mn}\right)d\sigma_{kl}\right\}\left(\sigma_{ij} - \alpha_{ij}\right) - \left(\frac{dR}{dW^p}\right)\left(\sigma_{ij} - \alpha_{ij}\right)d\bar{\varepsilon}^p \tag{3}$$

where dW^p is the modified plastic work increment. The hardening or softening parameter κ is assumed to be a scalar proportional to the modified plastic work:

$$d\kappa = dW^p = \bar{\sigma}d\bar{\varepsilon}^p = \left(\sigma_{ij} - \alpha_{ij}\right)d\varepsilon_{ij}^p \tag{4}$$

To represent the nonlinearity or the roundness of the stress–strain curve, the modified Ramberg–Osgood law (Eq. 5) is employed:

$$\varepsilon_t - e_t = \frac{\sigma_t - \alpha_t}{E}\left[1 + K\left\{\frac{\bar{\sigma}}{\sigma_{0(n)}}\right\}^{m_{(n)}}\right] \tag{5}$$

where σ_t, ε_t, α_t, and e_t are the uniaxial stress, uniaxial strain, the center of the yield surface, and the strain at the center, respectively. E is Young's modulus and K is the material constant represented by $K = E\varepsilon_0/\sigma_{0(n)}$ where $\sigma_{0(n)}$ and $m_{(n)}$ are the stress at the proof strain ε_0 and the exponent of hardening or softening after the

(n −1)th inversion of loading, respectively. They depend on the modified plastic work according to the following Eqs. 6 and 7:

$$\sigma_{0(n)} = \sigma_{0(\infty)} \left[1 - \alpha \, \exp\left\{ -\frac{W^p_{(n-1)}}{W_0} \right\} \right], \quad (n \geq 2) \tag{6}$$

$$m_{(n)} = m_{(\infty)} \left[1 - \beta \, \exp\left\{ -\frac{W^p_{(n-1)}}{W_1} \right\} \right], \quad (n \geq 2) \tag{7}$$

where $\sigma_{0(\infty)}$, α, W_0, $m_{(\infty)}$, β, and W_1 are material constants prescribed by the history of loading or effected by a strain path memory. $W^p_{(n-1)}$ is the accumulated plastic work until the $(n-1)$th inversion of loading.

The flow stress R after the $(n-1)$th inversion of loading is assumed to be represented by Eq. 8, following Eq. 6:

$$R_{(n)} = R_{(\infty)} \left[1 - \lambda \, \exp\left\{ -\frac{W^p}{W_2} \right\} \right] \tag{8}$$

where W^p is the accumulated plastic work, which is equal to $W^p = W^p_{(n-1)} + dW^p$ with the modified plastic work increment dW^p during loading in the current stage of deformation. $R_{(\infty)}$, λ, and W_2 are constants prescribed also by the history of loading or effected by a strain path memory. The material constants in Eqs. 6–8 are determined from both the experiment and the simulation, as shown later. The plastic deformation generally induces an anisotropy even in an initially isotropic material [16], but the anisotropy coefficient tensor C_{ijkl} in Eq. 3 is considered here to take the constant value of isotropy as a first approximation because a large number of experiments concerned with the subsequent yield surface are required to determine the coefficients. Then, these coefficients are to be $C_{1111} = C_{2222} = C_{3333} = 2/3$, $C_{1122} = C_{2233} = C_{3311} = -1/3$, and $C_{1212} = 1/2$. From Eqs. 1–8, the components of the plastic strain increments and the motion of the center of the yield surface are represented as follows for the plane strain state with $\Sigma_x = \sigma_x - \alpha_x$, and so on:

$$d\varepsilon^p_x = B \left\{ \frac{\bar{\sigma}}{\sigma_{0(n)}} \right\}^{m(n)} \frac{3}{2\bar{\sigma}^2} F \left(\frac{2}{3}\sum_x - \frac{1}{3}\sum_y - \frac{1}{3}\sum_z \right)$$

$$d\varepsilon^p_y = B \left\{ \frac{\bar{\sigma}}{\sigma_{0(n)}} \right\}^{m(n)} \frac{3}{2\bar{\sigma}^2} F \left(\frac{2}{3}\sum_y - \frac{1}{3}\sum_z - \frac{1}{3}\sum_x \right)$$

$$d\gamma^p_{xy} = 2B \left\{ \frac{\bar{\sigma}}{\sigma_{0(n)}} \right\}^{m(n)} \frac{3}{2\bar{\sigma}^2} F \sum_{xy} \tag{9}$$

$$d\alpha_x = \frac{3G}{2\bar{\sigma}^2}\sum_x - R_{(\infty)}\frac{\lambda}{W_2}\exp\left(-\frac{W^p}{W_2}\right)B\left\{\frac{\bar{\sigma}}{\sigma_{0(n)}}\right\}^{m_{(n)}}\frac{F}{\bar{\sigma}}\sum_x$$

$$d\alpha_y = \frac{3G}{2\bar{\sigma}^2}\sum_y - R_{(\infty)}\frac{\lambda}{W_2}\exp\left(-\frac{W^p}{W_2}\right)B\left\{\frac{\bar{\sigma}}{\sigma_{0(n)}}\right\}^{m_{(n)}}\frac{F}{\bar{\sigma}}\sum_y$$

$$d\alpha_z = \frac{3G}{2\bar{\sigma}^2}\sum_z - R_{(\infty)}\frac{\lambda}{W_2}\exp\left(-\frac{W^p}{W_2}\right)B\left\{\frac{\bar{\sigma}}{\sigma_{0(n)}}\right\}^{m_{(n)}}\frac{F}{\bar{\sigma}}\sum_z$$

$$d\alpha_{xy} = \frac{3G}{2\bar{\sigma}^2}\sum_{xy} - R_{(\infty)}\frac{\lambda}{W_2}\exp\left(-\frac{W^p}{W_2}\right)B\left\{\frac{\bar{\sigma}}{\sigma_{0(n)}}\right\}^{m_{(n)}}\frac{F}{\bar{\sigma}}\sum_{xy} \qquad (10)$$

where B, F, and G in Eqs. 9 and 10 are as follows.

$$B = \frac{3K}{2E}\left\{m_{(n)}+1\right\}$$

$$F = \frac{2}{3}\left(\sum_x d\sum_x + \sum_y d\sum_y + \sum_z d\sum_z\right) + 2\sum_{xy}d\sum_{xy}$$
$$-\frac{1}{3}\left(\sum_x d\sum_y + \sum_x d\sum_z + \sum_y d\sum_x + \sum_y d\sum_z + \sum_z d\sum_x + \sum_z d\sum_y\right)$$

$$G = \frac{2}{3}\left(\sum_x d\sigma_x + \sum_y d\sigma_y + \sum_z d\sigma_z\right) + 2\sum_{xy}d\sigma_{xy}$$
$$-\frac{1}{3}\left(\sum_x d\sigma_y + \sum_x d\sigma_z + \sum_y d\sigma_x + \sum_y d\sigma_z + \sum_z d\sigma_x + \sum_z d\sigma_y\right) \qquad (11)$$

2.3 Cyclic Tension–Compression Test and Simulation

The material properties $\sigma_{0(\infty)}$, α, W_0, $m_{(\infty)}$, β, W_1, $R_{(\infty)}$, λ, and W_2 in Eqs. 6–8 were determined from the second response for uniaxial cyclic stress and the approach to the stable response following almost the same procedure as in Drucker and Palgen [18].

The open circles, triangles, and squares in Fig. 6 show the experimental results of cyclic tension–compression straining with strain amplitude $\Delta\bar{\varepsilon} = 3\%$ where the strain rate is 0.01%/s at room temperature. This stress–strain curve was stabilized at the third cycle. From these experimental results, shown in Fig. 6, $\sigma_{0(1)} = 15.0$ (MPa) and $m_{(1)} = 3.0$ could be evaluated directly where the proof strain ε_0 is 2.5%. After several trials with a computer (PC-9801DA, NEC, Tokyo, Japan), the stress–strain curves shown by the solid lines in Fig. 6 were depicted using $\sigma_{0(\infty)} = 18.5$ (MPa), $\alpha = \beta = \lambda = 0$, $W_0 = W_1 = W_2 = 1.0$ (MPa), $m_{(\infty)} = 2.2$, and $R_{(\infty)} = 14.6$ (MPa). Comparison between the experimental results and the numerically simu-

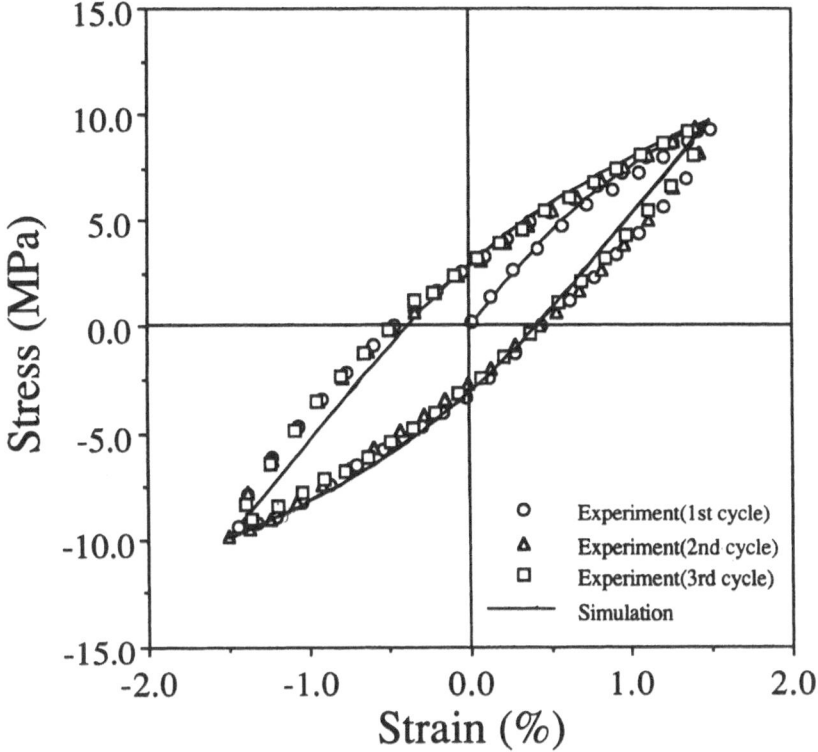

FIG. 6. Cyclic tension–compression loading with constant strain amplitude of 3%

lated ones shows a good agreement except for the slight swelling in experiments during the unloading process, as in Fig. 6.

The material properties $\sigma_{0(\infty)}$, α, W_0, $m_{(\infty)}$, β, W_1, $R_{(\infty)}$, λ, and W_2 were represented in the general form from the three cyclic loading tests including two more additional cyclic straining conditions, $\Delta\bar{\varepsilon} = 2\%$ and 4%. The relationship between the material property $R_{(\infty)}$ and the strain amplitude was represented by the following equation, while other properties maintained their constant values.

$$R_{(\infty)} = 9.55 + 1.69\Delta\varepsilon^p \left(MPa \right) \tag{12}$$

where $\Delta\varepsilon^p$ is shown as a percentage (%).

2.4 Analytical Model

For the basic analytical model, the anatomical posterior cruciate ligament retention-type artificial knee joint (LFA-III) developed in the Department of Orthopaedic Surgery at the Hokkaido University School of Medicine was employed. The whole view of the knee joint is shown in Fig. 7, and the detailed shape of the contact surface of the joint in the sagittal plane is shown in Fig. 8 (model I). This artificial knee joint is composed of an alumina ceramic femoral component, a UHMWPE articular plate, and a titanium alloy tray with stem for fixation as a tibial component. To simplify the analysis, the contact behavior of the joint was replaced by a two-dimensional plane strain model in the sagittal plane because knee motion occurs mostly in the sagittal plane and the shapes of the two condylar contact surfaces of this artificial knee joint are the same.

The contact surface of the alumina ceramic femoral component comprises three circular arcs in the sagittal plane, and the radius of the bottom of the component is the largest (Fig. 8). This shape of contact surface was designed imitating the shape of the contact surface of the femur. The contact surface of the UHMWPE articular plate has the shape of a circular arc in the anterior region, which prevents the luxation of the femur to the anterior direction, and has the shape of a straight line in the posterior region, which easily produces rollback movement and permits the rotating movement of the femoral component. Moreover, to consider the effect of the shape of the contact surface of the joint on the wear of the plate, two more modified contact surface models are introduced. These shapes of contact surface are shown in Fig. 9a (model II) and Fig. 9b (model III), respectively. Model II has the plain UHMWPE articular plate with the same femoral component as model I, and model III has more conformity between the contact surfaces of the two components in a wide range of knee flexion using the same radius of R40.0.

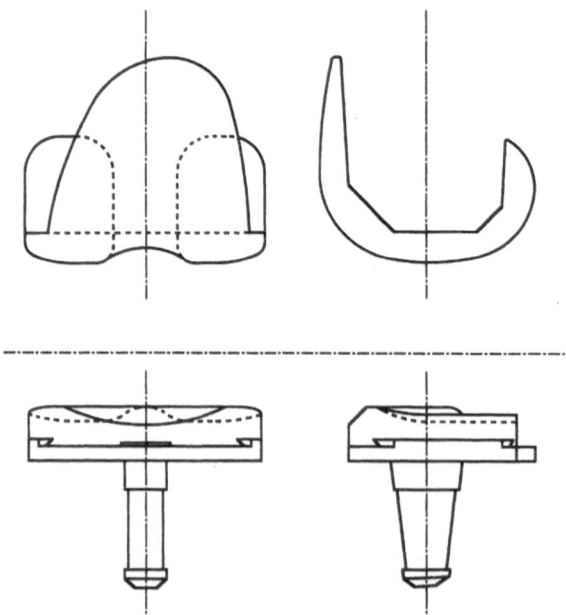

FIG. 7. Posterior cruciate ligament retention-type artificial knee joint LFA-III: femoral (*upper*) and tibial (*lower*) components

FIG. 8. Shape of the contact surface of the LFA-III in the sagittal plane (model I). *UHMWPE*, Ultrahigh molecular weight polyethylene

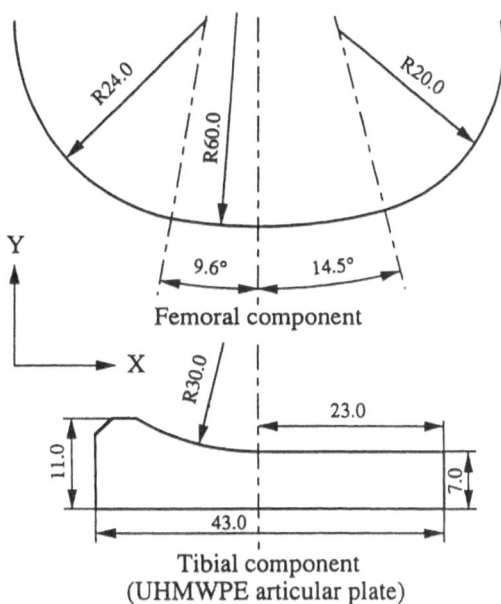

Femoral component

Tibial component
(UHMWPE articular plate)

Table 1 and Fig. 10 show the basic material properties and the FEM model of the UHMWPE articular plate of model I, which consists of 688 rectangular, isoparametric, eight-noded (total, 2253 nodes) elements. The size of a minimum mesh is 0.5 mm × 0.3 mm. In this artificial knee joint, the UHMWPE articular plate is fixed on the titanium tray. Then, as the boundary condition, the bottom of this UHMWPE articular plate model is fixed toward the vertical and the horizontal directions. In the case of models II and III, only the contour shape of the contact surface of the FEM model is modified and the number of nodes and elements, the size of the minimum mesh, and the boundary condition are the same as those of model I.

2.5 Analytical Procedure

In the artificial knee joint, the contact load and the contact position between the femoral and the tibial components and the shape of the contact surface of the two components at the contact point change in a complicated way during walking. The distribution and the position of the contact stress to which the UHMWPE articular plate is subjected change in a similar complicated fashion and, in addition, the plate is subjected to cyclic loading with the number of walking cycles. To analyze the contact behavior of the plate under this condition, two analytical methods were employed. First, the contact stress distributions at each point of the walking cycle were determined by FEM contact analysis (general-purpose finite-element program MARC K-5), and then cyclic elastoplastic analysis for the transition of contact stress on the UHMWPE articular plate was conducted

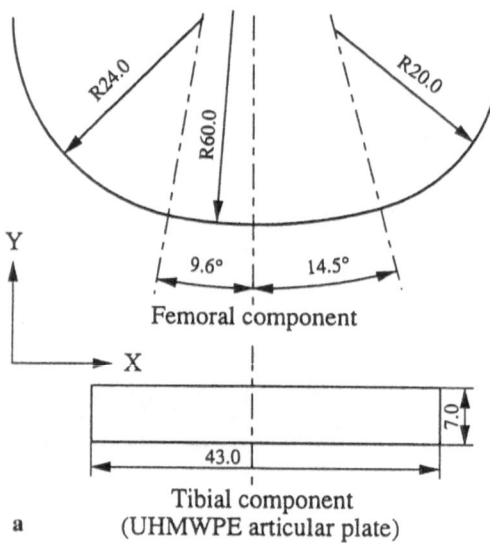

FIG. 9a,b. Shape of the modified contact surface in the sagittal plane. **a** Plain UHMWPE articular plate model (model II). **b** Conformed contact surface model (model III)

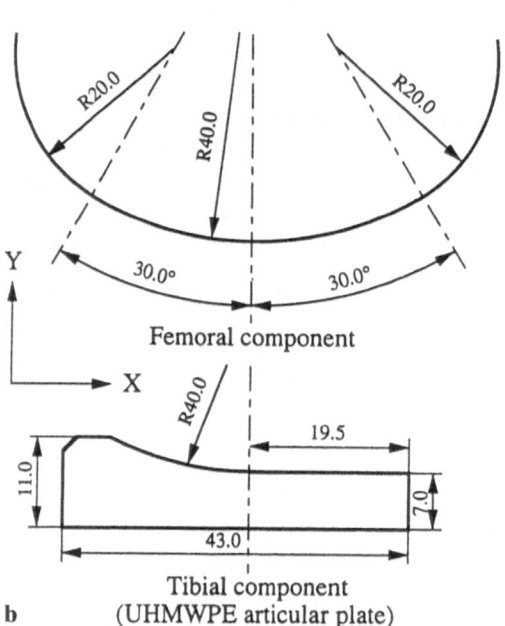

TABLE 1. Material properties of alumina ceramic and ultrahigh molecular weight polyethylene (UHMWPE).

Property	Alumina ceramic	UHMWPE
Young's modulus, E (MPa)	350 000	900
Poisson's ratio, ν	0.2	0.4

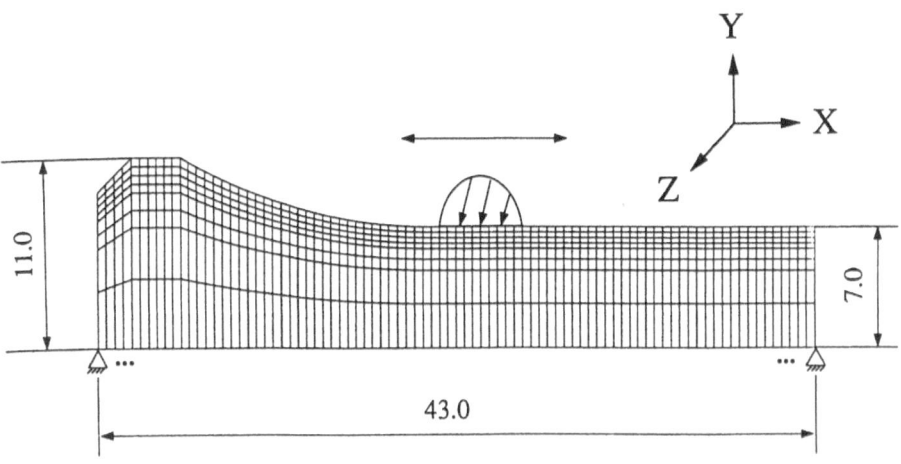

FIG. 10. Finite-element method (FEM) model of UHMWPE articular plate

with the implementation of the proposed constitutive model to computer code.

Figure 11 shows the pattern of load [19], to which the UHMWPE articular plate is subjected, and the flexion angle of the knee joint [20] during normal walking. The maximum load reaches about three times body weight, and the flexion angle changes with two peaks during the walking cycle. The relative position of the two components is obtained from the flexion angle of the knee joint and the anteroposterior movement of the tibial component. Figure 12 shows the variation of tibia movement with flexion angle. Tibia movement is defined as the anteroposterior distance moved of the tibial component observed from the lowest point of the femoral component. The experimental data shown in Fig. 12 were obtained from X-ray film of total knee arthroplasty using this artificial knee

FIG. 11. Pattern of load and flexion angle in knee joints during normal walking.
Solid line, load; *dashed line,* flexion angle (from [19], [20] with permission)

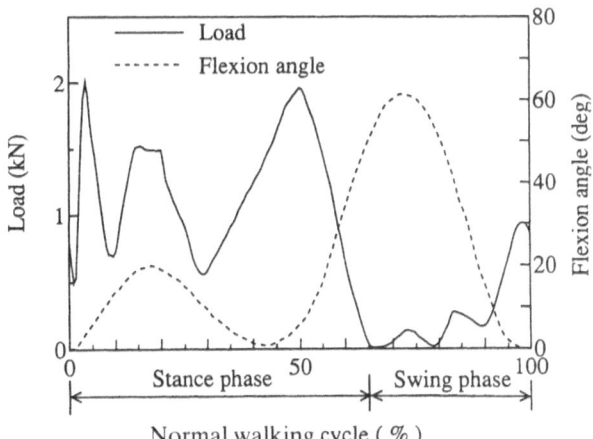

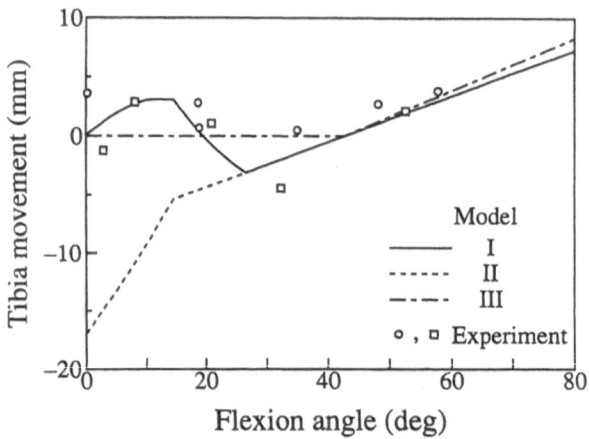

FIG. 12. Variation of tibia movement with flexion angle

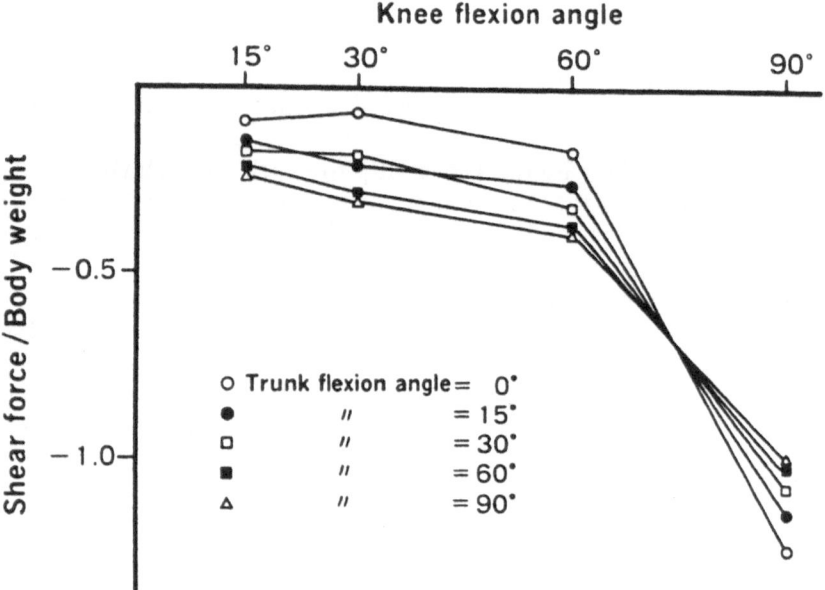

FIG. 13. Shear force per body weight while standing on both legs at various flexion angles of the knee and the trunk (from [21] with permission)

joint. The X-ray was performed in a standing position with the knee flexed at a constant angle and was photographed from the direction perpendicular to the sagittal plane confirmed by the naked eye. The static gravity forces and some muscle forces related to knee joint occurred, but real dynamic forces during walking did not. It is very difficult, however, to determine the correct forces that occurred in and around knee joint during the walking cycle; thus, the method mentioned earlier was employed as a first approximation in this analysis. These data have errors of a few millimeters in tibia movement or a few degrees in flexion angle because the rotation of knee joint from knee flexion was not considered; the direction of photographing is not as accurate, and the image on the film is not clear. The solid line shows the value calculated considering the interference between the femoral component and the anterior protuberance of the UHMWPE articular plate and the posterior cruciate ligament. The tibial component is assumed here to be always subjected to posterior drawer force.

Figure 13 shows the shear force per body weight while standing on both legs at various flexion angles of the knee and trunk as determined by Ohkoshi et al. [21].

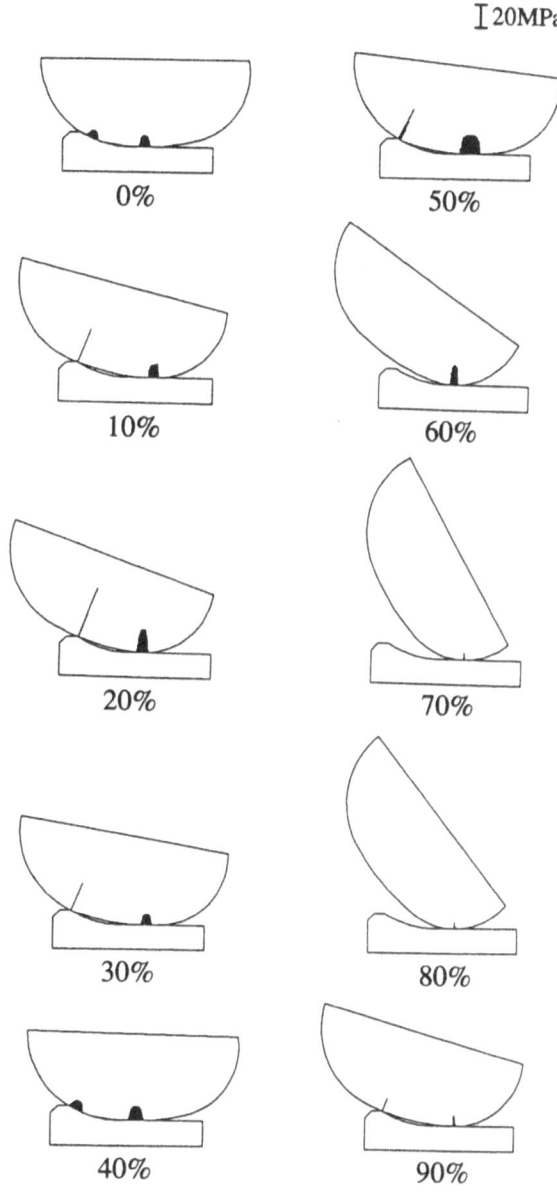

FIG. 14. Example of calculated contact stress distribution in model I

The values of shear force exerted on the tibia in the standing position were negative, revealing posterior drawer forces at every knee flexion angle. Therefore, the previous assumption is considered to be reasonable. The broken line and the dash-dotted line in Fig. 12 show the tibia movement calculated for model II and model III using the same method just mentioned. The tibia moves widely in model II, but in models I and III it does not move as widely in the range of small flexion angles because of the interference of the two components.

The contact stress distribution was determined from simple indentation analysis of the femoral and the tibial components at every 0.5% of the walking cycle considering the load and the relative position of the two components, where the friction between the two components was neglected. Figure 14 shows the example of the calculated contact stress distribution at every 10.0% of the walking cycle in model I. In this artificial knee joint, contact occurs in two regions because of the shape of the contact surface of the two components. The contact stress was then translated on the UHMWPE articular plate as the normal load to simulate the realistic gait of the knee joint. Moreover, the frictional force calculated with the coefficient of friction μ was employed as the tangential traction. In all the analyses, the coefficient of friction between two components was assumed to be 0.1 [8].

3 Results

As the mechanical factor that affects the wear behavior of the UHMWPE articular plate, the following stress components are considered: (1) equivalent stress $\bar{\sigma}$, which initiates the micro-cracks by fatigue of the material [9,15,22]; (2) contact stress p, which initiates and propagates the micro-cracks at the contact surface by the adhesion and micro-fatigue of the material [9,17] according to the direct contact of two components. In the anatomical artificial knee joint, the direct contact of the femoral and the tibial components occurs because of material properties and nonconformity of the shape of the contact surface [7]. (3) Tensile stress σ_x, which propagates the micro-cracks as mode I in the fracture mechanics [15]; σ_y was always compressive stress in this analysis; and (4) shear stress τ_{xy}, which propagates the micro-cracks as mode II in fracture mechanics [15].

Figure 15 shows the variation in sliding velocity of the three models during the walking cycle. The sliding velocities of models I and III vary similarly but that of model II is smaller throughout the cycle because of the wide anteroposterior movement of the femoral component. In all models, however, there are very narrow regions where the sliding velocity takes the values between ±35 mm/s. It is then considered that the amount of wear from the surface, that is, adhesive and abrasive wear, is dependent only on the contact stress, as mentioned in the Introduction.

Figure 16 shows the distribution of the maximum equivalent stress $(\bar{\sigma})_{max}$, the maximum tensile stress $(\sigma_x)_{max}$, and the maximum shear stress $(\tau_{xy})_{max}$ at each

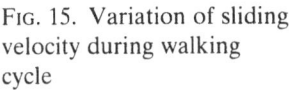

FIG. 15. Variation of sliding velocity during walking cycle

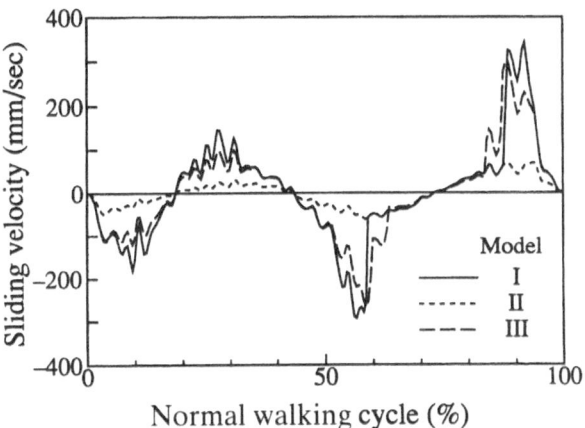

point for the first complete walking cycle in model I. The maximum shear stress $(\tau_{xy})_{max}$ is shown in the absolute value because shear stress τ_{xy} takes plus and minus values. In this analysis, the cyclic calculation was continued until the fifth cycle, but only the analytical results during the first cycle are indicated because the difference between the results of the first cycle and those of subsequent cycles was not remarkable. The equivalent stress $\bar{\sigma}$ becomes larger at two regions, at the surface of the plate in the anterior region and at the subsurface in the middle region. Therefore, the micro-crack initiation caused by material fatigue at these regions is predicted. Also, the plate is subjected to large tensile stress σ_x around the contact surface and to large shear stress τ_{xy} at the surface in the anterior region and at the subsurface in the middle region during walking. The contact stress p also occurs at two regions and becomes vary much larger at the corner of the protuberance of the plate in the anterior region when the corner is in contact with the femoral component.

To study the effect of the shape of the plate, Fig. 17 shows the comparison of the maximum values of these stresses $\bar{\sigma}$, σ_x, τ_{xy}, and p in the whole plate during the first walking cycle. In comparison with model I and model II, the maximum equivalent stress $(\bar{\sigma})_{max}$ and the maximum shear stress $(\tau_{xy})_{max}$ are almost the same, but the maximum tensile stress $(\sigma_x)_{max}$ is larger and the maximum contact stress $(p)_{max}$ is smaller in model II. In model III, all stresses become the smallest of all the models throughout the walking cycle.

4 Discussion

As regards model I, the contact of two components occurs in two regions because of the shape of the contact surface. In the middle region, the equivalent stress $\bar{\sigma}$ and the shear stress τ_{xy} become the largest at the subsurface of the plate, but the tensile stress σ_x becomes the largest at the surface of the plate where the contact stress p also occurs. Therefore, it is considered that the wear of the plate should

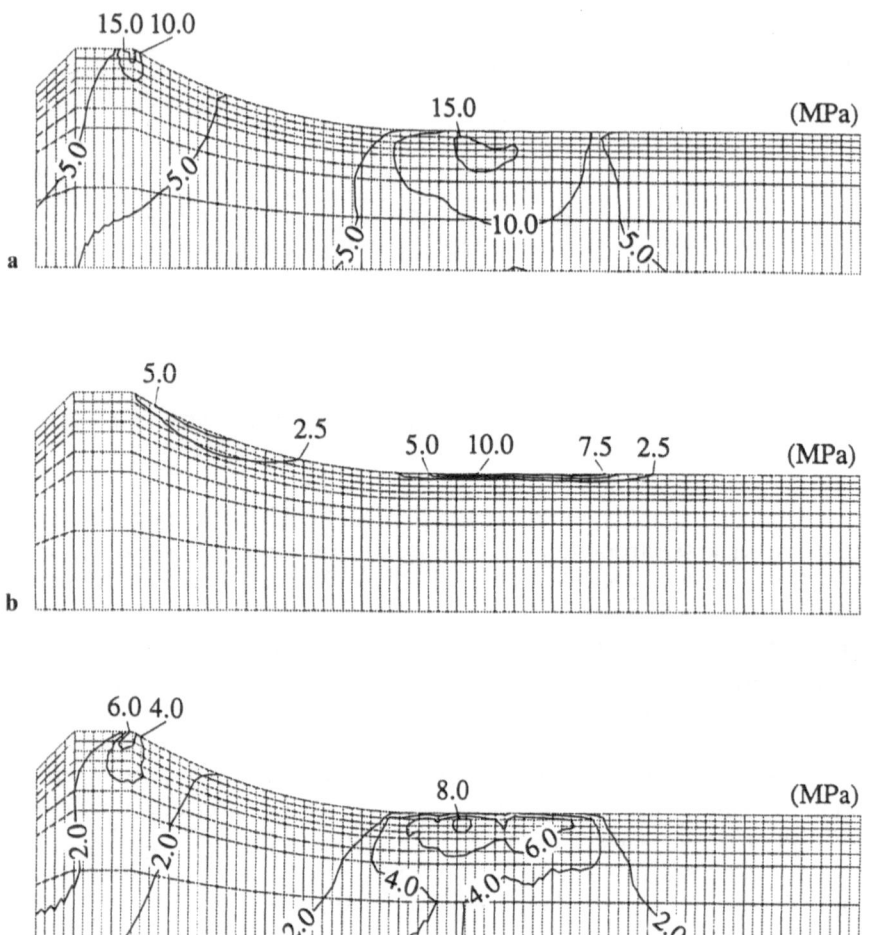

FIG. 16a–c. Distribution of the maximum values of stresses at each point for the first complete walking cycle in model I. **a** Maximum equivalent stree $(\overline{\sigma})_{max}$. **b** Maximum tensile stress $(\sigma_x)_{max}$. **c** Maximum shear stress $(\tau_{xy})_{max}$ (the absolute value)

be initiated from both the subsurface and the surface of the plate. In the evaluation of the retrieved UHMWPE articular plate [13] and in the wear test of the UHMWPE plate, supposing an artificial knee joint [9], wear from the subsurface of the plate caused by material fatigue and from the surface of the plate was observed, and it is considered that the wear appearance is deeply related to these stresses. On the other hand, in the anterior region all stresses become the largest at the surface of the plate; it is thus considered that wear particularly occurs from the surface.

As a result, in model I, from the shape of the contact surface of the UHMWPE articular plate, the anteroposterior movement of the tibial component that causes

FIG. 17. Comparison of maximum values of stresses in the whole plate during the first walking cycle. *Solid bars*, model I; *hatched bars*, model II; *shaded bars*, model III

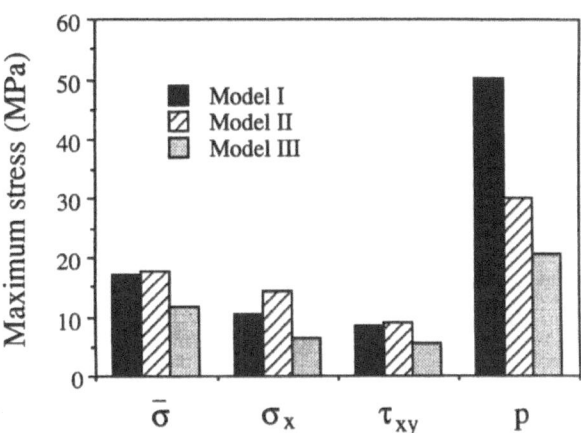

the luxation of the femur is controlled but contact occurs between the femoral component and the corner of the protuberance of the plate. Wear of the plate is then predicted to appear especially from the corner, which is observed only in model I, and it is made clear that the wear of the plate is closely related to the shape of the contact surface.

By modification of the shape of the contact surface, different results were obtained. Because distribution of the contact stress is not divided into two parts and contact occurs in the flat area in model II, maximum tensile stress $(\sigma_x)_{max}$ is larger and maximum contact stress $(p)_{max}$ is smaller than those in model I. In model III, which is designed to prevent luxation and to provide more conformity of the two components in the wider range of the flexion angle, contact stress is dispersed in a wider contact area because of conformity of the contact surface, and all stresses associated with wear of the plate then become the smallest of the three models throughout the walking cycle. Thus it is considered that wear of the plate in model III is reduced. Furthermore, this analysis assumed a constant coefficient of friction and did not consider the effect of lubrication. Actually, the level of the contact surface lubrication varies according to the contact stress [7]. The condition in model III therefore, becomes better than other models because of the smaller contact stress, and thus wear of the plate would be further reduced in model III.

Landy and Walker [23] and Blunn et al. [24] have pointed out that in retrieved articular plates a subsurface crack that causes delamination is initiated by fusion defects produced during manufacture of the UHMWPE articular plate. Delamination is never seen when the articular plate does not contain any defects, as confirmed in articular plates containing no defects that were retrieved for other reasons. Stress concentration obviously occurs around the defects and the subsurface cracks propagate from these defects. If there are defects in the UHMWPE from the beginning of implantation, delamination of the articular plate occurs in a short period. In the long term, however, pure fatigue of the material of the articular plate should be also considered. Thus, including wear from the surface and propagation of subsurface cracks, it is considered important that the amplitude of stress history in the articular plate should be as small as possible.

In this analysis, the shape of the contact surface in model III was employed as an example of the improved conformity model. However, many other shapes of the contact surface that have conformity are expected. Therefore, the shape in model III is not necessarily the optimal shape. To consider the optimal shape of the contact surface in detail, it is necessary to investigate many other models, but the strategy for decreasing wear of the artificial knee joint was obtained from this analysis.

5 Conclusions

Contact analysis of the UHMWPE articular plate used in artificial knee joints during walking was performed using the finite-element method based on the constitutive model of cyclic plasticity. In particular, the effect of the shape of the contact surface on the wear mechanism of the plate was investigated. As a result, it is clear that the appearance of wear from both the subsurface and the surface of the plate is expected. Only at the anterior contact region in model I, however, did all stresses become larger at the surface; wear then would occur especially at the surface region. In comparison with model I, model II was improved from the aspect of contact stress. Conversely, however, the wider anteroposterior tibia movement, which might cause the luxation of the femoral component to occur in the anterior direction, is not controlled and the tensile stress σ_x at the contact surface becomes bigger. In model III, all stresses concerned with wear of the plate became the least of these three models throughout the walking cycle because of the greater conformity of the contact surface. It is thus considered that wear of the plate in model III is reduced. The shape of the contact surface of an artificial knee joint strongly affects the wear behavior of the UHMWPE articular plate, and optimization of the shape for the property of wear can be performed using this method.

During normal walking the movement of the knee joint, the load, and the moment change according to the shape of the contact surface of the artificial knee joint. Evaluation of the artificial knee joint including dynamic gait analysis should then be performed to examine more rigorously the effect of the shape of the component on the life of the joint. Evaluation of the stresses at the fixation interface could also be obtained by this dynamic analysis. Furthermore, we expect to develop an analysis including viscosity of the UHMWPE in the future.

Acknowledgments. The authors thank K. Yasuda, Hokkaido University School of Medicine, for comments from the orthopedic point of view. This research was supported by a Grant-in-Aid for Scientific Research on Priority Area [Biomechanics] from the Ministry of Education, Science and Culture in Japan (No. 04237101).

References

1. Amstutz HC, Campbell P, Kossovsky N, Clarke IC (1992) Mechanism and clinical significance of wear debris-induced osteolysis. Clin Orthop 276:7–18
2. Yasuda K, Miyagi N, Kaneda K (1993) Low friction total knee arthroplasty with the alumina ceramic condylar prosthesis. Bull Hosp Jt Dis 52:15–21
3. Lausmaa J, Rostlund T, McKellop H (1991) Wear of ion implanted pure titanium and Ti6A14V alloy against ultrahigh molecular weight polyethylene. Surf Eng 7:311–317
4. Wright TM, Rimnac CM, Faris PM, Bansal M (1988) Analysis of surface damage in retrieved carbon fiber-reinforced and plain polyethylene tibial components from posterior Stabilized total knee replacements. J Bone Joint Surg 70A:1312–1319
5. Tateishi T, Fukubayashi T (1988) Advanced biocomposite material and application to the artificial joint. Bioceramics 1:48–53
6. Oka M, Noguchi T, Kumar P, Ikeuchi K, Yamamuro T, Hyon SH, Ikada Y (1990) Development of an artificial articular cartilage. Clin Mater 6:361–381
7. Murakami T, Ohtsuki N, Higaki H (1993) The adaptive multimode lubrication in knee prostheses with compliant layer during walking motion. In: Dowson D, Taylor CM, Childs THC, Godet M, Dalmaz G (eds) Thin films in tribology. Elsevier, Amsterdam, pp 673–682
8. McKellop H, Clarke I, Markolf K, Amstutz H (1981) Friction and wear properties of polymer, metal, and ceramic prosthetic joint materials evaluated on a multichannel screening device. J Biomed Mater Res 15:619–653
9. Blunn GW, Walker PS, Joshi A, Hardinge K (1991) The dominance of cyclic sliding in producing wear in total knee replacements. Clin Orthop 273:253–260
10. Fisher J, Dowson D, Hamdzah H, Lee HL (1994) The effect of sliding velocity on the friction and wear of UHMWPE for use in total artificial joints. Wear 175:219–225
11. Rose RM, Ries MD, Paul IL, Crugnola AM, Ellis E (1984) On the true wear rate of ultrahigh molecular weight polyethylene in the total knee prosthesis. J Biomed Mater Res 18:207–224
12. Hood RW, Wright TM, Burstein AH (1983) Retrieval analysis of total knee prostheses: a method and its application to 48 total condylar prostheses. J Biomed Mater Res 17:829–842
13. Engh GA, Dwyer KA, Hanes CK (1992) Polyethylene wear of metal-backed tibial components in total and unicompartmental knee prostheses. J Bone Joint Surg 74B:9–17
14. Bartel DL, Burstein AM, Toda MD, Edwards DL (1985) The effect of conformity and plastic thickness on contact stresses in metal-backed plastic implants. Trans ASME J Biomech Eng 107:193–199
15. Bartel DL, Bicknell VL, Wright TM (1986) The effect of conformity, thickness, and material on stresses in ultra-high molecular weight components for total joint replacement. J Bone Surg 68A:1041–1051
16. Ishikawa H, Sasaki K (1987) Constitutive model of cyclic plasticity considering induced anisotropy. In: Desai CS, Krempl E, Kiousis PD, Kundu T (eds) Constitutive laws for engineering materials. Elsevier, New York, pp 581–587

17. Atkinson JR, Brown KJ, Dowson D (1978) The wear of high molecular weight polyethylene. Part I: The wear of isotropic polyethylene against dry stainless steel in unidirectional motion. Trans ASME J Lubr Technol 100:208–218
18. Drucker DC, Palgen L (1981) On stress-strain relation suitable for cyclic and other loading. Trans ASME J Appl Mech 48:479–485
19. Morrison JB (1968) Bioengineering analysis of force actions transmitted by the knee joint. Biomed Eng (Berl) 3:164–170
20. Lafortune MA, Cavanagh PR, Sommer HJ III, Kalenak A (1992) Three-dimensional kinematics of the human knee during walking. J Biomech 25:347–357
21. Ohkoshi Y, Yasuda K, Kaneda K, Wada T, Yamanaka M (1991) Biomechanical analysis of rehabilitation in the standing position. Am J Sports Med 19:605–611
22. Cheng W, Cheng HS, Mura T, Keer LM (1994) Micromechanics modeling of crack initiation under contact fatigue. Trans ASME J Tribol 116:2–8
23. Landy MM, Walker PS (1988) Wear of ultra-high-molecular-weight polyethylene components of 90 retrieved knee prostheses. J Arthroplasty 3:S73–S85
24. Blunn GW, Joshi AB, Liley PA, Engelbrecht E, Ryd L, Lidgren L, Hardinge K, Nieder E, Walker PS (1992) Polyethylene wear in unicondylar knee prostheses: 106 retrieved Marmor, PCA, and St Georg tibial components compared. Acta Orthop Scand 63:247–255

Morphological Modeling and Growth Simulation of Idiopathic Scoliosis

SHIGERU TADANO[1], MASAHIRO KANAYAMA[2], TAKAYOSHI UKAI[1], and KIYOSHI KANEDA[2]

Summary. Scoliosis is defined as an appreciable lateral deviation with axial rotation in the normally straight vertical line of the spine. Idiopathic scoliosis is a deformity that develops during a period of rapid growth and is reduced after skeletal maturity. As a biomechanical approach to scoliosis, this chapter presents both a morphological modeling method to mathematically express the three-dimensional configuration of the scoliotic spine and a computer simulation method to examine the effect of asymmetrical local growth on scoliosis deformities of the spinal column. In morphological modeling, the three-dimensional location of the vertebral centroid was reconstructed from both fronal and sagittal roentgenograms. The Cobb angle, which is an important clinical index used for the evaluation of scoliosis curvature, could be calculated numerically and three-dimensionally from the proposed model. The other geometrical characteristics of the spatial curve of the scoliotic spine were also confirmed. In simulation of growth deformation, a three-dimensional, finite-element model of the normal skeletal spine was constructed. It consists of the vertebrae and the intervertebral disks of the thoracolumbar region from T-1 to L-5, the sacrum, the rib pairs 1–10, the sternum and costal cartilages, and the joint capsules. Bony growth deformation induced by growth force was defined as permanent deformation. When the axial asymmetrical growth force was applied to the lateral region from the left to posterior in the T-8 vertebral body, this model could simulate well a single scoliosis curvature toward the lateral direction with vertebral rotation, as seen in typical scoliosis deformities.

Key words: Biomechanics—Idiopathic scoliosis—Morphological modeling—Computer simulation—Growth analysis

[1]Department of Mechanical Engineering II, Faculty of Engineering, Hokkaido University, N13 W8 Kita-ku, Sapporo, Hokkaido, 060 Japan
[2]Department of Orthopaedic Surgery, Hokkaido University School of Medicine, N15 W7 Kita-ku, Sapporo, Hokkaido, 060 Japan

1 Introduction

The human spine is a complex structure that is principally composed of many vertebrae, intervertebral disks, and the rib cage, and has three main regions: cervical, thoracic, and lumbar. The normal geometry of the spine is straight frontally with a physiological sagittal curvature that shows kyphosis in the thoracic region and lordosis in the lumbar region. One of the most serious diseases of the spine is scoliosis, which is characterized as a lateral deformity of the spine in the frontal plane. Scoliosis is a three-dimensional spinal deformity with an appreciable lateral deviation. It also accompanies axial rotation of the vertebrae in the curve area of scoliosis [1,2]. Figure 1 shows a schematic configuration of the scoliotic spine of a single thoracic curvature.

A number of reports have described three-dimensional measurement and evaluation of the scoliosis deformity [3–6]. Deacon et al. [7] also emphasized the importance of three-dimensional evaluation of scoliosis deformity. Stokes et al. [6] mathematically expressed the scoliotic spine by a Fourier sine series that was applicable regardless of curvature and curve patterns, and also calculated Cobb angles in the frontal and sagittal planes from the approximation curve. However, their modeling of the scoliotic spine was performed two-dimensionally on the projections of the spine in specified planes. Because scoliosis is a three-dimensional spinal deformity, it should be evaluated in a three-dimensional reconstruction of the spine.

On the other hand, idiopathic scoliosis is a deformity that develops during a period of rapid growth and is reduced after skeletal maturity. The definite cause

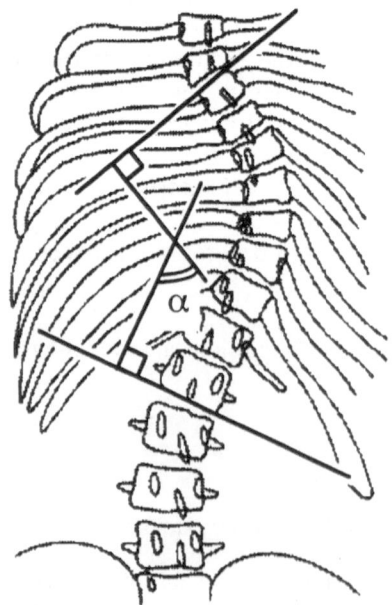

Fig. 1. Schematic configuration of idiopathic scoliotic spine of a single thoracic curvature (from [17], [18] with permission)

of idiopathic scoliosis, however, is unknown in spite of numerous clinical studies. Scoliosis is a condition defined by many mechanical terms, so biomechanical studies are relevant and have investigated various factors that induce the lateral curvature of the spine. Schultz [8] reviewed in detail articles on the use of mathematical and other types of models for the biomechanical study of scoliosis. The hypothesis of the growth factor is one of the strongest for the cause of idiopathic scoliosis. Some evidence of asymmetrical growth in spinal components have been reported to be responsible for causing scoliosis: asymmetrical growth in the vertebrae [9–11], in the upper arm [12], and in the rib [13,14].

These observations of asymmetries implicate asymmetrical growth in the etiology of scoliosis. However, they did not establish that asymmetrical growth is the primary cause of the spinal and other asymmetries, nor did they define the precise mechanisms responsible for the observed changes. Therefore, the biomechanical aspects of curve development and the mechanism of scoliosis were analyzed by mathematical modeling techniques. Stokes et al. [15] presented a finite osseoligamentous structural model of the human thorax to analyze the asymmetrical growth of the rib cage. Kawabata et al. [16] analyzed one-plane buckling deformation of the spinal column by the growth force analogous to a thermal stress.

As a biomechanical approach to idiopathic scoliosis, the intent of this chapter is to provide (1) a morphological modeling method to express mathematically the three-dimensional configuration of the scoliotic spine [17,18] and (2) a computer simulation method to examine the hypothesis that asymmetrical local growth in a vertebral body might initiate scoliosis deformities of the spinal column [25].

2 Morphological Modeling of the Scoliotic Spine

2.1 Morphological Curve of the Spine

To express numerically the whole spine, three-dimensional locations of each vertebra were determined from both frontal and sagittal roentgenograms. A coordinate system of the spinal column was defined as shown in Fig. 2. The origin of the axes is the midpoint between the upper edge lines of the sacrum (S-1) on both roentgenograms. The x-, y-, and z-axes are orthogonal to the frontal, the sagittal, and the horizontal plane, respectively. Positive directions of these axes are anterior, right side, and head side, respectively. The measuring points in a frontal roentgenogram were the right-upper corner (y_1^n, z_1^n), the right-lower corner (y_2^n, z_2^n), the left-upper corner (y_3^n, z_3^n), and the left-lower corner (y_4^n, z_4^n) at each vertebral body. The upper point (y_5^n, z_5^n) and the lower point (y_6^n, z_6^n) in the right pedicle, and the upper point (y_7^n, z_7^n) and the lower point (y_8^n, z_8^n) in left pedicle, were also measured. Similarly, the measuring points in a sagittal roentgenogram were the anterior-upper corner (x_9^n, z_9^n), the anterior-lower corner (x_{10}^n, z_{10}^n), the posterior-upper corner (x_{11}^n, z_{11}^n), and the posterior-lower corner (x_{12}^n, z_{12}^n); the superscript n indicates vertebral level. The positions of 12 points at each vertebra

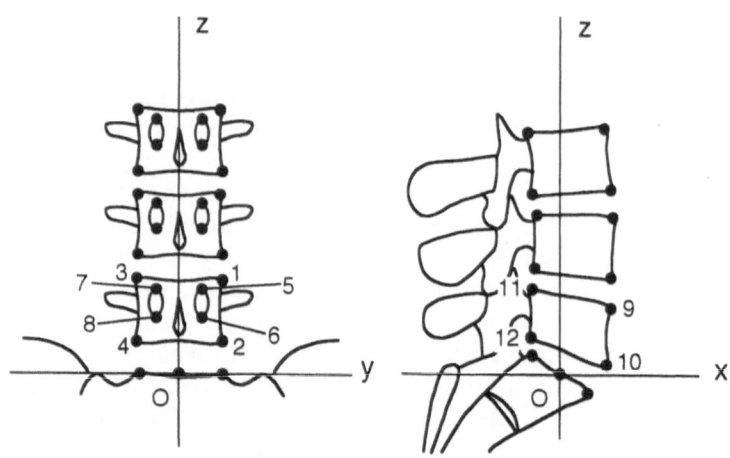

FIG. 2. Spinal coordinate system and measured points, frontal (*left*) and sagittal (*right*) views (from [17], [18] with permission)

from T-1 (first thoracic vertebra, $n = 1$) to L-5 (fifth lumbar vertebra, $n = 17$) were measured carefully and precisely on both roentgenograms using a digitizer (KD5050L, Graphtec, Tokyo, Japan).

The morphological curve of the spine was reconstructed as a spatial curve that was connected with each center position of the vertebral body. The curve was also defined as the vertebral centroid by Stokes and Laible [15]. The position of the vertebral center, $C_n(x_C^n, y_C^n, z_C^n)$, is obtained by Eq. 1 from measuring points in Fig. 2.

$$x_C^n = \left(x_9^n + x_{10}^n + x_{11}^n + x_{12}^n\right)/4$$
$$y_C^n = \left(y_1^n + y_2^n + y_3^n + y_4^n\right)/4$$
$$z_C^n = \left(z_1^n + z_2^n + z_3^n + z_4^n\right)/4 = \left(z_9^n + z_{10}^n + z_{11}^n + z_{12}^n\right)/4 \qquad (1)$$

In general, a spatial curve is mathematically represented as Eq. 2, where the position vector of an arbitrary point on the curve is defined as $\boldsymbol{r} = (x, y, z)$.

$$\boldsymbol{r} = x(t)\boldsymbol{i} + y(t)\boldsymbol{j} + z(t)\boldsymbol{k} \qquad (2)$$

In Eq. 2, $(\boldsymbol{i}, \boldsymbol{j}, \boldsymbol{k})$ are the unit vectors for x-, y-, and z-directions, respectively. Parameters of $x(t)$ and $y(t)$ represent alignments of the vertebral centroid in the yz-plane (frontal plane) and the xz-plane (sagittal plane) under $z(t) = t$. They were approximated by quintic polynomials passing through the origin of the axes and were represented as Eqs. 3 and 4:

$$x = a_1 z^5 + a_2 z^4 + a_3 z^3 + a_4 z^2 + a_5 z \qquad (3)$$
$$y = b_1 z^5 + b_2 z^4 + b_3 z^3 + b_4 z^2 + b_5 z \qquad (4)$$

Both Eq. 3 and Eq. 4 geometrically indicate each curved surface in space. The intersection between both curves forms a three-dimensional curve. Therefore, parameters of Eq. 2 were represented by Eq. 5. These equations are defined as a morphological curve of the spine.

$$x(t) = a_1 t^5 + a_2 t^4 + a_3 t^3 + a_4 t^2 + a_5 t$$
$$y(t) = b_1 t^5 + b_2 t^4 + b_3 t^3 + b_4 t^2 + b_5 t$$
$$z(t) = t \tag{5}$$

2.2 Estimation of Axial Rotation Angle of Each Vertebra

It is difficult to measure accurately the axial rotation of vertebrae in the xy-plane because we have no xy-plane roentgenograms. However, the axial rotation can be estimated by using a semicylindrical model of the vertebral body. Figure 3 shows the axial and frontal views of the model geometry. The angle of vertebral rotation can be calculated from the value of deviation between the sagittal center line and the relative position of both pedicles where the geometric center of vertebral body is assumed to coincide with the center of vertebral rotation [2]. In this figure, d indicates the minimum distance in the x-direction between the vertebral centroid (C) and the posterior wall of the vertebra. The pedicle offsets from the sagittal center line are a on the left side and b on the right side. W is the distance in the y-direction between the midpoint (M) of both pedicles and the sagittal center line. Using the geometric relation of $W = b - (a + b)/2 = (b - a)/2$, the angle of axial vertebral rotation ($\theta'' = \theta''_{xy}$) is calculated as Eq. 6. The positive direction of θ'' is counterclockwise viewed from the top.

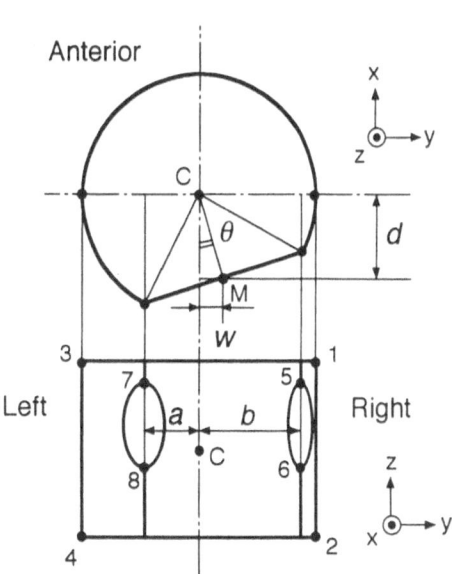

FIG. 3. Model geometry to calculate vertebral rotation (from [17], [18] with permission)

$$\tan\theta'' = \frac{W''}{d''} = \frac{b'' - a''}{2d''} \tag{6}$$

The values of a'', b'', and d'' in Eq. 6 are obtained from the coordinates of measuring points, as Eq. 7:

$$a'' = \left| \frac{y_7'' + y_8''}{2} - \frac{y_1'' + y_2'' + y_3'' + y_4''}{4} \right|$$

$$b'' = \left| \frac{y_5'' + y_6''}{2} - \frac{y_1'' + y_2'' + y_3'' + y_4''}{4} \right|$$

$$d'' = \left| \frac{x_{11}'' + x_{12}''}{2} - \frac{x_9'' + x_{10}'' + x_{11}'' + x_{12}''}{4} \right| \tag{7}$$

Consequently, θ'' is represented as Eq. 8:

$$\tan\theta'' = \frac{\left|2y_5'' + 2y_6'' - y_1'' - y_2'' - y_3'' - y_4''\right| - \left|2y_7'' + 2y_8'' - y_1'' - y_2'' - y_3'' - y_4''\right|}{2\left|x_{11}'' + x_{12}'' - x_9'' - x_{10}''\right|} \tag{8}$$

2.3 Formulation of the Three-Dimensional Cobb Angle

Magnitude of scoliosis curvature is clinically evaluated by the Cobb angle, measured on a frontal roentgenogram of the whole spine. The Cobb angle is defined as the angle between both lines drawn on the end plates of end vertebrae in the curve area, which means the maximum tangent angle between two vertebrae in the whole spine (see Fig. 1). In this method, the Cobb angle can be calculated not only in two dimensions but in three dimensions from the mathematical morphological curve.

A tangent vector ($\dot{r}$) at an arbitrary point on the morphological curve of Eqs. 2 and 5 is obtained as Eq. 9:

$$\dot{r} = \left(\frac{\partial x}{\partial t}, \frac{\partial y}{\partial t}, \frac{\partial z}{\partial t} \right) = \left(x'(z), y'(z), 1 \right) \tag{9}$$

The three-dimentsional Cobb angle is the angle formed in three dimensions by normals of the end plates of end vertebrae. The angle α_{kl} between the tangent vectors at the end vertebrae can be obtained from Eq. 10, where $\dot{r}_k$ and $\dot{r}_l$ are the tangent vectors at the upper and lower end vertebrae.

$$\alpha_{kl} = \cos^{-1}\left(\frac{\dot{r}_k \cdot \dot{r}_l}{|\dot{r}_k| \cdot |\dot{r}_l|} \right) \tag{10}$$

The three-dimensional Cobb angle α is defined as the maximum value calculated from Eq. 10 in the curve area of scoliosis. Figure 4 shows a geometric description of the three-dimensional Cobb angle. To determine the curve area of scoliosis,

FIG. 4. Geometrical description of three-dimensional Cobb angle side (from [17], [18] with permission)

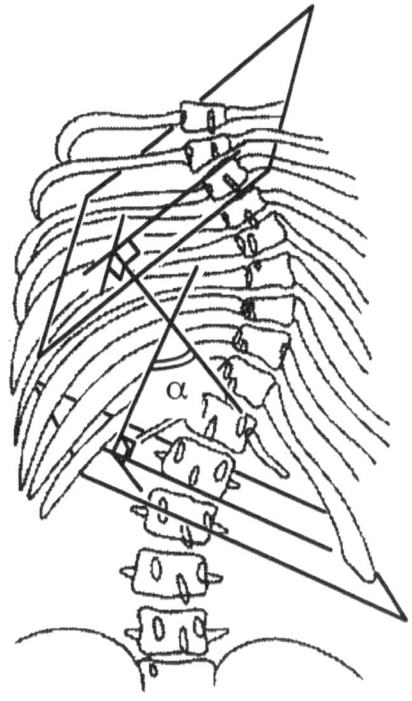

the upper and the lower end vertebrae must be specified. The end vertebrae are regarded as the inflection points of the frontal curve of Eq. 4. Therefore, the three-dimensional Cobb angle can be calculated from two tangent vectors at the points where the value of $\partial^2 y/\partial z^2$ becomes nearest to zero. Eliminating the x-component in Eqs. 9 and 10, the value of α calculated from Eq. 10 is equivalent to the clinical Cobb angle in the frontal plane.

2.4 Geometric Torsion in the Scoliotic Spine

Geometric torsion T represents the amount of deviation from a plane curve, which is calculated according to Frenet's formulae as follows [19,20]:

$$T = \rho^2 \frac{\dfrac{d\boldsymbol{r}}{dt} \dfrac{d^2\boldsymbol{r}}{dt^2} \dfrac{d^3\boldsymbol{r}}{dt^3}}{\left|\left(\dfrac{d\boldsymbol{r}}{dt}\right)^2\right|^3} = \rho^2 \frac{\begin{vmatrix} x' & y' & z' \\ x'' & y'' & z'' \\ x''' & y''' & z''' \end{vmatrix}}{\left(x'^2 + y'^2 + z'^2\right)^3} = \rho^2 \frac{\left(\dfrac{d^2x}{dz^2}\dfrac{d^3y}{dz^3} - \dfrac{d^2y}{dz^2}\dfrac{d^3x}{dz^3}\right)}{\left(\left(\dfrac{dx}{dz}\right)^2 + \left(\dfrac{dy}{dz}\right)^2\right)^3} \quad (11)$$

where ρ is the radius of curvature, and is calculated as follows:

$$\rho^2 = \frac{\left|\left(\dfrac{d\mathbf{r}}{dt}\right)^2\right|^3}{\left(\dfrac{d\mathbf{r}}{dt}\right)^2\left(\dfrac{d^2\mathbf{r}}{dt^2}\right)^2 - \left(\dfrac{d\mathbf{r}}{dt}\dfrac{d^2\mathbf{r}}{dt^2}\right)^2}$$

$$= \frac{\left(x'^2 + y'^2 + z'^2\right)^3}{\left(x'^2 + y'^2 + z'^2\right)\left(x''^2 + y''^2 + z''^2\right) - \left(x'x'' + y'y'' + z'z''\right)^2}$$

$$= \frac{\left(\left(\dfrac{dx}{dz}\right)^2 + \left(\dfrac{dy}{dz}\right)^2 + 1\right)^3}{\left(\left(\dfrac{dx}{dz}\right)^2 + \left(\dfrac{dy}{dz}\right)^2 + 1\right)\left(\left(\dfrac{d^2x}{dz^2}\right)^2 + \left(\dfrac{d^2y}{dz^2}\right)^2\right) - \left(\dfrac{dx}{dz}\dfrac{d^2x}{dz^2} + \dfrac{dy}{dz}\dfrac{d^2y}{dz^2}\right)^2} \tag{12}$$

Because the normal spine has no curvature in the frontal plane, the morphological curve can be regarded as a plane curve on the sagittal plane. Then, the geometric torsion of Eq. 11 becomes constantly zero. The scoliotic spine will produce some deviation from the plane curve according to lateral curvature; the geometric torsion then becomes some value other than zero. Therefore, geometric torsion is a significant index that shows a morphological property of the scoliotic spine.

2.5 Evaluation of the Morphology of Scoliosis

Forty-five spines of adolescent idiopathic scoliosis were analyzed with this method. Figure 5 shows a typical configuration of right thoracic scoliosis (T-5–T-12; Cobb angle = 47°). The ordinate of the figure indicates the nondimensional spinal height from the sacrum (h/H), where H is the height of the upper surface at the T-1 vertebra. The closed circles represent the position of each vertebral centroid. The left side of Fig. 5 shows the nondimensional value of frontal displacement (Dx/H), the middle is the nondimensional value of sagittal displacement (Dy/H), and the right side is the axial rotation angle of each vertebra. It is clear from these figures that the clinical configuration of scoliosis is lateral deviation on the right, disappearance of the physiological sagittal curve, and the appearance of vertebral axial rotation, where the maximum rotation occurs at the T-8 vertebra. The frontal and sagittal alignments of the vertebral centroid were very closely approximated by Eq. 5 (correlation coefficients, $r = 0.998$), and are shown by solid lines in these figures. The r value in each approximation was more than 0.96 in all cases of this examination. Therefore, it was confirmed that the three-dimensional configuration of the scoliotic spine could be represented by the morphological curve of Eqs. 2 and 5.

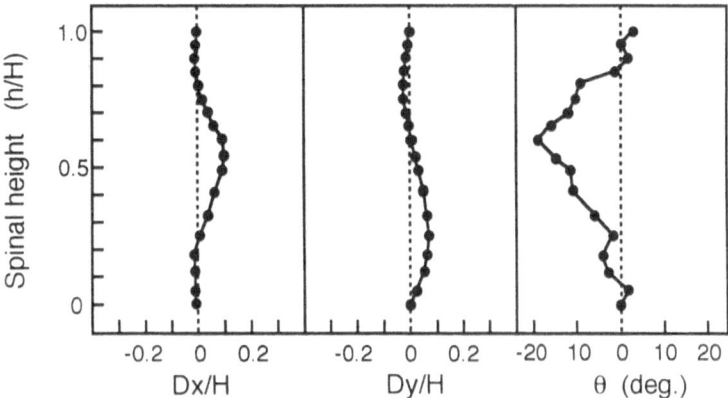

F_{IG}. 5. A Typical configuration of idiopathic scoliosis with a right thoracic curve. *Left*, frontal view; *middle*, sagittal view; *right*, vertebral rotation (from [18] with permission)

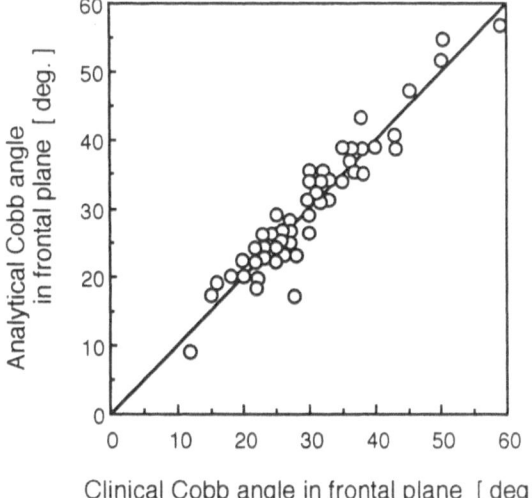

F_{IG}. 6. Relationship between frontal-plane Cobb angle calculated from the morphological curve and Cobb angle measured on frontal roentgenogram (from [17], [18] with permission)

Figure 6 shows the relationship between the frontal-plane Cobb angle calculated from the morphological curve (defined as analytical Cobb angle) and the Cobb angle measured on the frontal roentgenogram (defined as clinical Cobb angle). The two Cobb angles were almost equivalent. This result also validated this mathematical model for the scoliotic spine. Figure 7 shows the relationship between frontal-plane and three-dimensional Cobb angles. In most cases, the three-dimensional Cobb angle was larger than the Cobb angle in the frontal plane

Figure 8 shows the distribution of geometric torsion with the curve area of scoliosis indicated by shading. These data were calculated from the result shown

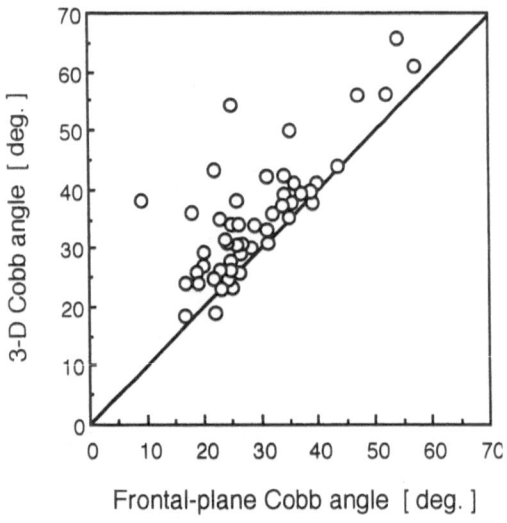

FIG. 7. Relationship between three-dimensional (3-D) Cobb angle and frontal-plane Cobb angle (from [17], [18] with permission)

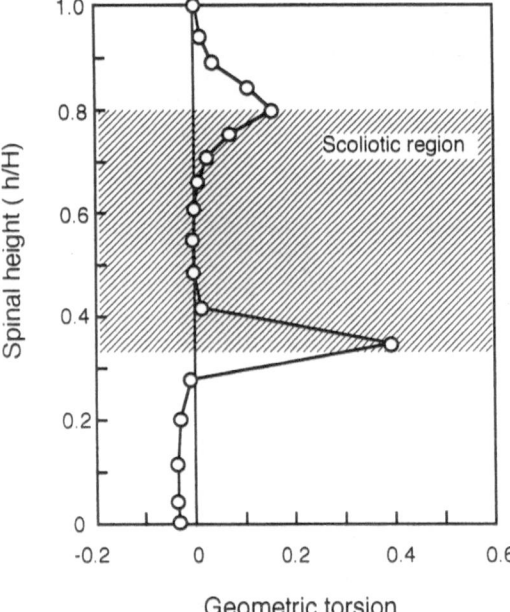

FIG. 8. Distribution of geometric torsion. *Shaded area* is the scoliotic region (from [17], [18] with permission)

in Fig. 5. The geometric torsion had extreme values at the levels of upper and lower end vertebrae and was nearly zero within the curve area of scoliosis. These results were also confirmed in most cases of this study. Therefore, it is revealed that the scoliotic spine swerves from a plane curve only at the levels of end vertebrae and shows a plane curve within the curve area of scoliosis. That is, the

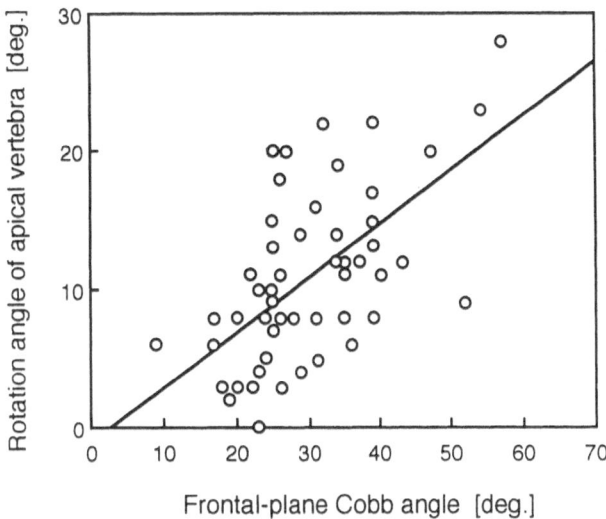

FIG. 9. Relationship between vertebral axial rotation and frontal-plane Cobb angle (from [17], [18] with permission)

vertebrae within the curve area were arranged on a specified plane. The three-dimensional Cobb angle is measured in this plane, and as the three-dimensional Cobb angle indicates maximum curvature of the spine, this plane can be regarded as the plane of maximum curvature, as pointed out by Stokes [21].

The three-dimensional Cobb angle can quantify the spinal curvature, but is unable to qualify the deformity because the physiological curvature is included in the sagittal plane. As a property of spinal deformity, the spatial orientation of the plane of maximum curvature can be calculated as inclinations of this plane to the frontal, sagittal, and horizontal planes (β_{yz}, β_{xz}, β_{xy}). In Fig. 5, these values of β_{yz}, β_{xz}, and β_{xy} were 33°, 59°, and 81°, respectively.

The inclination to the horizontal plane (β_{xy}) in all measurements was 81.4° ± 6.2° (SD). The relationship was investigated between vertebral axial rotation and inclinations of the plane of maximum curvature to the coordinate planes. It was confirmed that the plane of maximum curvature was orthogonal to the horizontal plane regardless of the amount of vertebral axial rotation. However, inclinations to the frontal and sagittal planes (β_{xy} and β_{xz}) had no statistical correlation with vertebral axial rotation ($r = 0.126$ and 0.141, respectively). There was also no significant relationship between froznal-plane, three-dimensional Cobb angles and sagittal inclination (β_{xz}) of the maximum curve plane ($r = 0.407$ and 0.094).

Figure 9 shows the relationship between vertebral rotation and frontal-plane Cobb angle. Positive correlation between these values was found ($r = 0.607$); however, the correlation between the three-dimensional Cobb angle and vertebral rotation was not clear ($r = 0.497$).

3 Computer Simulation for the Scoliotic Spine

3.1 Three-Dimensional Structural Modeling of the Whole Spine

The finite-element model of the normal skeletal spine consists of the vertebrae and the intervertebral disks of the thoracolumbar region from T-1 to L-5, the sacrum, the rib pairs 1–10, the sternum, the costal cartilages, and the joint capsules. The initial geometry of the model was created by reflecting the data of many anatomical features; the physiological curves of the spinal column in the sagittal plane, the complex shape of vertebrae, and rib pairs with level-to-level variations. Figure 10 shows the overall geometry of the model in frontal and sagittal view. This model has 2002 three-dimensional isoparametric solid elements. Each vertebral body has the substructures of cortical and cancellous bone; each intervertebral disk has the substructures of annulus fibrosus and nucleus pulposus.

Material properties are much more difficult to determine, because biological tissue is well known as a material with severe nonlinearity and inhomogeneity. Therefore, the linear elastic properties of each component in this model were taken from the reference data in many published papers. Table 1 lists Young's modulus E (MPa) and the Poisson ratio v at each structural part. Sacrum, lamina, spinal process, rib, and sternum were modeled by cortical bone tissue; facet joints

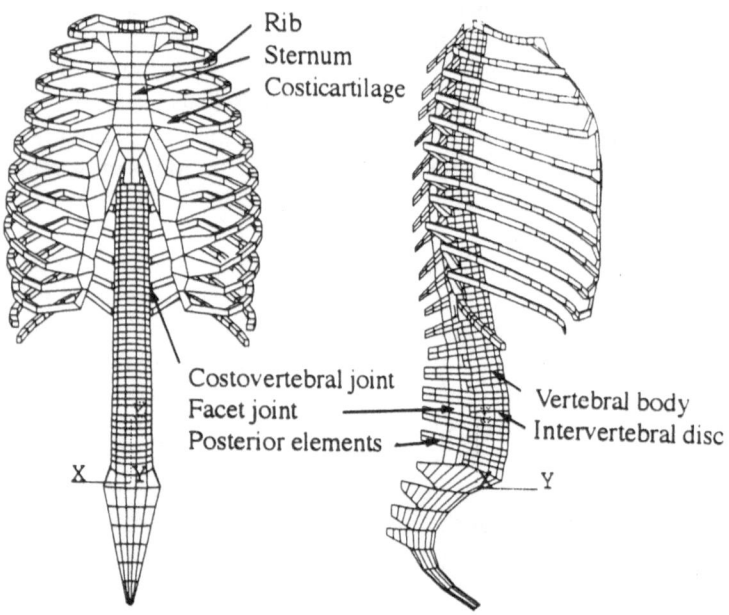

FIG. 10. Initial geometry of three-dimensional finite-element model. *Left*, frontal view; *right*, sagittal view (from [25] with permission)

TABLE 1. Material constants. (From [25] with permission)

Parts	Tissue	E(MPa)	γ
Vertebral body	Cortical bone	12 000	0.3
	Cancellous bone	1 500	0.2
Sacrum	Cortical bone	12 000	0.3
Lamina and spinal process	Cortical bone	12 000	0.3
Rib and sternum	Cortical bone	12 000	0.3
Facet joint	Articular tissue	1.0	0.4
Intervertebral disk	Annulus fibrosus	10	0.4
	Nucleus pulposus	0.13	0.49
Costocartilage	Cartilage	480	0.49
Costovertebral joint	Articular tissue	1.0	0.4

and costovertebral joints were modeled by a solid element having the lowest elastic modulus to represent an articular tissue; and costicartilage was modeled by a cartilage tissue.

3.2 Growth Analysis

It can be assumed, in the macroscopic and mechanical aspects, that growth of a living tissue is analogous to deformation with an increase in volume. A stress may then occur in the living tissue so that it is itself deformed. The stress is considered as a growth stress that induces self-swelling and acts externally to outer tissue. To simplify these phenomena in this analysis, growth force was defined as an equivalent external load acting at nodal points in an element where growth stress occurred.

The purpose of this analysis was to investigate the effect of local asymmetrical growth force on the curve configuration of scoliosis. Therefore, the growth deformation of only the spinal column was analyzed by applying a growth force at cortical bone on the lower and upper surfaces of vertebral bodies. The force is assumed to be tensile and is always applied for the axial direction on the local coordinate system set in a vertebral body. Bony growth deformation induced by growth force was defined as permanent deformation, which was analyzed by introducing the constitutive laws of incremental stress–plastic strain, which permits the volume change in a loading direction. The material matrix representing the relationship between stress and plastic strain under growth deformation is unknown. Therefore, the $[D]$ matrix of elasticity was used except for the values of the Poisson ratio on the axial direction of cortical bone in a vertebral body. These values of the Poisson ratio were 0.1. This computational procedure is analogous to a rigid-plastic analysis that is often used in a metal-forming analysis.

The configuration of scoliotic spine with a single thoracic curve as shown in Fig. 5 was simulated in this analysis. Because it was observed that actual scoliotic spines with a single thoracic curve often had the apical vertebra as the T-8 vertebra, the asymmetrical growth force was applied at the T-8 vertebral body only. At the vertebrae other than T-8, uniform growth force was applied to be deformed symmetrically. Figure 11 shows distribution of both uniform and asymmetrical growth force applied at a vertebral body. The maximum value in the distribution of the asymmetrical growth force was located at the anterior region of the T-8 vertebra (case 1), the anterolateral right (case 2), the right (case 3), the posterolateral right (case 4), the posterior (case 5), and the left (case 6). All rotations and three translations were constrained at the sacrum and T-1 vertebra of the upper and lower bound in the model. In the less constrained model, all rotations and only vertical translation were permitted at the T-1 vertebra.

3.3 Procedure of Computer Simulation

The solution was obtained by using the ANSYS three-dimensional finite-element package (ANSYS, Houston, PA, USA). Linearity of both material properties and geometry of small displacements were assumed. To simulate geometric nonlinearity from large displacements, the model was calculated in reiteration with increments of varying growth force. Figure 12 shows a flow chart of this calculation. This calculation starts from setting the initial geometry of the model. Local coordinate systems in each vertebral body are set up. Next, one vertebral level at which to apply growth force is selected at random. If the T-8 vertebra is selected, asymmetrical growth force is applied; to any other vertebra, uniform growth force is applied. End constraints are determined and the model is analyzed in succession. The geometric data of the deformed spine are obtained and are used as the initial geometry for the next step in the calculation. This loop is iterated. One step is the calculation that growth force is loaded in one vertebral body. One cycle is iterated in 16 steps, which means one round calculation from the T-1 to L-5 vertebra in the whole spine. The increment magnitude of uniform growth force was defined as an equivalent value of external load when the height of the model increased in 1% at one cycle of iteration. The maximum force in local asymmetrical distribution was twofold that of the uniform force. The calculation was carried out for five cycles of 80 steps. An example of the iteration schedule is shown in Fig. 13. The run time for one solution cycle was 90 min when run on an HP-712/80 workstation (Hewlett-Packard, Palo Alto, CA, USA).

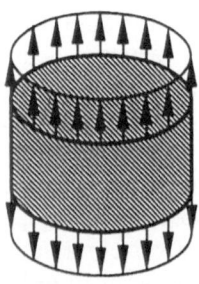 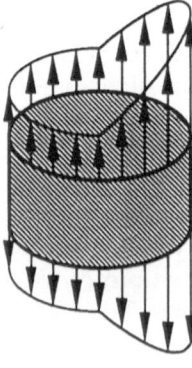

FIG. 11. Distribution of growth force in a vertebral body. *Left*, loading condition of uniform growth force; *right*, loading condition of asymmetrical growth force (from [25] with permission)

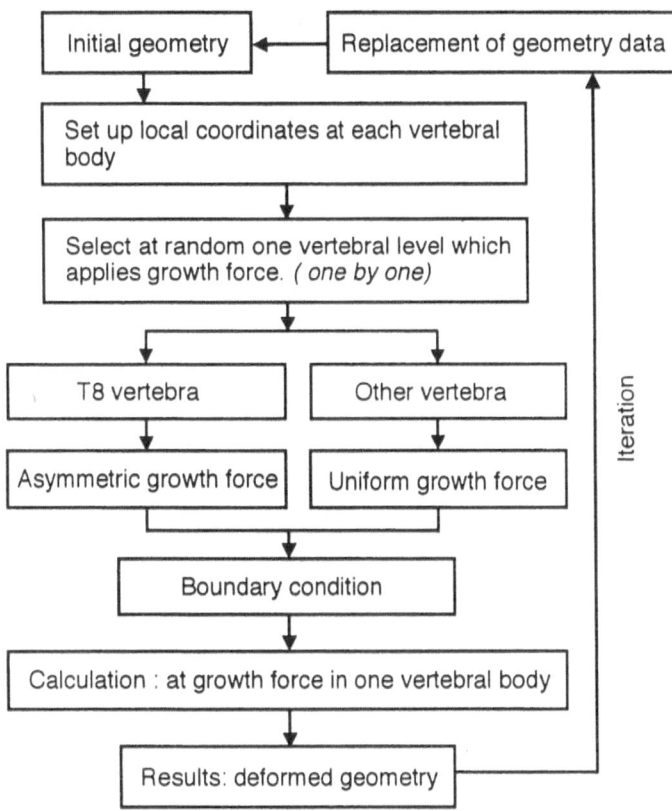

FIG. 12. Flow chart of calculation for growth simulation (from [25] with permission)

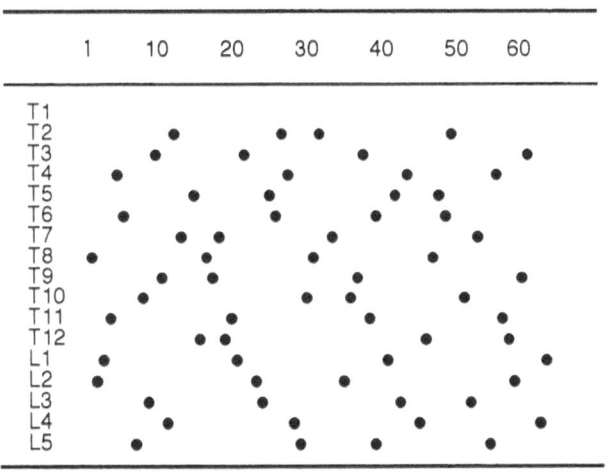

FIG. 13. An example of the iteration schedule

3.4 Effect of Asymmetrical Growth Force on Scoliotic Deformity

The result of the computer simulation from this growth analysis was obtained at each condition of asymmetrical growth force. The result of case 1 is shown in Fig. 14, where the maximum asymmetrical growth force was located in the anterior region of the T-8 vertebral body. Roaf [10] pointed out that asymmetrical growth induced a morphological feature of scoliosis. Somerville [9] developed "rotational lordosis," a theory which proposed that accelerated anterior growth or constrained posterior growth forces the spine into a combination of lordosis, rotation, and lateral deviation. In Fig. 14, however, no lateral deviation except back deviation appears. There is also no vertebral rotation. These results are much different from the clinical configuration shown in Fig. 5. Case 2 shows maximum growth force in the anterolateral right region. Slight lateral deviation occurred on the right. However, no deviation and no vertebral rotation appeared (Fig. 15).

Figure 16 shows the results of case 4, which has maximum growth force in the posterolateral right region. Lateral deviation occurred on the left; forward deviation and vertebral rotation also occurred. The result shows a deformation opposite to clinical configuration. However, because this model has symmetrical geometry, the opposite result of this case can be obtained at maximum growth force in the posterolateral left region, which is similar to the clinical configuration.

Case 6 is maximum growth force in the left region (Fig. 17), where T-1 is constrained in three directions. Large lateral deviation occurred on the right. It should be noted that the deviation appeared in the opposite side of the region to which the maximum force was applied. Moreover, sagittal deviation decreased

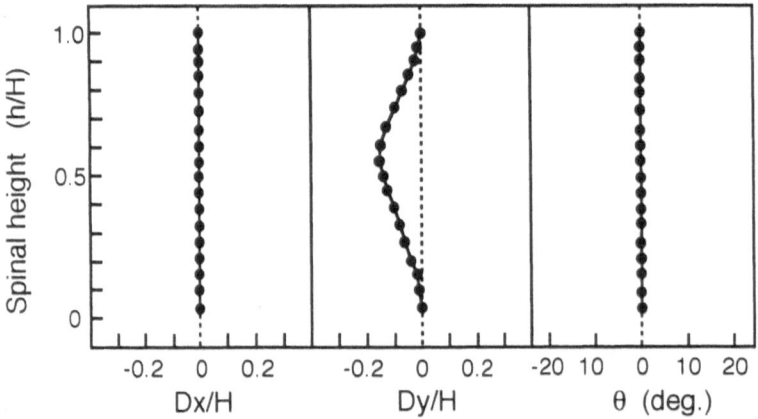

FIG. 14. Results of computer simulation. Maximum value of asymmetrical growth force was located at the anterior region in the T-8 vertebral body (case 1). *Left*, frontal view; *middle*, sagittal view; *right*, vertebral rotation (from [25] with permission)

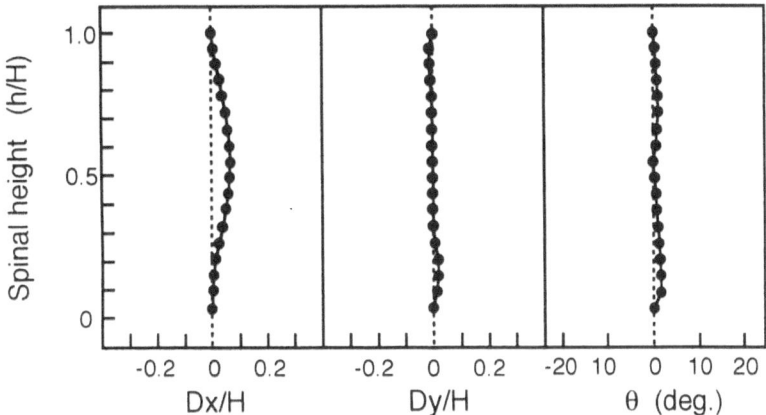

FIG. 15. Results of computer simulation. Maximum value of asymmetrical growth force was located at the left region in the T-8 vertebral body (Case 2). *Left*, frontal view; *middle*, sagittal view; *right*, vertebral rotation

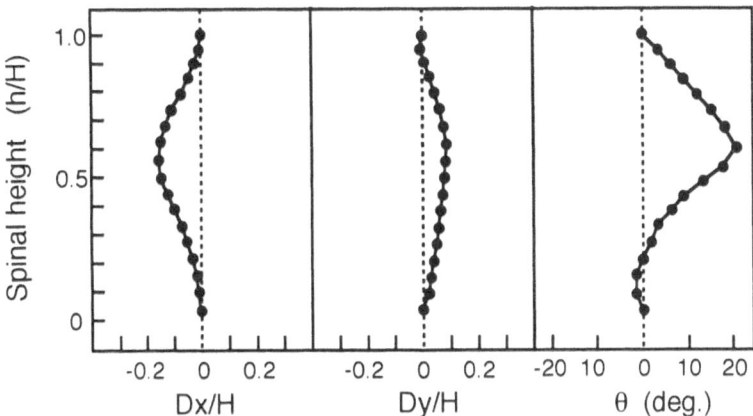

FIG. 16. Results of computer simulation. Maximum value of asymmetrical growth force was located at the posterolateral right region in the T-8 vertebral body (case 4). *Left*, frontal view; *middle*, sagittal view; *right*, vertebral rolation

and much vertebral rotation occurred. These results simulated well the character-istics of the clinical configuration. When the T-1 constraint was free in only the axial direction, the result for the same loading condition as case 6 was obtained such that the lateral deviation and vertebral rotation became much greater than in case 6.

Figure 18 shows the geometry of case 6 obtained by the computer simulation. The lateral deviation with axial rotation can be seen clearly. Figure 19 shows the deformity increasing as the iteration cycle progressed. The lateral deviation

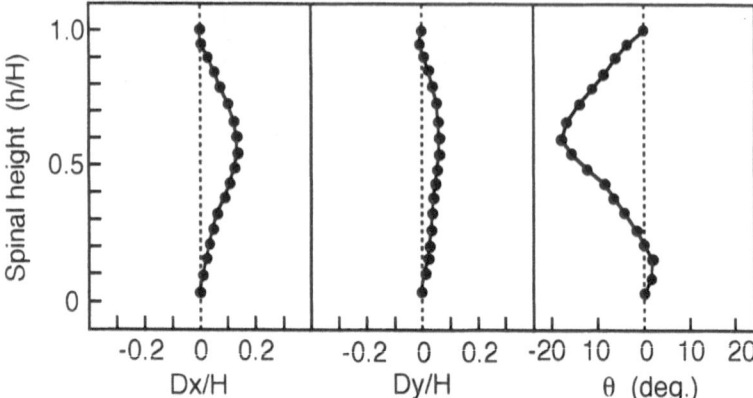

FIG. 17. Results of computer simulation. Maximum value of asymmetrical growth force was located at the left region in the T-8 vertebral body (case 6). *Left*, frontal view, *middle*, sagittal view; *right*, vertebral rotation (from [25] with permission)

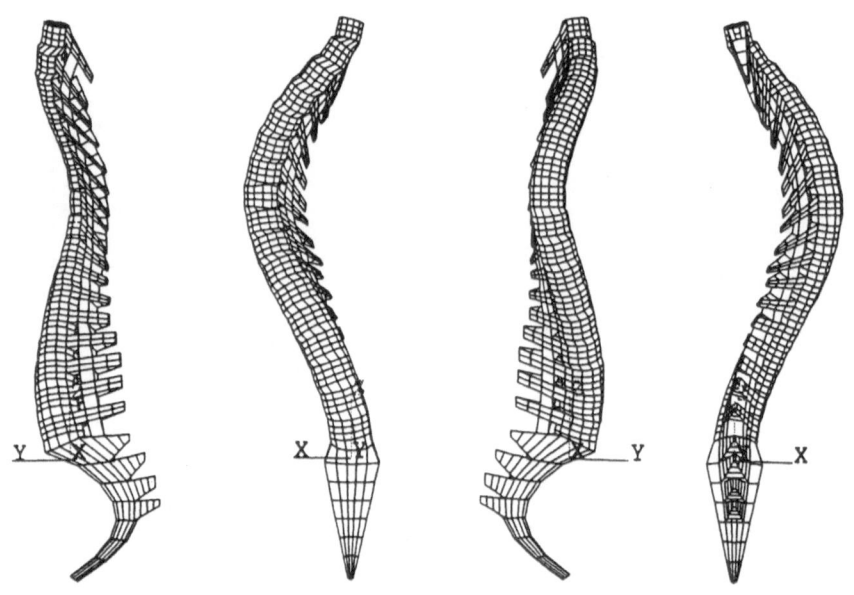

FIG. 18. Deformed geometry of case 6. The views from *left* to *right* are: left side, anterior, right side, posterior

increases gradually with the iteration cycle, but the vertebral rotation is almost unchanged until three cycles have been completed. After that, it becomes much higher.

Figure 20 shows the geometric torsion of case 6 calculated by Eq. 12. The tendency of geometric torsion was also confirmed to be similar to the clinical case

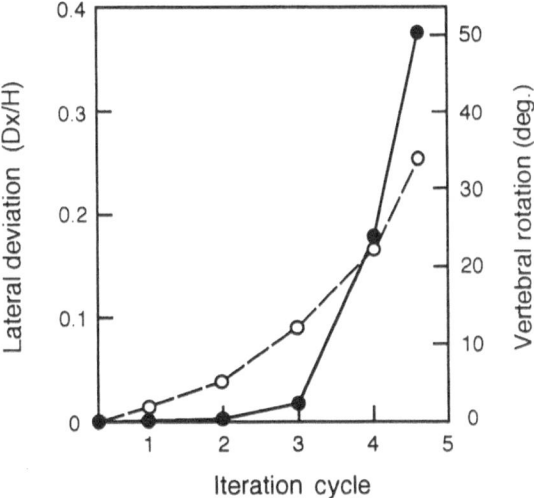

FIG. 19. The deformity progression with increasing iteration. *Open circles*, maximum lateral deviation (*Dx/H*); *closed circles*, maximum vertebral rotation

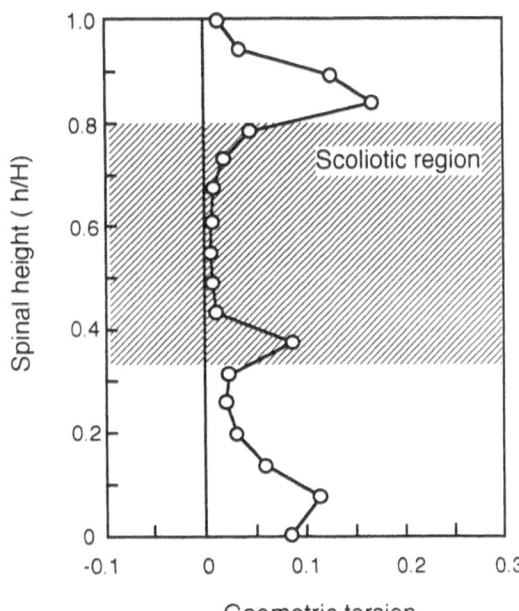

FIG. 20. Geometric torsion of case 6

of Fig. 4; that is, in the scoliotic region, this value was nearly equal to zero. From these results, it was confirmed that the proposed method of computer simulation is very effective for the analysis of the progression of the scoliotic spine. Configurations similar to those seen clinically could be obtained.

If the axial asymmetric growth force was applied to the lateral region from the left to the posterior in the T-8 vertebral body, the deformation from the normal

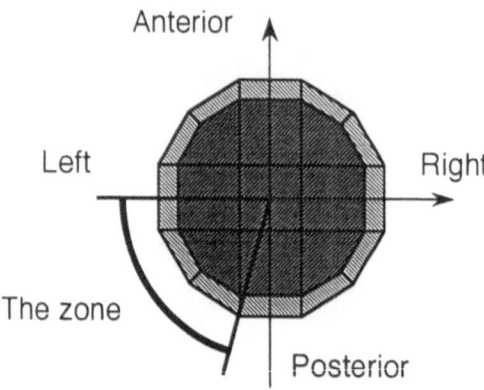

FIG. 21. The zone where the maximum vertical growth force is applied in the T-8 cross section to induce the configuration of scoliosis (from [25] with permission)

spine was similar to the configuration of typical scoliosis with a thoracic curve. That is, scoliosis with a single thoracic curve might be induced by the maximum asymmetrical growth force applied at the zone in the T-8 vertebral body (Fig. 21). In addition, when T-1 constraints were set as free in the axial direction only, greater lateral deviation and vertebral rotation in the scoliotic spine than in case 6 resulted.

The model developed here can also be used to study correction of scoliosis deformity by incorporating the actual geometry of a patient into the model node list and applying forces to simulate those occurring in surgery or brace treatment, thus individualizing the kind of pretreatment simulations done previously [22–24].

4 Conclusions

Based on measurements on the plain roentgenograms of the whole spine, the configuration of the scoliotic spine was reconstructed mathematically by a spatial curve. The frontal-plane Cobb angle calculated from this mathematical model (morphological curve) was equivalent to that measured clinically on the sagittal roentgenogram. The morphological curve showed a plane curve in the area of scoliosis. As the parameters to evaluate the configuration of the scoliotic spine, the three-dimensional Cobb angle and plane of maximum curvature were mathematically calculated.

From the computer simulation using the structural model of the whole spine, the effect of varying distribution of growth force and the end constraints on deformation from the normal spine were investigated. This model could simulate the modulation of growth in the osseous tissues, as well as a single thoracic scoliosis curvature convex toward the lateral direction with axial rotation, as seen in typical scoliosis deformities.

Acknowledgments. This study was supported by a Grant-in-Aid for Scientific Research on Priority Area [Biomechanics] from the Ministry of Education, Science and Culture in Japan.

References

1. Nash CL, Moe JH (1969) Study of vertebral rotation. J Bone Joint Surg 51A:223–229
2. Stokes LAF, Bigalow LC, Moreland MS (1986) Measurement of axial rotation of vertebrae in scoliosis. Spine 11:213–218
3. DeSmet AA, Asher MA, Cook LT, Goin JE, Scheuch H, Orrick JM (1984) Three-dimensional analysis of right thoracic idiopathic scoliosis. Spine 9:377–381
4. Hierholzer E, Luxmann G (1982) Three-dimensional shape analysis of the scoliotic spine using invariant shape parameters. J Biomech 15:583–598
5. Raso J, Gillespie R, McNeice G (1980) Determination of the plane of maximum deformity in idiopathic scoliosis. Orthop Trans 4:23
6. Stokes IAF, Bigalow LC, Moreland MS (1987) Three-dimensional spinal curvature in idiopathic scoliosis. J Orthop Res 5:102–113
7. Deacon P, Flood BM, Dickson RA (1984) Idiopathic scoliosis in three dimensions. a radiographic and morphometric analysis. J Bone Joint Surg 66B:509–512
8. Schultz AB (1991) The use of mathematical models for studies of scoliosis biomechanics. Spine 16:1211–1216
9. Somerville EW (1952) Rotational lordosis: the development of the single curve. J Bone Jt Surg 69B:421–427
10. Roaf R (1963) The treatment of progressive scoliosis by unilateral growth-arrest. J Bone Jt Surg 45B:637–651
11. Roaf R (1966) The basic anatomy of scoliosis. J Bone Joint Surg 48B:786–792
12. Dangerfield PH, Burwell RG, Vernon CL (1980) Anthropometry and scoliosis. In: Roaf R (ed) Spinal deformities. Pitman, London, pp 259–280
13. Stokes IAF, Dansereau J, Moreland MS (1989) Rib cage asymmetry in idiopathic scoliosis. J Orthop Res 7:102–113
14. Agadir M, Sevastik B, Sevastik JA, Persson A, Isberg B (1988) Induction of scoliosis in the growing rabbit by unilateral rib-growth stimulation. Spine 13:1065–1069
15. Stokes IAF, Laible JP (1990) Three-dimensional osseo-ligamentous model of the thorax representing initiation of scoliosis by asymmetric growth. J Biomech 23:589–595
16. Kawabata H, Ono K, Seguchi Y, Tanaka M (1988) Idiopathic scoliosis and growth— a biomechanical consideration. J Jpn Orthop Assoc 62:161–170
17. Kanayama M, Tadano S, Kaneda K, Ukai T, Abumi K (1995) A mathematical expression of three-dimensional configuration of the scoliotic spine. J Biomech Eng ASME (in press)
18. Tadano S, Kanayama M, Ukai T, Kaneda K (1995) Three-dimensional morphologic modeling of scoliotic spine (in Japanese). Trans Jpn Soc Mech Eng 61:1682–1688
19. Aleksandrov AD, Kolmogorov AN, Lavrent'ev MA (1984) Mathematics. Its content, methods, and meaning. Part 3. MIT Press, Cambridge, pp 57–117
20. MacLane S (1986) Mathematics: form and function. Springer, Berlin Heidelberg New York, pp 219–258
21. Stokes IAF (1994) Three-dimensional terminology of spinal deformity. Spine 19:236–242

22. Schultz A, Haderspeck K, Takashima S (1981) Correction of scoliosis by muscle stimulation—biomechanical analysis. Spine 6:468–476
23. Patwardhan AG, Bunch WH, Meade KP, Vanderby R, Knight GW (1986) A biomechanical analog of curve progression and orthotic stabilization in idiopathic scoliosis. J Biomech 19:103–117
24. Subbaraj K, Ghista DN, Viviani GR (1989) Presurgical finite element simulation of scoliosis correction. J Biomed Eng 11:9–18
25. Tadan S, Kanayama K, Ukai T (1995) Computer simulation of idiopathic scoliosis initiated by local asymmetric growth force in a vertebral body. In: Power H, Hart RT (eds) Computer Simulations in Biomedicine. Computational Mechanics Publications, Southampton, pp 369–376

Molecular Dynamics Simulation of Skeletal Muscle Contraction

EIJI NAKAMACHI[1], JUN TSUKAMOTO[2], and YOJIRO TAMURA[3]

Summary. Investigation of the contractile mechanism of skeletal muscle at the molecular level will contribute to development of the design technology of living material and nano-machines. Earlier micromechanical models to elucidate the relative sliding of actin and myosin filaments were proposed by Hill, Huxley, and Zahalak. First, we applied the phenomenological macromolecular potential theory, initially proposed by Mitsui, to study myosin head sliding and the isotonic and isometric contraction of a sarcomere. The equation of motion of each myosin head under the viscosity dominant condition was solved. The numerical results show good agreement with experimental data obtained by Yanagida, Hill, and Gordon. Second, the three-dimensional structural and dynamic properties of G-actin, which constitutes the actin filament, were analyzed by using the atomic/molecular mechanics analysis code AMBER. These studies demonstrate that this numerical model is a powerful tool for analyzing the atomic and macromolecular dynamics of skeletal muscle contraction.

Key words: Molecular mechanics analysis—Skeletal muscle—Acto-myosin—Isotonic contraction—Isometric contraction

1 Introduction

Two numerical analysis schemes were employed to investigate skeletal muscle contraction mechanism on the basis of macromolecular and atomic/molecular mechanics.

1.1 Macromolecular Mechanics

The basic event that underlies muscle contraction has been elucidated as a cyclic interaction of cross-bridges (myosin head) between the thick myosin and thin

[1] Department of Mechanical Engineering, Osaka Institute of Technology, 5-16-1 Omiya, Asahi-ku, Osaka, Osaka, 535 Japan
[2] Toshiba Co. Ltd., 3-22 Kakamachi, Fuchu, Tokyo, 183 Japan
[3] Suzuka College of Technology, Shiroko-cho, Suzuka, Mie, 510-02 Japan

actin filaments [1] because muscle is a molecular machine that transfers chemical energy to work with high energy efficiency. The investigation of this mechanism will contribute to the development of the optimal design technology of artificial micro- and nanomachines and the constitutive equation of living tissues. However, the nature of the exact molecular process that generates the inter-filamentary force by attached cross-bridges remains a matter of debate and speculation. The functional formulation employing state variables, such as the viscoelasticity model, has been adopted for the constitutive equation of living tissues [2,3]. In these models, the generation and dissipation processes of energy and the zero-stress state have not been made clear. A muscle contraction model based on molecular structure has been proposed by Huxley and Simmons [4,5] and by Zahalak and Ma [6] according to electron microscope observations of the cross-bridge [7,8], and tension response to the sudden length change [9]. Recent experimental results of the sliding length during one adenosine triphosphate (ATP) hydrolysis [10,11], however, conflict with these models.

In this chapter, the constitutive relationship based on the phenomenological macromolecular potential theory initially proposed by Mitsui and Oshima [12] is developed to interpret skeletal muscle contraction. The biochemical energy of ATP hydrolysis generates the self-induced potential between the myosin heads and the actin filament, and forces the myosin heads to slide along the actin filament. The equation of motion of each myosin head is solved under the condition of the viscosity dominant state. The numerical results of one myosin head sliding along an actin filament are compared with the experimental results of a motility assay in vitro [10,11]. The movement of 20 myosin heads is also simulated to study the isotonic and isometric contraction of a sarcomere. In this case, we also compare simulation results with experimental data obtained using a muscle fiber [13–18].

1.2 Atomic/Molecular Mechanics [19–22]

In 1990, the group of Holmes revealed the three-dimensional (3-D) structure of G-actin of rabbit skeletal muscle by using X-ray crystalline experimental analysis [23–25]. Actin and myosin molecules combine to construct the actomyosin system, which generates the motility to induce the whole skeletal muscle contraction. We focused on analyzing the molecular structure of G-actin and its dynamic properties to elucidate the contraction mechanism at the molecular level by using the molecular mechanics (MM) simulation scheme. The MM calculations have been performed in four cases for normal G-actin and proK-actin (cut off between Met-47 and Gly-48) under conditions with ATP or without ATP [26].

First, we determined the minimum energy conformation of G-actin atoms by employing the steepest descent method and the conjugate gradient method in MM calculation. It was determined that G-actin with ATP has less energy than the other three cases. This means it has the most stable structure, and also shows the heterogeneous potential energy field, which might concern the intrinsic features of protein and also its functional ability. Next, the normal mode analyses were executed in four cases of G-actin. Root mean square of atomic fluctuation (rms fluctuation) determined by normal mode analysis revealed the atomic flexibility [27–35]. The compressibility results showed that G-actin with ATP is the most compressible and the binding site with the myosin head S1 is the most compressible at the atomic level. This means that this region should be the most flexible and the most easily activated.

2 Macromolecular Potential Model

Figure 1 is a schematic drawing of skeletal muscle, which consist of large and thin muscle fibers. Muscle fiber is mainly made up of myofibrils, long cylindrical elements 1–2 μm in diameter that extend over the entire length of the fiber. The contractile units of myofibril are visible under the light microscope, giving the myofibril a striated appearance. Each of the regular repeating units, called a sarcomere, is about 2.4 μm long. Each sarcomere was found to contain two sets of protein filaments: thick myosin and thin actin filaments [16,17]. The actin filament composed principally of actin is about 1.0 μm long and 8 nm in diameter, having a helical structure [24,25,27]. A myosin filament is composed mainly of myosin and is about 1.6 μm long and 15 nm in diameter, also having a helical structure. The myosin molecules aggregate together by using their tail part; their heads are

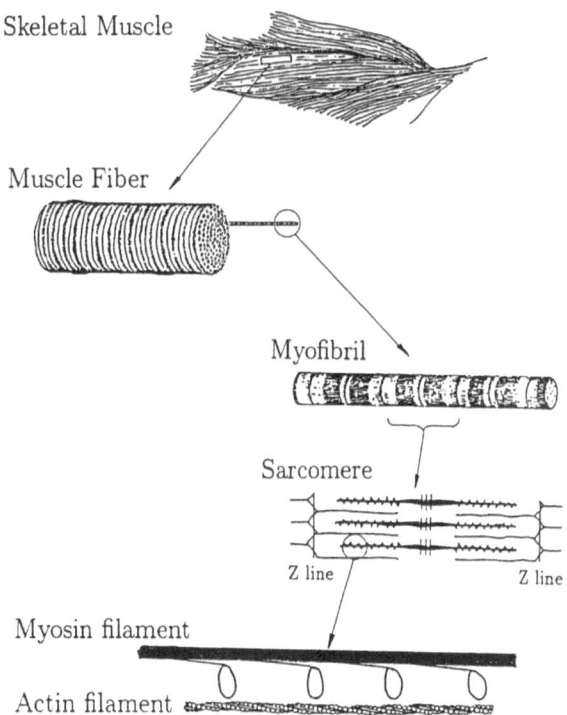

Skeletal Muscle

Muscle Fiber

Myofibril

Sarcomere

Z line   Z line

Myosin filament

Fig. 1. Muscle organization   Actin filament

projected to the actin side and are responsible for "walking" along an adjacent actin filament, resulting in muscle contraction.

2.1 Three Potentials

To interpret muscle contraction, we assumed three macromolecular potentials defined by a one-dimensional function along the sliding direction [12] (Fig. 2a).

The periodic potential Uo along the actin filament has the period of G-actin alignment. We simplify the noncovalent bonding potential between myosin heads and actin filament as a sinusoidal relationship. Uo is given by

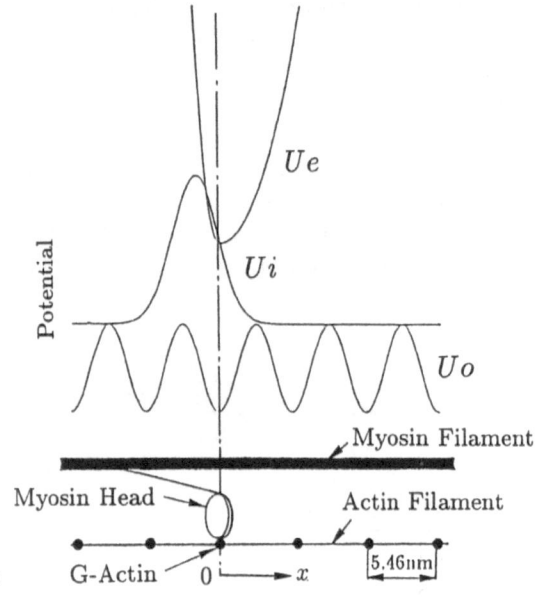

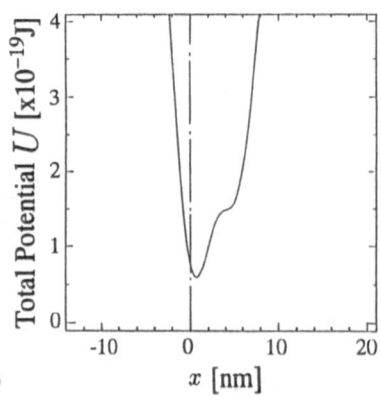

FIG. 2a,b. Macromolecular potential theory. **a** Molecular potential model. **b** Total potential

$$Uo(x) = \frac{Ho}{2}\left[\cos\left(\frac{2\pi x}{L}\right) - 1\right] \tag{1}$$

where x is the coordinate along actin filament, L is the helix period of the actin filament (5.46 nm in frog skeletal muscle) [12], and Ho is the amplitude of this potential.

The self-induced potential Ui is generated by ATP hydrolysis, which is activated by the increasing concentration of ionized calcium emitted from the sarcoplasmic reticulum. This potential forces myosin heads to slide along the actin filament, causing muscle contraction. The biochemical reaction of ATP hydrolysis is expressed as

$$M + ATP \xrightarrow{k_1:fast} M \cdot ADP \cdot Pi \xrightarrow{k_2:slow} M + ADP + Pi \tag{2}$$

where k_1 and k_2 are the fast and slow chemical reaction rate constants, respectively and ATP, ADP, Pi, and M indicate adenosine triphosphate, adenosine diphosphate, inorganic phosphate, and a myosin head, respectively. The self-induced potential Ui is assumed to be obtained by the product of two functions of the coordinate of myosin heads X and of time t, defined independently.

$$Ui = v(t) \cdot u(X) \tag{3}$$

The time-dependent function $v(t)$ and the coordinate dependent function $u(X)$ are expressed as follows:

$$v(t) = v_0 \cdot \exp(-k_1 t) \cdot \left[1 - \exp(-k_2 t)\right] \tag{4}$$

$$u(X) = \frac{1}{\sqrt{2\pi\sigma}} \exp\left(-\frac{X^2}{2\sigma^2}\right) \tag{5}$$

where σ is a standard deviation of normal distribution. To force myosin heads to slide in the right direction of the contraction, the spatial distribution of potential $u(X)$ is expressed by a normal distribution probability function. Parameters k_1 and k_2 are evaluated by

$$\frac{\int_0^{\Delta t} v(t)dt}{\int_0^{\infty} v(t)dt} = 0.995 \tag{6}$$

under the assumption that one ATP hydrolysis reaction saturates after $\Delta t = 0.1$ S. We also assumed that the self-induced potential exerts no influences on adjoining actin molecules, so the following expression is obtained:

$$\frac{u(L)}{u(0)} = 0.005 \tag{7}$$

where $L (= 5.46\,nm)$ is the helix period of actin filament [12]. From Eq. 7 we can obtain $\sigma = 1.812 \times 10^{-9}\,m$; Further, we assume that the time integration of the self-induced potential through Δt has the value of Gibbs free energy, ΔG, of ATP hydrolysis [12] as follows:

$$\int_0^{\Delta t} Ui\,dt = u(0)\int_0^{\Delta t} v(t)\,dt \equiv \Delta G \cdot \Delta t \tag{8}$$

where ΔG can be estimated by the following equation of chemical energetics in the process of chemical reaction in Eq. 2:

$$\Delta G = \Delta G^0 + RT \ln \frac{[ADP][Pi]}{[ATP]} \tag{9}$$

where ΔG^0 is the standard free energy change written with the equilibrium constant K_{eq} of ATP hydrolysis, as follows:

$$\Delta G^0 = -RT \ln K_{eq} \tag{10}$$

[ATP], [ADP], and [Pi] indicate the concentrations of ATP, ADP, and Pi, respectively, R represents the gas constant, and T expresses temperature. In this model, ΔG is set as $1.0 \times 10^{-19}\,J$ at room temperature (300 K) [12]. Using Eq. 8, the parameter v_0 can be evaluated by the following equation:

$$v_0 = \Delta G \cdot \Delta t \sqrt{2\pi} \sigma \frac{k_1}{k_2}(k_1 + k_2) \tag{11}$$

Consequently, the self-induced potential Ui can be calculated with these parameters.

The elastic potential Ue is associated with heavy meromyosin. Ue works as the spring that transmits the force generated on the myosin heads by ATP hydrolysis to the thick myosin filament. The potential Ue is given by

$$Ue = \begin{cases} A_1 \Delta l^2 + A_2 \Delta l & : \Delta l \geq 0 \\ A_3 \Delta l^2 & : \Delta l \leq 0 \end{cases} \tag{12}$$

where A_1, A_2, and A_3 are constants and Δl is the deviation from the zero tension position. In the simulation, we adopted elastic constants as follows: $A_1 = 1.14 \times 10^{-2}\,N/m$, $A_2 = 6.72 \times 10^{-11}\,N$, and $A_3 = 3.85 \times 10^{-2}\,N/m$. The total potential U on a myosin head can be derived by assembling these three potentials as shown in Fig. 2b.

$$U = Uo + Ue + Ui \tag{13}$$

2.2 The Equation of Motion

We assume that the energy of ATP hydrolysis is larger than the thermal energy. Furthermore, the relative sliding motion in vivo occurs in the viscosity dominant environment. Therefore, the forces of fluctuation and inertia are ignored in the derivation of the equation of motion of each myosin head, expressed as follows:

$$C\frac{dx}{dt} = -\frac{dU}{dx} = F$$

$$= -\frac{d(Uo + Ue + Ui)}{dx} = Fo + Fe + Fi \tag{14}$$

where C is the viscosity coefficient. The driving force F is obtained by the derivation of the total potential U. Execution of the time integration leads the time evolution of position of each myosin head along the sliding axis (Fig. 2a).

3 Atomic/Molecular Mechanics Analysis

Atomic potential energy is introduced to study the atomic mechanical properties of protein, which constitutes the skeletal muscle. The minimum conformation energy search is executed to find the 3-D atomic structure under the defined conditions of the molecule and its environment [21,22].

3.1 Potential Field Functions

The potential energy functions were determined by ab initio calculation and parameter fitting, employing the experimental data.

$$V = V_r + V_\theta + V_\phi + V_{el} + V_{vdW} + V_{hb} \tag{15}$$

Here V_r, V_θ, and V_ϕ mean bonded energies, namely, bending, and torsion; V_{el}, V_{vdW}, and V_{hb} are nonbonded energies, namely, electrostatic, van der Waals, and hydrogen bonding energies.

$$V_r = \sum k_r (r - r_e)^2$$

$$V_\theta = \sum k_\theta (\theta - \theta_e)^2$$

$$V_\phi = \sum \frac{1}{2} k_\phi \{1 + \cos(n\phi - \gamma)\}$$

$$V_{el} = \sum \frac{q_i q_j}{\varepsilon r_{ij}}$$

$$V_{vdW} = \sum_{i,j} \left(\frac{A_{ij}}{r_{ij}^{12}} - \frac{B_{ij}}{r_{ij}^{6}} \right)$$

$$V_{hb} = \sum_{ij} \left(\frac{C_{ij}}{r_{ij}^{12}} - \frac{D_{ij}}{r_{ij}^{10}} \right) \tag{16}$$

3.2 Minimum Conformation Energy

The conformation of minimum potential energy is searched for using combination of the steepest descent methods at the beginning stage and the conjugate gradient methods at the final stage [23]. We adopted the united atom modeling. The initial coordinate of 375 C^{α} obtained from the Protein Data Bank (PDB) was employed in the analysis [24,25]. Because there are water molecules around G-actin atoms, the total became 7821 atoms, 3621 from G-actin and 4200 from water.

3.3 Normal Mode Analysis

3.3.1 Root Mean Square Fluctuation

Normal mode analysis is basically understood as the perturbation method to find the fluctuation at the equilibrium state, which means the configuration with the minimum potential energy [28–30]. The fluctuation of each atom corresponds to the eigen vibration. The potential energy can be expressed as

$$V(q) = \frac{1}{2} \sum_{i,j=1}^{N} F_{ij} (q_i - q_i^0)(q_j - q_j^0) \tag{17}$$

where q_i means the coordinate of atom and F_{ij} the second derivative of the potential. The kinetic energy E is

$$E = \frac{1}{2} \sum_{i,j=1}^{N} \left(\sum_{l=1}^{N} m_l \frac{\partial r_l}{\partial q_i} \cdot \frac{\partial r_l}{\partial q_j} \right) \dot{q}_i \dot{q}_j \tag{18}$$

Here, N means atom number, m_l the mass, and r_l the position vector, respectively.

By solving the Lagrange equation of motion, the general solution is obtained by superposing harmonic functions:

$$q_j = q_j^0 + \sum_{k=1}^{N} A_{jk} Q_k$$

$$Q_k = \alpha_k \cos(\omega_k t + \delta_k) \tag{19}$$

Here, α_k means the amplitude, ω_k the eigen frequency, and δ_k the phase deviation. The eigen equation leads to the rms fluctuation of atomic vibration.

$$\sqrt{\left\langle (\Delta q_i)^2 \right\rangle} = \sqrt{\sum_{k}^{n} A_{ik}^2 \frac{k_B T}{\omega_k^2}} \tag{20}$$

Here, k_B is the Boltzman constant and T is the absolute temperature [31–34].

3.3.2 Isothermal Compressibility

The Isothermal compressibility of G-actin β_T can be given by

$$\beta_T = \frac{\left\langle (\Delta V)^2 \right\rangle}{k_B V T} \tag{21}$$

Here, $T = 300\,\text{K}$ and V means the volume. The volume fluctuation $\sqrt{\langle(\Delta V)^2\rangle}$ can be obtained by the rms fluctuation $\sqrt{\langle(\Delta r_i)^2\rangle}$ as follows:

$$\sqrt{\left\langle\left(\Delta V\right)^2\right\rangle} = 4\pi r_g^2 \sqrt{\left\langle\left(\Delta r_g\right)^2\right\rangle} \tag{22}$$

$$\sqrt{\left\langle\left(\Delta r_g\right)^2\right\rangle} = \frac{\sqrt{\sum_{i=1}^{n}\left(r_i + \sqrt{\left\langle\left(\Delta r_i\right)^2\right\rangle} - r_c\right)^2}}{\sqrt{n}}$$
$$- \frac{\sqrt{\sum_{i=1}^{n}\left(r_i - r_c\right)^2}}{\sqrt{n}} \tag{23}$$

4 Numerical Results of Macromolecular Analyses

We now determine the parameters of the three potentials that can predict the experimental results. Parameters are chosen to adjust the sliding distance of a myosin head obtained in an in vitro motility assay [10]. The isotonic shortening and the length–tension relationship of a half-sarcomere in the isometric contraction are shown and compared with experimental results [13,15].

4.1 Sliding of One Myosin Head

We analyzed the motility assay in vitro. The total execution time was 0.1 s, which means the average interval of one ATP hydrolysis cycle as has been observed in this assay [12]. The Euler method was adopted as the time integration scheme; 10000 time increments were devoted to each numerical analysis. The parameters employed for simulations are shown in Table 1; t_0 is the time when the time integral Ui, from 0 to t_0, becomes one-half its value until Δt, described in Eq. 8. In case 1, we set $k_2 = 1.0$, and derived k_1 and t_0 by using Eqs. 6 and 8. The time courses of the coordinate, the total potential $U(= Ui + Uo)$, and the driving force $F(= Fi + Fo)$ are demonstrated in Fig. 3a. Because of overriding the sinusoidal potential, oscillations of these values were observed. The myosin head slides for a distance of 60 nm, which agrees with the experimental results obtained by Yanagida et al. [10]. Thus, this model can interpret the multistep sliding.

TABLE 1. Parameters of potential model.

Parameter	Case 1	Case 2	Case 3	Case 4
k_1 (s^{-1})	75.87	58.43	75.87	75.87
k_2 (s^{-1})	1.00	90.0	1.00	1.00
t_0 (s)	0.0220	0.0192	0.0220	0.0220
Ho ($\times 10^{-19}$ J)	0.914	0.986	1.059	0.914
C ($\times 10^{-5}$ kg/s)	2.8	2.8	2.8	3.5

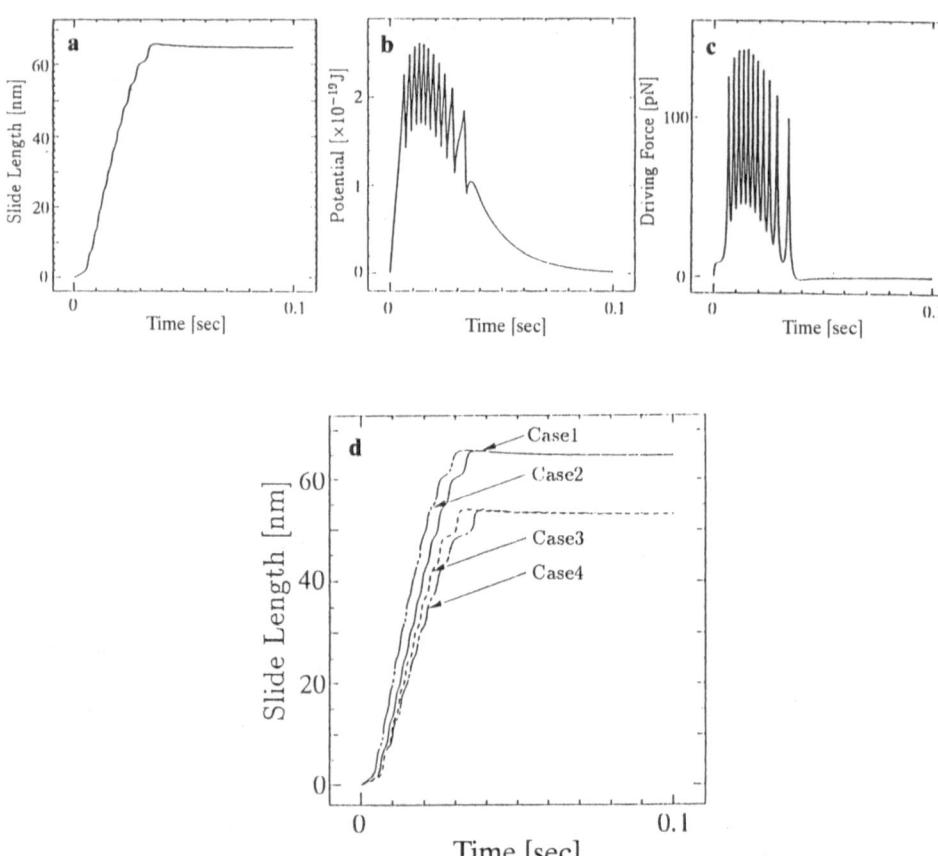

FIG. 3a–d. One myosin head sliding. **a–c** Time courses of coordinate, potential, and force in case 1. **d** Comparision of slide motions in cases 1, 2, 3, and 4

Next, we investigated the influences of parameters that are related to features of the potential, and compared these with the results of case 1 (see Fig. 3b). In case 2, the smaller value of the fast chemical reaction rate constant k_1 of Ui, gave the same slide length, but faster arrival to the final distance. In Case 3, the deeper well of the periodic potential Uo, shows a shorter slide distance. Case 4, with the same potentials as case 1 but a higher viscosity, C, produced the shortest distance and the slowest arrival time. These results show that the larger value for k_1 of Ui causes faster sliding, the deeper Ho of Uo gives a shorter slide length, and the higher viscosity C leads to a slower sliding speed. Hereafter, we employ the parameters of case 1 for numerical simulations.

4.2 Isotonic Contraction

Experiments with isotonic contraction are conducted by maintaining a specified constant force against the contraction at both ends of a half-sarcomere and then measuring the contraction velocity. Twenty myosin heads, assumed to be contained in a half-sarcomere (Fig. 4), slide under the constant force P applied at both ends, the Z and M lines. We assume that ATP hydrolysis occurs randomly during the total calculation time, 1.0 s, and has the average occurrence period of $\frac{1}{30}$ s at each myosin head. In this simulation, we set the load as $P/20$ at each

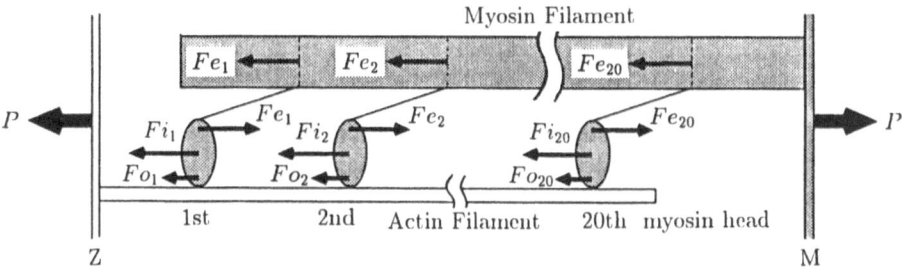

FIG. 4. Analyzing the model of a half-sarcomere

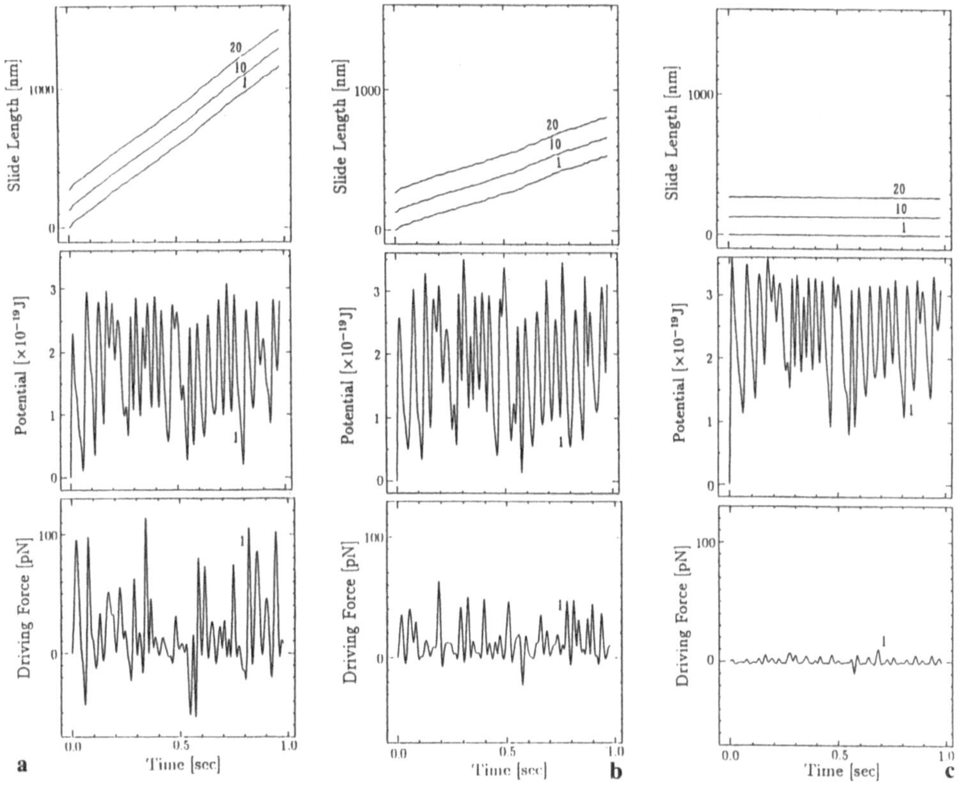

FIG. 5a–c. A half-sarcomere isotonic contraction: slide length, potential, and force vs. time. **a** $P/P_0 = 0.0$. **b** $P/P_0 = 0.27$. **c** $P/P_0 = 1.0$ where P is constant force and $P_0 = 55$ pN

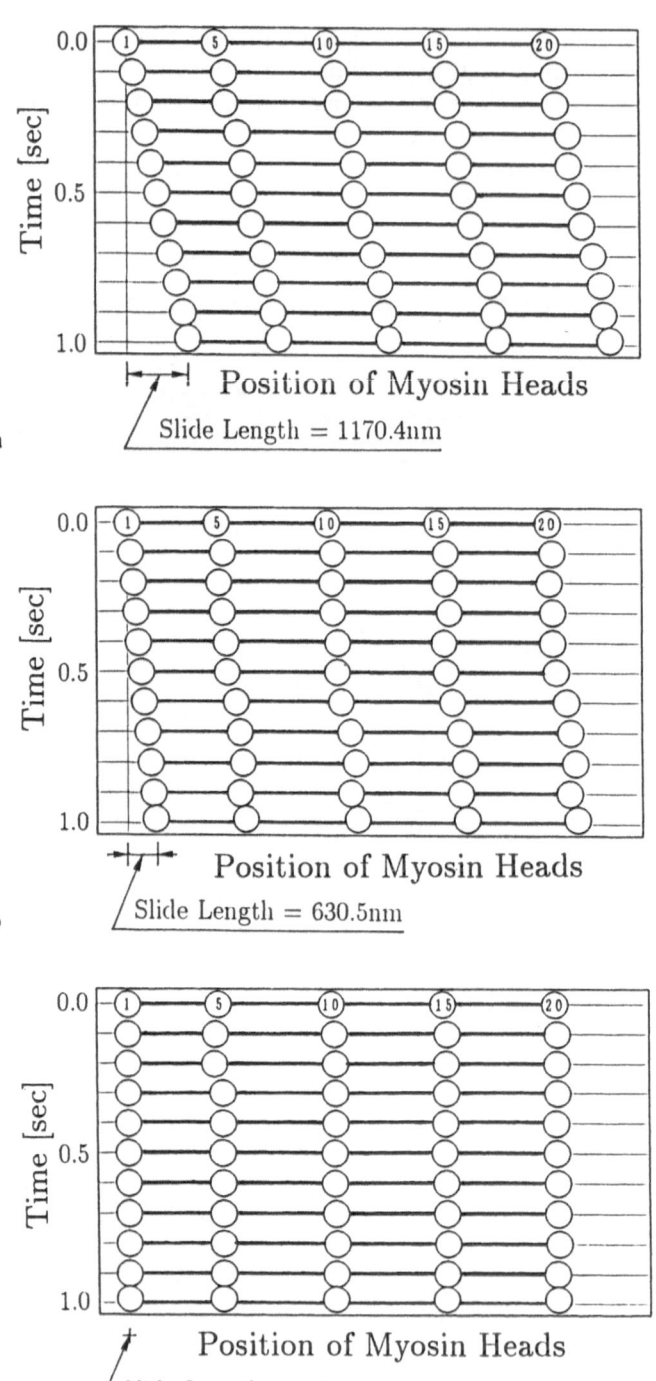

FIG. 6a–c. Sliding motion of a half-sarcomere under isotonic contraction. **a** $P/P_0 = 0.0$. **b** $P/P_0 = 0.27$. **c** $P/P_0 = 1.0$

FIG. 7. Tension–sliding velocity
relationship

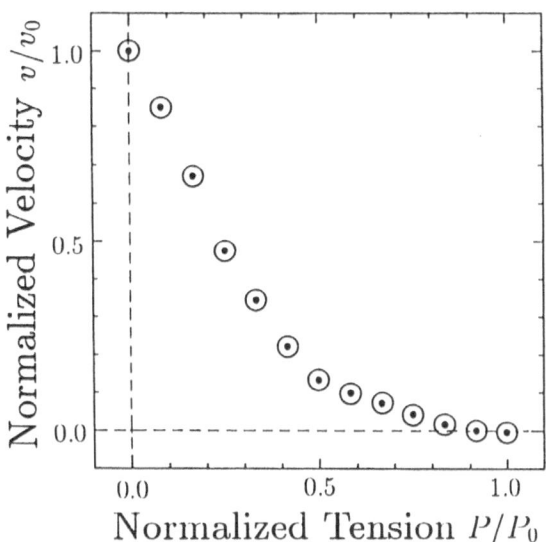

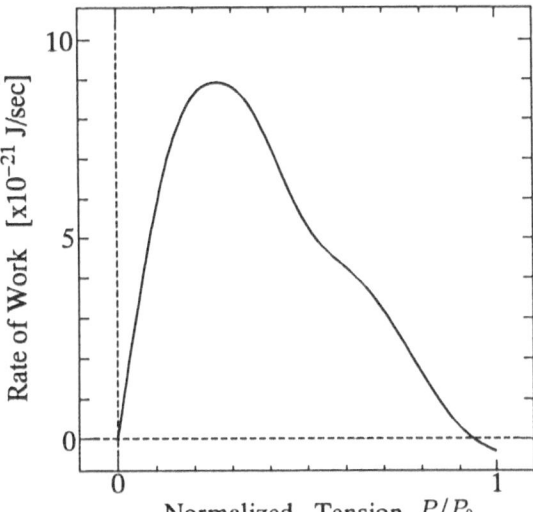

FIG. 8. Rate of work

myosin head and assumed that the thick (myosin) filament slides with the average
velocity of the 20 myosin heads.

Figure 5 shows time courses of the slide length of the first, tenth, and twentieth
myosin heads, and the potential and the driving force ($Fi + Fo + Fe - P/20$) of the
first mysoin head in the case of normalized forces, $P/P_0 = 0.0, 0.27$, and 1.0 where
$P_0 = 55$ pN. The total time for the analyses was 1.0 s. The lower the applied force
P, the more smoothly the myosin filament slides and for a longer distance.
Because of the resistance force caused by the elastic spring in the case of the
larger force P, the driving force was the smallest when $P/P_0 = 1.0$ (see Fig. 5c).

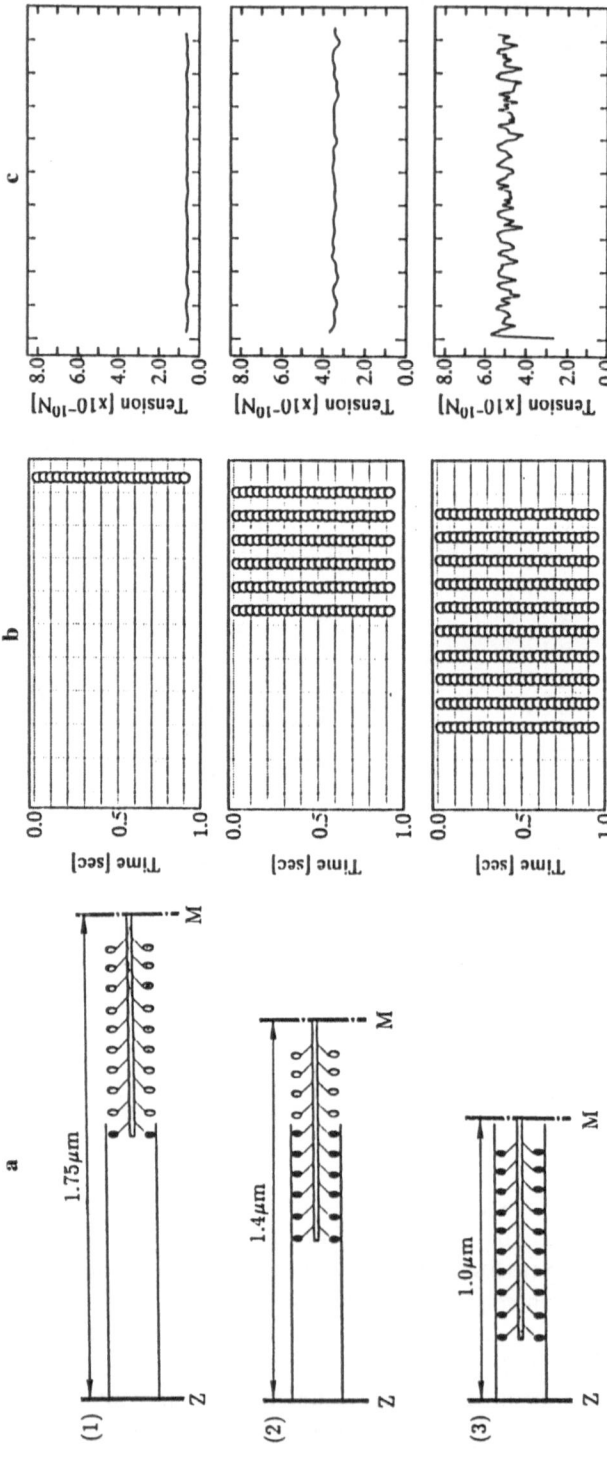

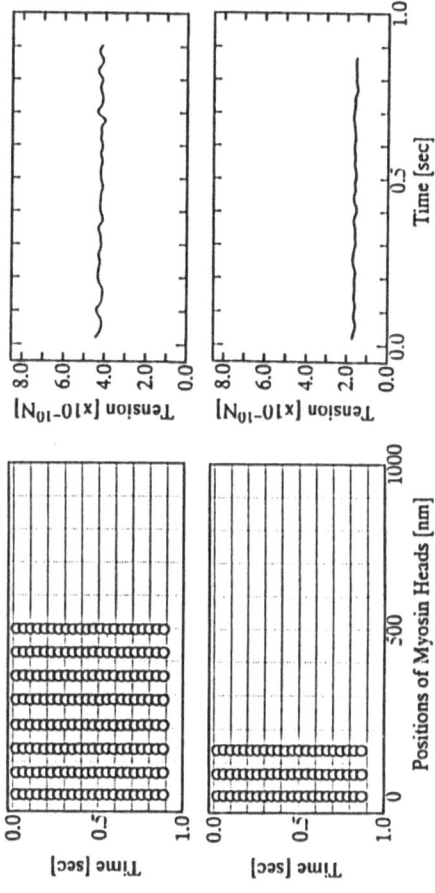

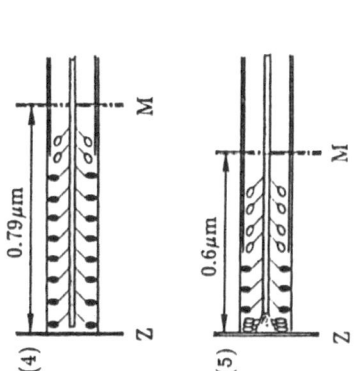

FIG. 9a–c. Isometric contraction model and the time course of positions of myosin heads and tension. **a** Schematic views of filaments. **b** Positions of myosin heads. **c** Tension, P

The amplitude of fluctuation of the total potential when $P/P_0 = 0.27$ is larger than at the other conditions. The actual timing and location of ATP hydrolysis generation cannot be determined, but it seems that this random generation assumption of ATP hydrolysis can predict the sliding motion reasonably well. Figure 6 shows the positions of the numbered myosin heads contained in the thick filament at 0.1-s intervals. In the case of $P/P_0 = 0.27$, the relative distances between myosin heads fluctuate more than in the other cases because the elastic spring is contending with the self-induced force generated by ATP hydrolysis. On the other hand, when $P/P_0 = 1.0$ the self-induced force cannot initiate sliding because the elastic spring potential is dominant. In Fig. 7, the force–velocity relationship and Hill's experimental results of isotonic contraction [13,14] show a good agreement.

In our model, the excess Gibbs free energy supplied by ATP hydrolysis is liberated to generate myosin heads sliding along actin filaments. Each myosin head will slide under the constant resistant force $P/20$. Therefore, the rate of work is obtained by the product of the force and the sliding velocity, which is the average value of 20 myosin heads in the period of 1 s. Figure 8 shows the relationship between this rate of work and the normalized force. The peak of this rate appears about $P/P_0 = 0.25$. This might explain the experimental observation reported by Yamada and Homsher [18], which shows the peak at $P/P_0 \cong 0.2$.

4.3 Isometric Contraction: Length–Tension Relationship

In this numerical simulation, the isometric tension is tested when the length of a half-sarcomere is kept constant, as shown schematically in Fig. 9a. The tension is generated by ATP hydrolysis, which happens randomly during steady state. The number of activated myosin heads is evaluated by obtaining the sum of purely overlapped actomyosin pairs, marked by solid ellipsoids in parts (1)–(5) of Fig. 9a. We did not count the suppressed actomyosin pairs, as shown in the left-hand side in (5) of Fig. 9a, or take account of the suppression-resistant force proportional to the length of the collapsed part. Figure 9b shows the activated myosin head positions at 0.04-s intervals. The slight relative fluctuation between neighboring myosin heads can be observed. The tension P applied at both ends, the Z and M lines, is in equilibrium with the force generated by ATP hydrolysis. The force P is evaluated by the sum of elastic spring forces Fe of each activated myosin head:

$$P = -\sum_j Fe_j \tag{24}$$

where Δj is the number of myosin heads. Figure 9c shows time courses of tension P in five cases of a half-sarcomere length. We averaged the tension P during the period 1.0 s. As more myosin heads are actived, the amplitude of tension P increases and its fluctuations are faster. The length–tension relationship obtained by this numerical simulation (solid line) shows a good agreement with Gordon's experimental results (dashed line) of muscle fiber in isometric contraction [15] (Fig. 10).

FIG. 10. Length–tension relationship. *Solid line*, simulation; *dashed
line*, experiment

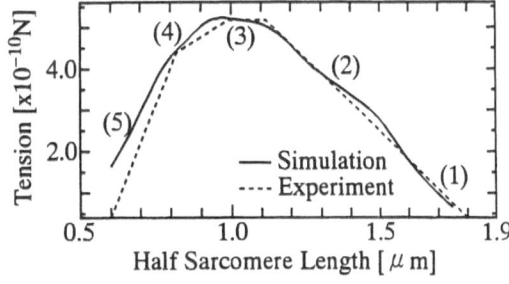

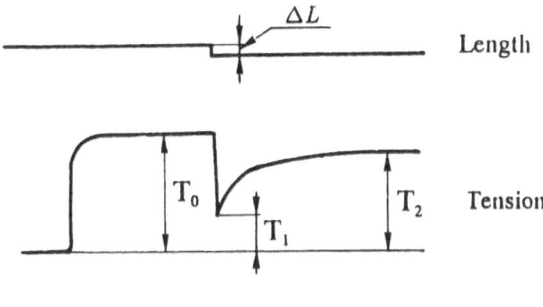

FIG. 11. Experimental observation of quick release

4.4 Quick Release

During isometric contraction, the length of the fiber is instantaneously altered
and the time course of the resulting tension changes is recorded. This experiment
is called quick release (Fig. 11). The experimental tension of quick release shows
a relatively large alteration with the step change of length. After that, tension
recovers quickly toward a level closer to that which existed before the step. The
response to these stepwise length changes is regarded as the viscoelastic feature
of muscle fiber, and suggests the presence of a structural element that would be
an elastic element whose length is altered simultaneously with the change of
length that is applied to the whole fiber. The transient process of force generation
is simulated by employing the same numerical algorithms as for isometric contraction. In our simulation, the initial length of a half-sarcomere is set as $1.0\,\mu m$,
and quick release occurs at time $t = 0.5\,s$. The number of myosin heads that are
activated by ATPase is assumed to increase with time; that is, 20% ($0 \le t \le 0.005$,
$0.5 \le t \le 0.505$), 45% ($0.005 \le t \le 0.125$, $0.505 \le t \le 0.625$), 90% ($0.125 \le t \le 0.25$,
$0.625 \le t \le 0.75$), and 100% ($0.25 \le t \le 0.5$, $0.75 \le t \le 1.0$) of the total number of
myosin heads which correspond to the length of overlap of two different filaments. The numerical results for the tension are shown in Fig. 12 under the
described length alternation conditions. These show good qualitative agreement
with experimental results [5].

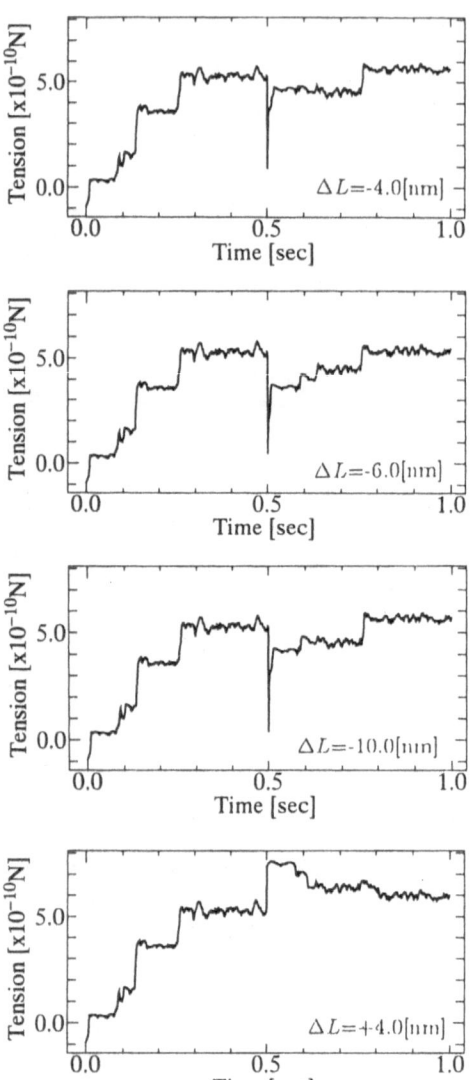

FIG. 12. Time course of tension force in the quick-release response at various step lengths. Quick release at time = 0.5 s; ΔL, length of step

5 Numerical Results of Atomic/Molecular Analyses

Figures 13–16 show the conformations, 3-D atom coordinates, at the minimum potential energy in four cases, i.e., G-actin and proK-actin [26] with or without ATP in water or in vacuo. From the comparison among the four cases, the role of ATP for structure stability was confirmed. If there is no ATP, the differences of atom coordinates between proK-actin and G-actin are exaggerated. It means that

Fig. 13. Minimum energy conformation
of G-actin in water

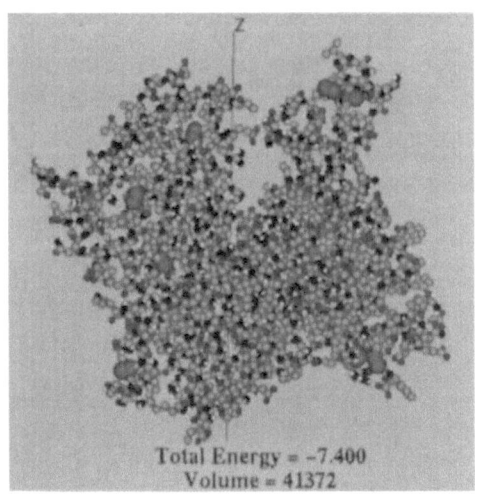

Total Energy = −7.400
Volume = 41372

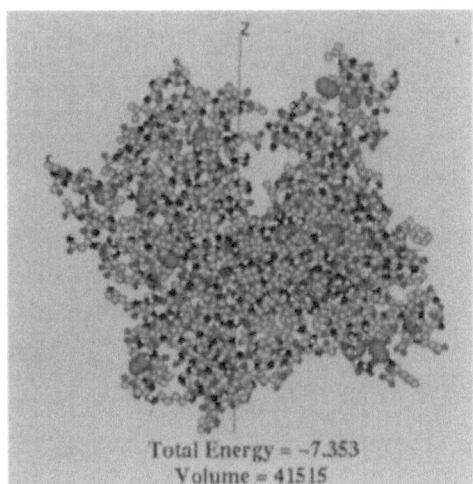

Fig. 14. Minimum energy conformation
of G-actin without adenosine triphosphate (ATP) in water

Total Energy = −7.353
Volume = 41515

ATP contributes to the stability of actin. Further, the 3-D structures in water or
in vacuo show the influence of environment.

Figures 17–20 also show the isothermal compressibilities at $T = 300\,\mathrm{K}$ of four
cases. The values of isothermal compressibility are 32.764 and $28.602 \times 10^{-11}\,\mathrm{m^2/N}$
for G-actin and proK-actin. Total values of root mean square (r.m.s) are shown
in Table 2. Comparison of the four cases shows that G-actin with ATP the most
compressible protein. G-actin has four subdomains (see Fig. 21). Comparison
with these four compressibilities, as shown in Table 3, also demonstrated that the
first subdomain, which has the binding site with myosin head S1, has the largest

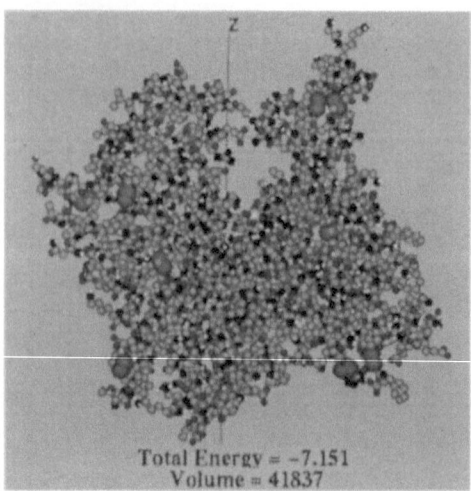

Total Energy = –7.151
Volume = 41837

FIG. 15. Minimum energy conformation
of proK-actin in water

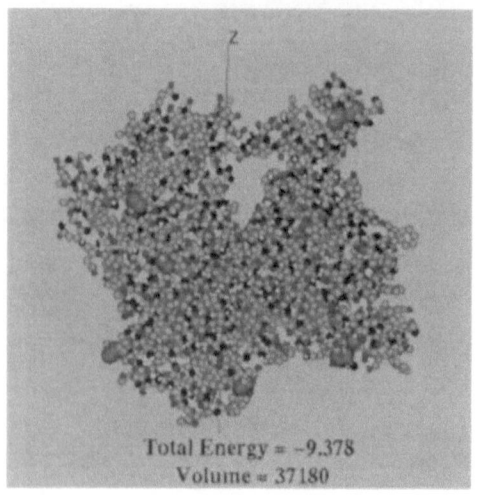

Total Energy = –9.378
Volume = 37180

FIG. 16. Minimum energy conformation
of G-actin without ATP in vacuo

TABLE 2. Total value of rms fluctuation.

Condition	Total value
G-Actin with ATP	2168×10^{-10} m
G-Actin without ATP	1529
ProK-Actin with ATP	1552
ProK-Actin without ATP	1472

rms, root mean square; ATP, adenosine
triphosphate.

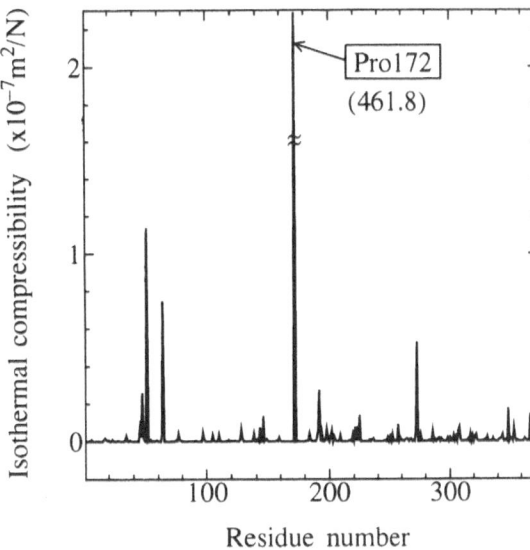

FIG. 17. Isothermal compressibilities of each residue of G-actin

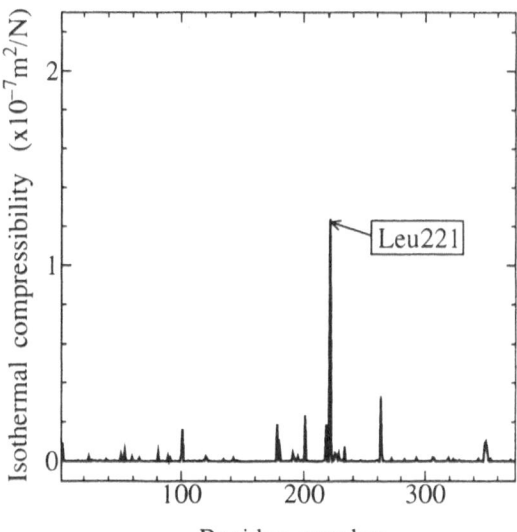

FIG. 18. Isothermal compressibilities of each residue of proK-actin

fluctuation, which means this subdomain is the most flexible and also the most easily activated. This suggests that the heterogeneous property of thermal compressibility and fluctuation leads to induction of contractile motion and the relative sliding motion between actomyosin filaments. The isothermal compressibility of G-actin with ATP shows a larger value than proK-actin with ATP. This suggests that normal G-actin has a higher activation function for generating muscle contraction (Table 4).

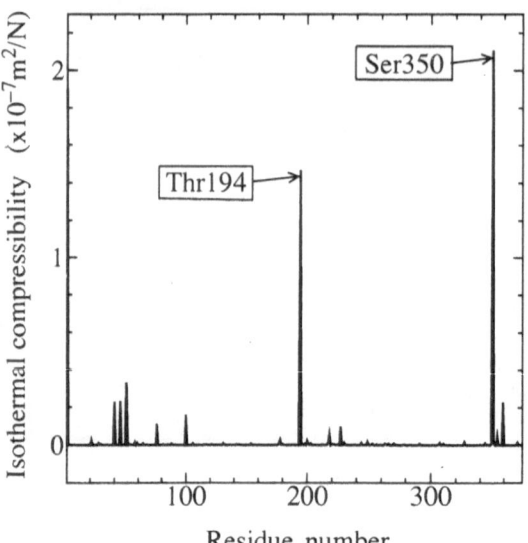

Fig. 19. Isothermal compressibilities of each residue of G-actin without ATP

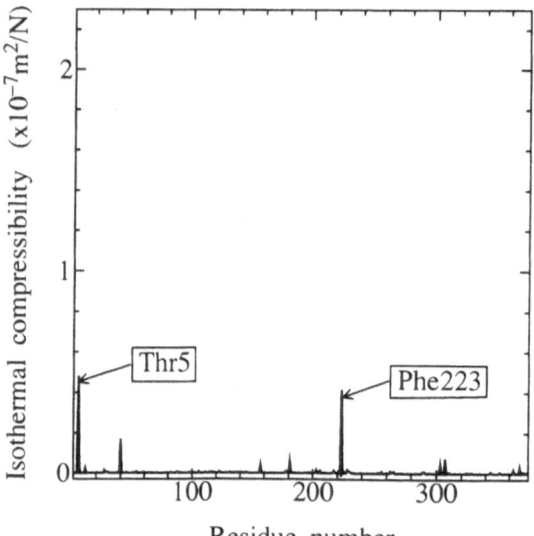

Fig. 20. Isothermal compressibilities of each residue of proK-actin without ATP

Table 3. Total fluctuation in each subdomain ($\times 10^{-10}$m).

Condition	SD1	SD2	SD3	SD4
G-Actin with ATP	805	231	560	574
G-Actin without ATP	630	177	342	380
ProK-Actin with ATP	607	168	352	426
ProK-Actin without ATP	596	153	352	372

SD, Subdomain.

FIG. 21. Domains of G-actin

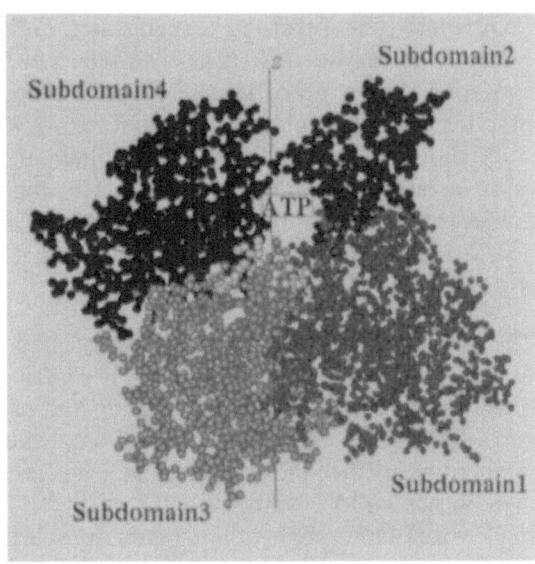

TABLE 4. Numerical results of isothermal compressibility of actin molecule.

Condition	Isothermal compressibility
G-Actin with ATP	$32.764 \times 10^{-11} \, m^2/N$
ProK-Actin with ATP	28.602

6 Conclusions

Studies employing the macromolecular and atomic/molecular numerical computation models reveal the basis of the skeletal muscle contractile mechanism at the microlevel.

6.1 Macromolecule Analyses

We proposed a numerical model based on the macromolecular potential theory to interpret different contractile events of skeletal muscle, and examined the applicability of this mathematical model by comparisons with experimental results. The numerical results from one myosin head can explain the result of the in vitro motility assay [10,11]. The calculation results of 20 myosin heads also agreed with the experimental result of the force–velocity relationship [13,14]. In the case of isometric contraction, the length–tension relationship is in good qualitative agreement with the experimental result [15]. Based on this agreement with experimental observations of whole muscle fiber, it can be emphasized that our macromolecular potential model is applicable to and might give some clues about the actin-myosin sliding motion mechanism in skeletal muscle contraction.

Obviously, the quantitative verification of the macromolecular potential itself is still to be provided. It is also necessary to understand the process from the excitation of the nerve system to muscle contraction, "excitation–contraction coupling," for designing the optimal micro- and nanomachines. However, this study shows the possibility that constitutive modeling of living tissue and design of an artificial machine that works with high efficiency may be achieved by numerical simulation based on the theory of actin-myosin molecular dynamics.

6.2 Atomic/Molecular Analyses

The studies of the G-actin molecule suggested that the heterogeneous properties of 3-D structure and compressibility are intrinsic features of proteins. The minimum energy conformations of G-actin and proK-actin, cut off between Met-47 and Gly-48, were determined by the steepest descent method and the conjugate gradient method of the molecular mechanics code AMBER. It is suggested that G-actin has a more stable structure with ATP than without ATP. The normal mode analyses elucidate the dynamic properties at the atomic/molecular level, which should involve actomyosin contraction motion. The distributions of root mean square atomic fluctuation and isothermal compressibility were also obtained by those analyses, which revealed that proK-actin has less fluctuation than G-actin. This means that proK has less functional ability for actomyosin sliding motion and binding with calcium ions, ATP, and the myosin head S1. In particular, the existence of ATP in G-actin exaggerates the fluctuation and makes the atomic structure "softer" at the binding site. We conclude that G-actin with ATP has the greatest functional ability for actomyosin sliding motion of our four cases.

References

1. Huxley HE (1985) The crossbridge mechanism of muscle contraction and its implications. J Exp Biol 115:17–30
2. Fung YC (1990) Biomechanics: motion flow stress and growth. Springer-Verlag, Berlin Heidelberg New York
3. Lamm G, Szabo A (1986) Langevin modes of macromolecules. J Chem Phys 85:7334–7348
4. Huxley AF (1957) Muscle structure and theories of contraction. Prog Biophys Biophys Chem 7:255–318
5. Huxley AF, Simmons RM (1971) Proposed mechanism of force generation in striated muscle. Nature 233:533–538
6. Zahalak GI, Ma SP (1990) Muscle activation and contraction: constitutive relations based directly on cross-bridge kinetics. Trans ASME J Biomech Eng 112:52–62
7. Heuser JE, Cooke R (1983) Actin-myosin interactions visualized by the quick-freeze, deep-etch replica technique. J Mol Biol 169:97–122
8. Reedy MK, Holmes RC, Tregear RT (1965) Induced changes in orientation of the cross-bridges of glycerinated insect flight muscle. Nature 207:1276–1281
9. Ford LE, Huxley AF, Simmons RM (1977) Tension responses to sudden length change in stimulated frog muscle fibers near slack length. J Physiol (Camb) 269:441–515

10. Yanagida T, Arata T, Oosawa F (1985) Sliding distance of actin filament induced by a myosin crossbridge during one ATP hydrolysis cycle. Nature 316:366–369
11. Uyeda TQP, Warrick HM, Kron SJ, Spudich JA (1991) Quantized velocities at low myosin densities in an in vitro motility assay, Nature 352:307–311
12. Mitsui T, Oshima H (1988) A self-induced translation model of myosin head motion in contracting muscle. I. Force-velocity relation and energy liberation. J Muscle Res Cell Motil 9:52–62
13. Hill AV (1938) The heat of shortening and the dynamic constants of muscle. Proc R Soc Lond Ser B Biol Sci 126:136–195
14. Oiwa K, Chaen S, Kamitsubo E, Shimmen T, Sugi H (1990) Steady-state force-velocity relation in the ATP-dependent sliding movement of myosin-coated beads on actin cables in vitro studied with a centrifuge microscope. Proc Natl Acad Sci USA 87:7893–7897
15. Gordon AM, Huxley AF, Julian FJ (1966) The variation in isometric tension with sarcomere length in vertebrate muscle fibers. J Physiol (Camb) 184:170–192
16. Huxley AF, Niedergerke R (1954) Structural changes in muscle during contraction-interference microscopy of living muscle fibers. Nature 173:971–973
17. Huxley HE, Hanson J (1954) Structural changes in muscle during contraction-changes in the cross-striations of muscle during contraction and stretch and their structural interpretation. Nature 173:973–976
18. Yamada T, Homsher E (1984) The dependence on the distance of shortening of the energy output from frog skeletal muscle shortening at velocities of V_{max}, $1/2V_{max}$ and $1/4_{vmax}$. In: Pollack GH, Sugi H (eds) Contractile mechanism in muscle Plenum, New York, pp 883–885
19. Shulz GE, Schirmer RE (1979) Principles of protein structure. Springer-Verlag, Berlin Heidelberg New York
20. Alberts B, Bray D, Lewis J, Raff M, Roberts K, Watson JD (1989) Molecular biology of the cell, 2nd edn. Garland, pp 613–623
21. Weiner SJ, Kollman PA, Case DA, Singh VC, Ghio C, A lagona G, Profeta S Jr, Weiner P (1984) A new force flied of molecular mechanics simulation of nucleic acids and proteins. J Am Chem Soc 106:765–784
22. Weiner SJ, Kollman PA, Nguyen DT, Case DA (1986) An all atom force field for simulations of proteins and nucleic acids. J Comput Chem 7:230–252
23. Nguyen DT, Case DA (1985) On finding stationary states on large-molecule potential energy surfaces. J Phys Chem 89:4020–4026
24. Kabsch W, Mannherz HG, Suck D, Pai EF, Holmes KO (1990) Atomic structure of the actin:DNase I complex. Nature 347:37–44
25. Holmes KC, Popp D, Gebhard W, Kabsch W (1990) Atomic model of the actin filament. Nature 347:44–49
26. Fujime SH, Suzuki M, Titani K, Hozumi T (1992) Muscle actin cleaved by proteinase K: its polymerization and in vitro motility. J Biochem 112:568–572
27. Tokunaga M, Sutoh K, Toyoshima C, Wakabayashi T (1987) Location of the ATPase site of myosin determined by three-dimensional electron microscopy. Nature 329:635–638
28. Brooks B, Karplus M (1983) Harmonic dynamics of proteins: normal modes and fluctuations in bovine pancreatic trypsin inhibitor. Proc Natl Acad Sci USA 80:6571–6575
29. van Gunsteren WF, Karplus M (1981) Effect of constraints, solvent and crystal environment on protein dynamics. Nature 293:677–678

30. van Gunsteren WF, Karplus M (1982) Protein dynamics in solution and in a crystalline environment: a molecular dynamics study. Biochemistry 21:2259–2274
31. Levitt M, Sander C, Stern PS (1985) Protein normal-mode dynamics: trypsin inhibitor,
   · crambin, ribonuclease and lysozyme. J Mol Biol 181:423–447
32. Levitt M, Sharon R (1988) Accurate simulation of protein dynamics in solution. Proc Natl Acad Sci USA 85:7557–7561
33. Gō N, Noguti T, Nishikawa T (1983) Dynamics of a small globular protein in terms of low-frequency vibrational modes. Proc Natl Acad Sci USA 80:3696–3700
34. Seno Y, Gō N (1990) Deoxymyoglobin studied by the conformational normal mode analysis. I. Dynamics of globin and the heme-globin interaction. J Mol Biol 216:95–109
35. Seno Y, Gō N (1990) Deoxymyoglobin studied by the conformational normal mode analysis. II. The conformational change upon oxygenation. J Mol Biol 216:111–126

Computational Analysis of Bone Remodeling in Orthodontics

KATSUYUKI YAMAMOTO[1], HAJIME MORIKAWA[2], YOSHIAKI SATOH[3], and SHINJI NAKAMURA[3]

Summary. When orthodontic force is applied to a tooth, alveolar bone remodeling occurs, resulting in tooth movement. The way in which an orthodontic force is transferred to the tooth root is of fundamental importance in orthodontics. It is believed that there is an optimal stress distribution to bring about efficient tooth movement. However, there is little information concerning the quantitative relationship between stress and alveolar bone remodeling. In this chapter, two kinds of studies concerning this relationship are described, preceded by a brief review on computational analysis of orthodontics. The resorption rate of the alveolar bone during orthodontic treatment was first investigated. The stress distributions around the canine tooth were analyzed using a three-dimensional (3-D) finite-element method (FEM) model. The amounts of alveolar bone resorption were obtained indirectly from 3-D tooth movement under various clinical treatments. From these results, the alveolar bone resorption rate from a unit stress was found to be $0.6\,\mu$m/(kPa·day), ranging from 0.4 to $0.8\,\mu$m/(kPa·day). The relationship between the appearance of osteoclasts and stress distribution was also investigated. Histological observations of tissue sections taken from animals subjected to experimental tooth movement were compared with the analytical findings obtained by specimen-specific FEM models. The results clearly demonstrated that there is a close correlation between the appearance of osteoclasts and the principal stress distribution in the periodontal ligament. The osteoclasts appeared at the specific sites where the compressive stress was within a relatively narrow range. The obtained stress level is discussed from the aspect of optimal stress.

Key words: Orthodontics—Remodeling—Alveolar bone—Finite-element model— Osteoclasts

[1] Division of Biomedical Engineering, Graduate School of Engineering, Hokkaido University, N13 W8 Kita-ku, Sapporo, Hokkaido, 060 Japan
[2] Asahikawa National College of Technology, Shinkoudai, Asahikawa, Hokkaido, 071 Japan
[3] Department of Orthodontics, Hokkaido University School of Dentistry, N13 W7 Kita-ku, Sapporo, Hokkaido, 060 Japan

1 Introduction

Orthodontic treatment utilizes the remodeling process of the alveolar bone in response to externally applied force to teeth to correct dental deformities in patients with malocclusion. When an orthodontic force is applied to a tooth, osteoclasts and osteoblasts appear in the pressure and tension areas, respectively, around the tooth root. These cells induce resorption and apposition of the alveolar bone, which is the supporting tissue of the tooth, thereby resulting in tooth movement.

Through studies on experimental tooth movement and clinical treatments, it is believed that there is an optimal force which is responsible for the most efficient tooth movement [1–4]. From a biomechanical point of view, the force has to be applied to the crown so as to provide the optimal stress distribution, which then generates maximum cellular activities [4–6]. However, in clinical orthodontics, force magnitude and direction at the crown of the tooth are the only controlling factors for tooth movement. It is therefore of fundamental importance to know how the force is transferred to the tooth root and the surrounding tissues. For studying the stress/strain distributions around the tooth, the finite-element method (FEM) was introduced into orthodontics in the mid-1970s. Since then, many studies have been published to clarify the force–stress relationships [7–25].

Tooth movement has also been widely studied from histological, histochemical, and physiological points of view [26]. Although the relationship between the mechanical factors and the biological response is not yet fully understood, it is known that osteoclasts appear at specific sites on the wall of the alveolar bone, depending on tissue geometry, mechanical stress, and vascularity around a tooth. The periodontal ligament (PDL), which is the connective tissue between a tooth and the alveolar bone, plays an important role in remodeling of the alveolar bone [26]. When the PDL is excessively compressed by orthodontic force, it degenerates to what is called a cell-free zone and efficient tooth movement does not occur. In such a situation, the front lines of osteoclasts become situated adjacent to the cell-free zone. This site-specific response results in undermining resorption; in contrast, direct resorption is generally accepted to be ideal. In general, these patterns of resorption are understood to correspond well qualitatively to the stress distribution around a tooth. However, until now there has been almost no quantitative verification of a close correlation between the appearance of osteoclasts and mechanical stress.

In this study, an attempt was made to estimate the alveolar bone resorption rate to a unit stress during orthodontic treatment, which may be one of the most fundamental factors for understanding tooth movement in orthodontics. In addition to this macroscopic approach to alveolar bone remodeling from clinical measurements, we also investigated the relationship between the appearance of osteoclasts and stress distribution by comparing histological observations from animal experiments with the analytical findings obtained by specimen-specific FEM models.

2 Overview of Computational Analysis in Orthodontics

The anatomical structure of a tooth is schematically shown in Fig. 1. The bulk of the tooth consists of a hard material known as dentine. Each tooth has a pulp chamber with blood vessels and nerves. The surface of the crown is covered with a dense enamel, which is the hardest material in the body, and the surface of the root is covered by a thin layer of another dense material, cementum. The tooth root is secured to the alveolar bone by a thin layer of connective tissue, called the periodontal ligament (PDL). The cells of the PDL are composed of fibroblasts, osteoblasts, and cementoblasts. The PDL is richly supplied by blood vessels, compared to other ligaments and tendons. In addition to its role in tooth support, the PDL is also essential for remodeling of the alveolar bone. This adaptability of the bone, in relation to the PDL, is important for the maintenance of optimal occlusion at the proper vertical dimension. Orthodontic treatments make use of this adaptability, although its mechanism at the cellular level is not fully understood.

When orthodontic force is applied to a tooth, it moves three-dimensionally with translations and rotations according to the geometry of the tooth and the position and direction of the force applied at the crown. The resulting tooth movement is often described in general terms, such as tipping and bodily move-ment (pure translation) (Fig. 2). When a horizontal force F is applied to a tooth, tipping occurs around the center of rotation, CR. To prevent the tipping, orth-odontists apply an appropriate moment M to the teeth by adjusting orthodontic appliances about once every month.

In daily practice, orthodontists analyze tooth movement during treatment in a one-dimensional (1-D) way by measuring the distance between two teeth using calipers or in a two-dimensional (2-D) way by tracing the movement of teeth on radiographs taken at different stages of treatment. However, for three-dimen-sional (3-D) measurement, only the instantaneous translation and rotation, ob-served immediately after applying a force to a tooth, has been measured using

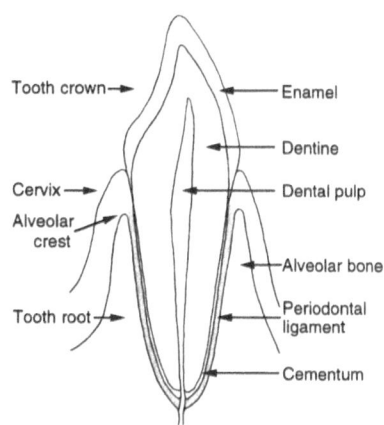

FIG. 1. Anatomical structure of the tooth

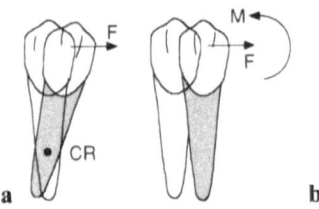

FIG. 2a,b. Movements of a tooth in response to orthodontic force. **a** Tipping caused by pure horizontal force F; CR is a center of rotation. **b** Bodily movement attained by the force combined with moment M

laser hologram interferometry [27,28]. This technique measures the movement with the highest possible degree of sensitivity, but is restricted to short-term observations, and therefore tooth movement during orthodontic treatment cannot be traced. The authors have developed a computer-controlled optical system for measuring 3-D profiles of dental casts and 3-D tooth movement during treatment. This method has been successfully applied in quantifying the differences in tooth movement resulting from orthodontic therapeutics [29].

As mentioned previously, the mechanism by which force is transferred to the tooth root is a very important subject of study in orthodontics. Before the introduction of FEM analysis, strain gauge techniques, photoelastic techniques, and mathematical solid geometry models were employed for analyzing stress/strain distributions and the center of rotation [8,30]. FEM analysis was introduced to orthodontics in the mid-1970s, using 2-D [7,9,10], axisymmetric [8] and 3-D models [11]. Since the introduction of FEM analysis, there have been many studies investigating how stresses are produced around the tooth root under various loading and geometric conditions. Not only stress distribution but many kinds of other analyses now have been performed: tooth mobility when changing load and bone structure [9], the instantaneous center of rotation under various loadings [10], the influence of material constants on the center of rotation and tip movement [14], the relationship between a moment-to-force ratio and the center of rotation [16], the dependence of the stress level and tooth displacement on root length and alveolar bone height [17,21,24], stress levels when the tooth is subjected to vertical forces [25], and FEM models based on morphology and material parameters measured from human autopsy specimens [19,20].

Although these studies have greatly contributed to an understanding of the initial cause of tooth movement, there have been almost no studies showing quantitatively the direct relationship between stress/strain and bone remodeling in orthodontics. Tanne et al. [22] investigated, in their preliminary study, the association between the stress in the PDL and bone remodeling by integrating analytical results with histological findings during experimental tooth movements. This approach to the process of bone remodeling seems to be a beneficial tool for a better understanding of orthodontics. In the subsequent sections, we focus on the relationship between stress and alveolar bone resorption during clinical treatment and the relationship between stress and the appearance of osteoclasts during experimental tooth movement.

3 Resorption Rate of the Alveolar Bone During Orthodontic Treatment

In this section, mechanical stress in the PDL is analyzed using a 3-D finite-element model of a tooth to determine the alveolar bone resorption rate during orthodontic treatment. The forces, produced by an orthodontic appliance and then applied to the tooth model, are also determined by a 3-D FEM model of the appliance. Because there are no quantitative tools for measuring the resorption of the alveolar bone, we calculated the resorption indirectly from 3-D tooth movement measured in clinical orthodontics. Based on the FEM analyses and clinical measurements, we ultimately estimated a resorption rate of the alveolar bone to a unit stress under various orthodontic treatments.

3.1 Materials and Methods

3.1.1 Stress Analysis

A canine tooth was chosen for the present analysis because in clinical treatments the canines are among the teeth most frequently mobilized. A 3-D finite element model for a canine was constructed as shown in Fig. 3. The average dimensions of a human maxillary canine were obtained from an impression of a canine replica, which was sliced at intervals of 1 mm for discretization of the FEM model. After taking enlarged photocopies of the slices, the profiles were fed into a workstation (SPARCstation IPX, Sun Microsystems, Mountain View, CA, USA) using a digitizer (KW4300, Graphtec, Tokyo, Japan). The model consists of 392 eight-noded solid elements, which are divided into three parts, the tooth of 28 mm in length, the PDL of 0.2 mm in thickness, and the bracket for an orthodontic

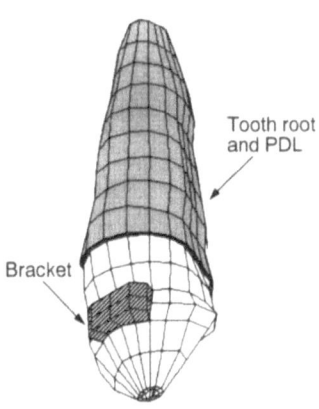

Tooth root
and PDL

Bracket

FIG. 3. Three-dimensional (3-D) finite-element method (FEM) model of a canine tooth with the periodontal ligament (PDL) and a bracket

appliance. For simplicity, the alveolar bone is not included in this model, because the PDL has an extremely low Young's modulus in comparison with alveolar bone. Thus, all the nodes on the external surface of the PDL are fixed, treating the bone as a rigid body.

Before analysis of the tooth model, the forces to be applied to the portion of the bracket should be determined. In this study, two kinds of orthodontic appliances were used, a simple open-loop wire and a power chain (also called elastic). We constructed 3-D finite-element models for the simple loop wire to determine the magnitude and direction of the force produced by this appliance (Fig. 4). This model consists of 41 beam elements and includes the gable and antirotation bends, which are incorporated to avoid tipping and rotation of a tooth and to maintain the bodily movement in clinical orthodontics. As loading conditions, a horizontal force and two kinds of forced deflections corresponding to an orthodontic force and the bends, respectively, were simultaneously applied to the wire model. The resulting forces at the nodes N_1 and N_2 to be attached to the bracket were obtained under a large deflection mode of FEM analysis. The calculated forces, including the moment, were then transferred to the bracket of the tooth model (Fig. 5). As for the power chain, only a point force produced by this appliance was directly applied to the bracket. However, as the effective force rapidly decreases and reaches a stable level within a few days after the appliance is activated, the force magnitude was reduced according to an experimentally determined rate of reduction.

The stress and force analyses were performed on the workstation (Sun Microsystems, SPARCstation IPX), using the ANSYS package (ANSYS, Houston, PA, USA). The mechanical properties of the tooth were determined from

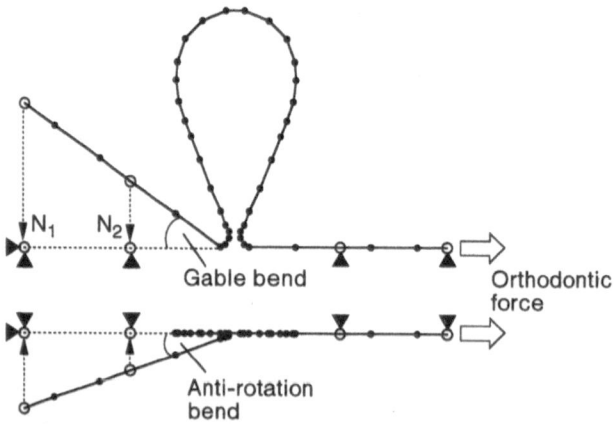

FIG. 4. A 3-D FEM model of an orthodontic appliance. This simple open-loop wire was incorporated with gable and antirotation bends of 35° and 20°, respectively. A horizontal orthodontic force and forced deflections corresponding to the bends were applied to the wire. The resulting forces at nodes N_1 and N_2 were transferred to the bracket, as shown in Fig. 5

FIG. 5. Forces produced by a simple open-loop wire and applied to the bracket of the tooth model. The gable bend produces F_1 and F_2. Another moment, not shown in this figure, is also produced by the antirotation bend. N_1, N_2, nodes

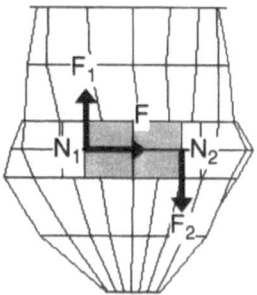

the literature values [13,18,20]: Young's modulus, 20 Gpa, and Poisson's ratio, 0.3, for the tooth; 0.67 MPa and 0.49 for the PDL; and 15 Gpa and 0.3 for the simple loop wire. We analyzed stress distributions of 13 maxillary canines during various orthodontic treatments (Table 1).

3.1.2 Bone Resorption

In our previous study [29], we developed a 3-D measurement system for profiles of dental plaster casts (Fig. 6), which consisted of an optical apparatus, a movable stage, and a personal computer. A dental plaster cast was set on the stage. A laser beam directed at a dental plaster cast formed a small spot of light, the vertical position of which was detected by a charge-coupled device (CCD) optical sensor. While the computer-controlled mechanical stage moved in a horizontal plane, profiles of the cast were automatically measured and stored into the computer (Fig. 7). Tooth profiles of the patients were taken at an interval of about once every month during the period of treatment. Tooth movements, represented by six variables (three translations and three rotations), were determined by means of a 3-D registration technique for tooth profiles, which were stored on the computer. With this technique, we can superimpose the profiles between casts serially taken at different stages of treatment and calculate the 3-D movements from the beginning to a certain stage. The accuracy of this measurement is about 0.1 mm and 0.5° in translations and rotations, respectively.

Using this system, we measured the movements of 13 upper canines of nine patients over periods up to 190 days. The 3-D movement obtained from this algorithm refers to the center of the crown. Therefore, from these movements at

TABLE 1. Clinical orthodontic treatment conditions.

Appliance	Gable bend (deg)	Antirotation bend (deg)	Force (gf)	Number of subjects
Simple loop wire	35	0	150	1
	35	20	150	2
	35	60	150	1
Power chain	—	—	150	3
	—	—	300	6

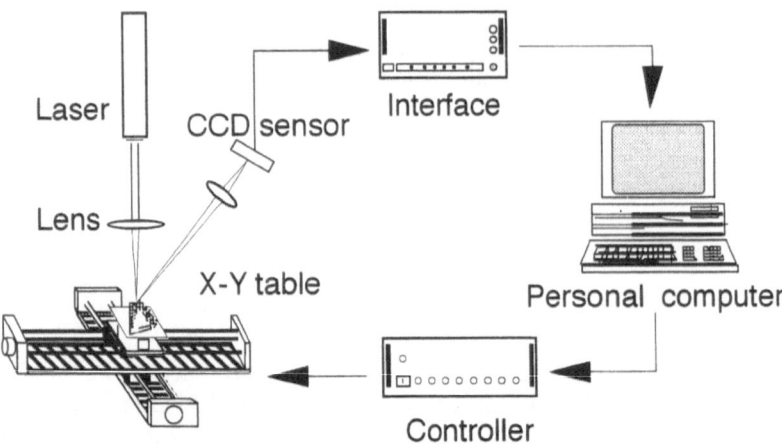

Fig. 6. A 3-D measurement system for a dental plaster cast. *CCD*, charge-coupled device

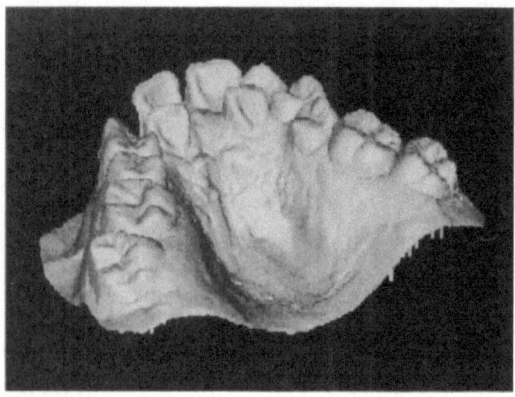

Fig. 7. Measured dental cast profiles displayed on a computer

the crown, we calculated the movement at the tooth root that gave us an estimate of bone resorption. In this calculation, we used the tooth model for the FEM analysis, assuming that the dimensions of a patient tooth root were identical with those of the tooth model.

3.2 Results

Before the stress analysis, we measured the decay of the initial force produced by a power chain and a simple loop wire. Power chains and simple loop wires were immersed into 37 °C water after activation, and their force was measured daily using a tension gauge for 3 weeks. The force produced by power chains decreased rapidly within a few days and reached a final stable level. Based on the results of this experiment, we applied a force of 110 and 200 gf to the tooth model for the stress analysis instead of the initial forces of 150 and 300 gf. In contrast, the force produced by the simple loop wire was not corrected because the results of the experiment showed no significant decrease.

Examples of the minimum principal stress distribution within the PDL in the distal aspect of the tooth are shown in Fig. 8. Only the minimum principal stress levels were plotted because three principal stresses resulted in almost identical stress levels in the PDL. The greatest compressive stress was observed near the alveolar crest, with a gradual decrease to zero and with tensile stress at the level of the apex. The maximum compressive stress ranged from about 30 to 55 kPa, depending on treatment conditions such as the magnitude of the orthodontic force and the configuration of the orthodontic appliances. Figure 8 also shows the alveolar bone resorption estimated from 3-D tooth movements at the crown. One of the crown movements, translation in the distal direction, is shown in Fig. 9. Other translations and rotations similar to this were also obtained. Because the degree of tooth movements changed almost linearly with time over the treatment period, we interpolated the 3-D movements per day using regression lines for each patient. Applying the movements to the tooth model at the crown, the bone resorption at the root was assessed by displacement of the nodes in the distal

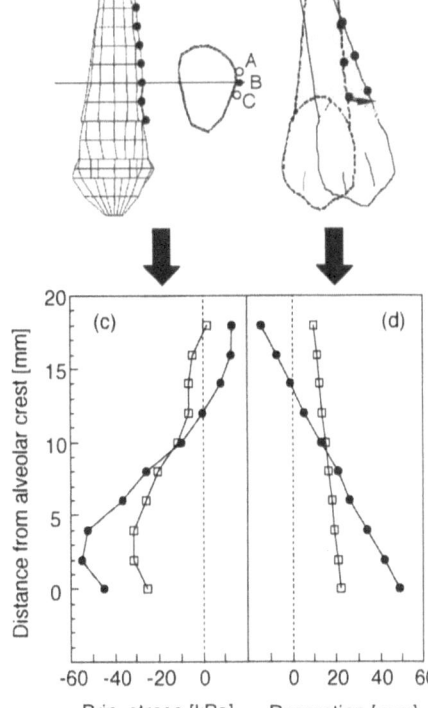

FIG. 8a–d. Examples of principal stress distributions within the PDL in the distal aspect (c) and bone resorptions (d), plotted along a longitudinal line through point B in **a**. The resorption was estimated from node movements as shown in **b**. *Closed circles* and *open squares* show distributions induced by a 300-gf power chain and a 150-gf open-loop wire, respectively

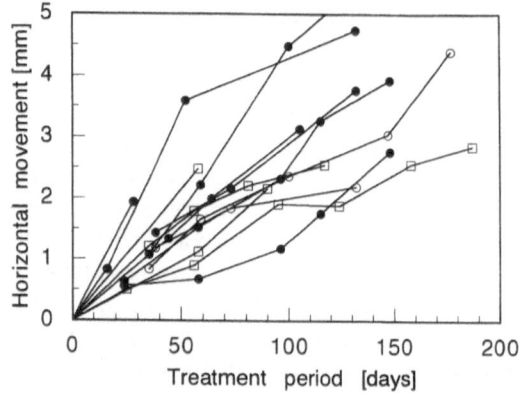

FIG. 9. Horizontal movements of 13 maxillary canines during orthodontic treatments shown in Table 1. *Closed circles, open circles,* and *squares* represent the treatments by 300-gf power chains, 150-gf power chains, and 150-gf open-loop wires, respectively

direction. Similar results for stress and resorption were also obtained in 11 other canines.

From the results obtained through this procedure, we plotted Fig. 10, which shows the relationship between the principal stress and resorption rate in all 13 cases. Because the horizontal and the vertical axes denote the stress and the resorption, respectively, the slope of the plots gives the alveolar bone resorption

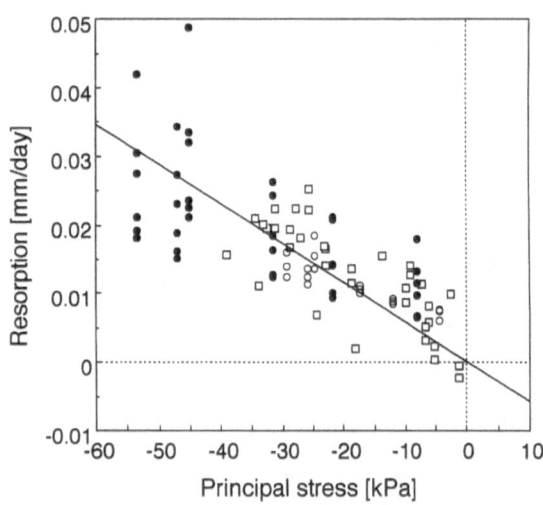

FIG. 10. Estimated alveolar bone resorption to compressive principal stress in the PDL. Distributions of stress and resorption in 13 canines were plotted from results as shown in Fig. 8. An averaged value of points A to C in Fig. 8 was plotted at each layers. Symbols are as in Fig. 9

rate to a unit stress. Although we plotted stress–resorption relationships for the various treatment conditions, most of the data were in the range 0.4–0.8 µm/(kPa·day). The mean value of the bone resorption rate to a unit stress was 0.58 ± 0.16 µm/(kPa·day).

The foregoing rate is based on clinical measurements of tooth movement. In other words, the rate is estimated from a macroscopic point of view, although the actual resorption is caused by the site-specific response to mechanical stress on a microscopic level. In the following section, site-specific absorption is investigated by integrating the stress analysis and histological study.

4 Mechanical Stress and Appearance of Osteoclasts

4.1 Materials and Methods

The maxillary canines of two cats were continuously retracted by an initial force of 100 and 200 gf for 1–2 weeks using a spring. After tissue fixation, the canine and the surrounding tissues were removed from the jaw and embedded in celloidin following decalcification. Tissue sections around the tooth root of 30 µm thickness were obtained and stained for histological analysis (Fig. 11). Then, the locations of osteoclasts in the PDL were observed using a light microscope.

To investigate the relationship between the appearance of cells and stress, we must construct a finite-element model at a microscopic level. Based on the morphological structures of each tissue section, we developed specimen-specific 2-D finite-element models. For this, the micrographs of the sections were traced and fed into a computer (Sun Microsystems, SPARCstation IPX) using a digitizer

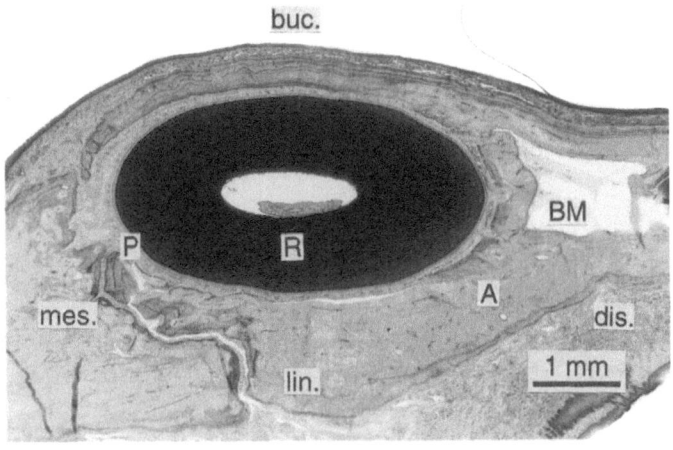

FIG. 11. A cross-sectional tissue section of a cat canine. *R*, *P*, *A*, and *BM* indicate tooth root, periodontal ligament, alveolar bone, and bone marrow, respectively; *buc.*, buccal; *dis.*, distal; *lin.*, lingual; *mes.*, mesial

(Graphtec, KW4300). The model, consisting of about 4000 eight-noded elements, was divided into the tooth, the PDL, and the alveolar bone, as shown in Fig. 12, and allowed us to model the morphological details such as the clefts of the alveolar wall and the marrow spaces. The following values of Young's modulus and Poisson's ratio were used: 20 GPa and 0.15 for the tooth, 10 MPa and 0.49 for the PDL, and 10 GPa and 0.3 for the bone, respectively. All stress analyses were performed using the ANSYS package (ANSYS).

To determine the force to be applied to the 2-D model, we also constructed a 3-D model (Fig. 13). The structure of this model was simpler than that of the 2-D model; for example, a constant thickness of 0.15 mm for the PDL and a smooth surface of the alveolar wall were assumed. We ascertained the shape of the 3-D model from longitudinal radiographs of the canine and the cross-sectional images of tissue sections. An initial force of 100 or 200 gf was applied to this model at the point where an orthodontic spring would be attached. Then, a stress component at every node in the direction of the spring's retraction was obtained on the external surface of the tooth root at a certain layer that corresponded to each of the 2-D models. Consequently, the sum of all the retraction components was applied to the point of loading in the 2-D model.

We conducted a plane strain analysis on the 2-D models, because the strain in the longitudinal direction in the PDL is considered to be much smaller than that of the cross-sectional direction. The stress distribution within the PDL obtained by each 2-D model was then compared with the appearance of osteoclasts observed by microscopy for each corresponding tissue section.

4.2 Results

Figure 14 shows a pressurized portion of a cross-sectional tissue section. Osteoclasts in the PDL appear on the side next to the alveolar bone, as denoted by the dots in the figure. Moreover, osteoclasts appeared mostly in the labial and lingual sides of the PDL adjacent to a cell-free zone and in the open clefts of the alveolar

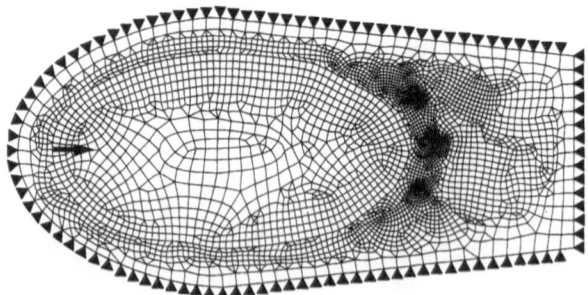

FIG. 12. A 2-D specimen-specific finite-element model of a tissue section. Point force was applied to a portion indicated by the arrow. The force magnitude was determined by a 3-D FEM model shown in Fig. 13

FIG. 13. A 3-D finite-element model of a cat canine to calculate a force to be applied to the 2-D model

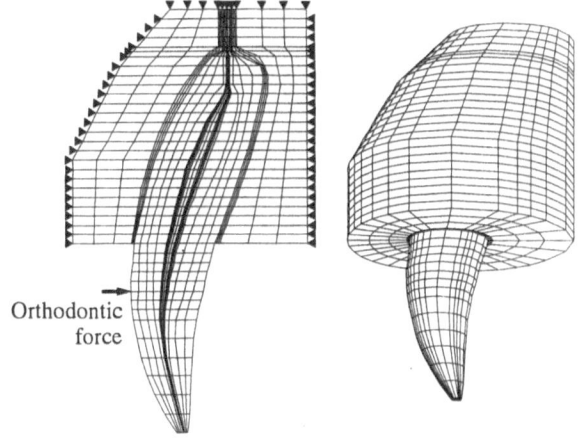

Orthodontic force

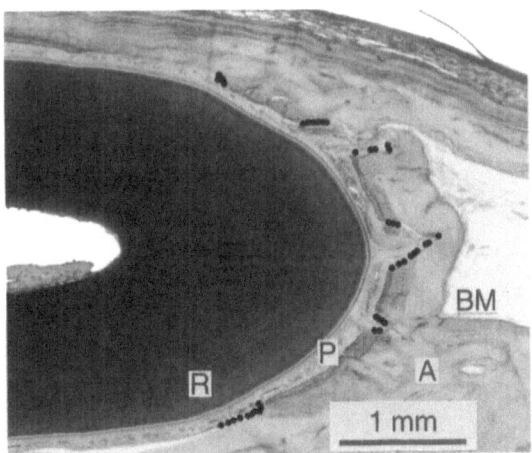

FIG. 14. A section of the canine sliced at 1.5 mm from the alveolar crest and the locations of osteoclasts denoted by the *dots*; *R, P, A,* and *BM* are as in Fig. 11

bone. This site-specific appearance is schematically depicted in Fig. 15. The calculated minimum principal stress distribution that corresponds to Fig. 14 is shown in Fig. 16, where only the distribution within the PDL is depicted for simplicity. The site-specific distribution of osteoclasts seems to coincide with that of the principal stress in the PDL (on the alveolar wall), as moderate stress is induced in the regions of the lateral wall and in the clefts while the highest stress is in the cell-free zone.

From the stress distribution of each tissue section, we read the stress levels at the sites where osteoclasts appeared. Nine tissue sections were examined; eight of them were taken from the portion near the alveolar crest and one near the apex. The results were plotted as histograms of the stress, which represents the relative frequency of osteoclasts appearance to stress level (Fig. 17). Even though each histogram was drawn according to different experimental conditions, it was

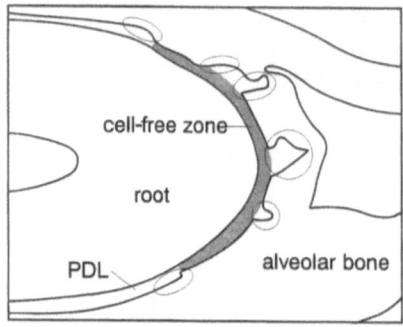

FIG. 15. A schematic drawing of the PDL divided into regions according to osteoclast existence. *Circles* and *ovals* indicate where these cells exist; *shaded area* is a cell-free zone

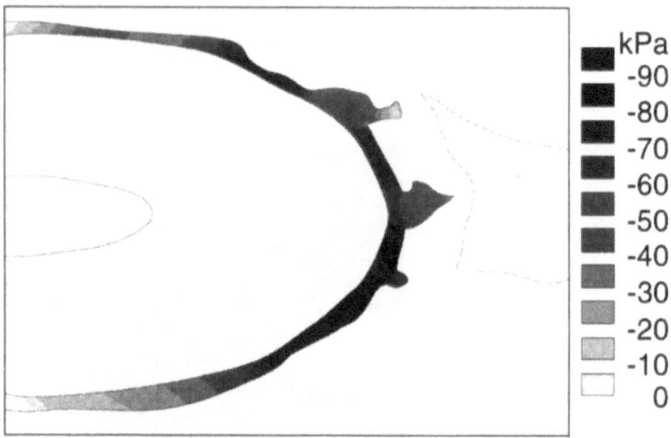

FIG. 16. Calculated principal stress distribution in the PDL

found that most of the osteoclasts appeared in the region of 40–50 kPa. The solid curve in this figure represents the relative frequency of stress over the entire region of the PDL, regardless of the existence of cells. This distribution was obtained by reading the stress level of any node selected at an interval of 0.1 mm along the interface between the PDL and the alveolar bone. By comparing these two distributions, it is clearly demonstrated that the cell appearance closely correlates with a certain level of principal stress. If there were no correlation between them, then the cells would disperse in a wider range.

5 Discussion

In this study, we first developed the 3-D FEM model of a human canine tooth to evaluate the alveolar bone resorption rate to a unit stress during orthodontic treatment. The resorption rate was estimated under various treatment conditions

FIG. 17. Histograms of minimum principal stress levels at sites where osteoclasts appeared. *Upper*, *middle*, and *bottom* panels show the results analyzed on tissue sections taken from the left and right canines of a cat and the left canine of a different cat, respectively. Each histogram was drawn from three tissue sections. All sections were taken from near the alveolar crest, except for one section in the bottom panel, taken from near the apex. *Solid curves* represent the relative frequency of stress over the entire region of the PDL, irrespective of cell existence. The total number of cells observed is shown by *n*

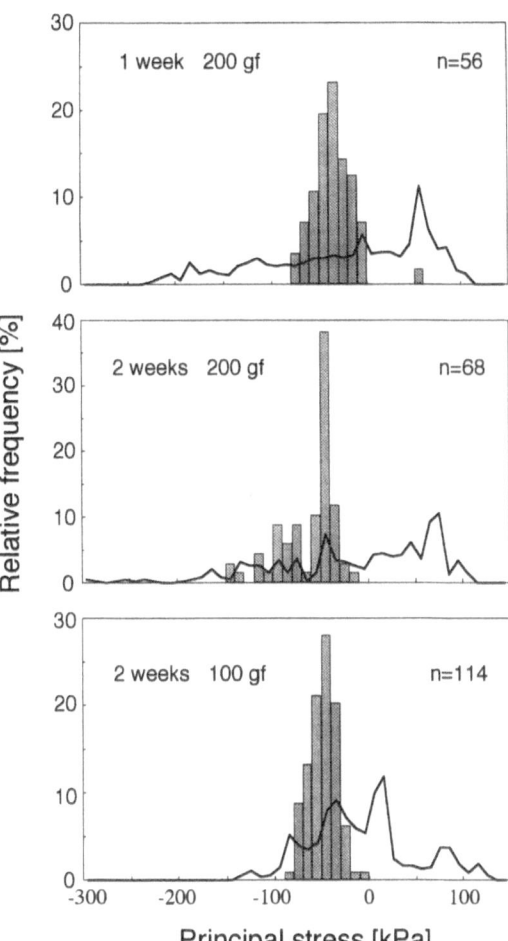

(see Table 1). Two kinds of orthodontic appliances were used, the simple open-loop wire and the power chain. As shown in the example of Fig. 8, the simple loop wire provided a moderate gradient of stress in the PDL along the tooth axis in comparison with the power chain because of the significant effect of the gable bend. Even though the stress distribution had various patterns, the resorption showed a relatively good correspondence to the stress distribution, from which we estimated the resorption rate of the alveolar bone. It should be emphasized that the resorption rate of $0.6\,\mu m/(kPa\cdot day)$ obtained in this study is one of the first estimates with respect to the rate per unit stress.

The results of the stress distribution in the PDL showed that the maximum levels of compressive principal stress were 30–55 kPa near the alveolar crest, depending on the different appliances and force magnitudes. These stress levels compare quantitatively with those of other investigators; for example, 72 kPa [23] and 100 kPa [18] at the alveolar crest by applying a 1-N horizontal force to the crown of a canine tooth model, 50 kPa at a level 5 mm distant from the apex of a lower canine by a 100-gf labiolingual force [24], 12 kPa at the cervix of a lower first premolar by a lingually directed 100-gf horizontal force [15], and 44 kPa at the apex of an upper central incisor by a 100-gf lingual force [17]. Although different appliances produce different stress distributions, the conventionally used orthodontic force, 100–200 gf, produces the principal stress of 10–100 kPa in the maximally compressed region of the PDL.

Storey and Smith [1] suggested that optimal movement of a canine occurred under an orthodontic force between 150 and 200 gf. Lee [2] reported the rate of tooth movement in relation to the forces for tipping and to the stress for bodily movement. He estimated the optimal force of 150–260 gf and the optimal stress of 100–200 gf/cm^2 (about 10–20 kPa), which resulted in the movement of 0.5–1 mm/week in a canine of a patient. Bench et al. [31] suggested 100 gf/cm^2 (10 kPa) as the optimal force, based on the evaluation of bioprogressive therapy, which produced a lighter continuous force being applied to teeth. In comparison with these values, the foregoing stress levels obtained in our study and by other researchers have shown significantly higher values. The reason for this difference lies in the fact that the optimal stress levels estimated from the conventional mathematical models were obtained by dividing the force by the projected area of tooth root; that is, a stress distribution was assumed to be uniform. The actual distribution inevitably has some stress concentration; the theoretical approach to the optimal stress level should therefore take account of the three-dimensional structures of a tooth. Only FEM analysis allows us to take an approach such as this.

The results in the animal experiments of this study might also suggest a higher optimal stress level because osteoclasts appeared at the specific sites whose stress level was 40–50 kPa. However, the high stress level contradicts the fact that osteoclasts are derived from hematogeneous cells. As is well known, when the stress level is too high for blood perfusion, the PDL changes its properties and degenerates to a cell-free zone (see Fig. 15). If we assume that the osteoclasts are directly carried with the blood, the stress level should not exceed the arterial blood pressure, which is several times less than the stress level obtained by the FEM analyses. Further investigations focusing on the optimal stress level in the PDL should be performed in association with studies on the histogenesis sequence of osteoclasts.

The validity of the models must also be examined. Although material constants, especially of the PDL in our case, are essential for the analysis, almost no experimentally determined values have been reported. Tanne [13] determined material parameters by comparing tooth displacement obtained by strain gauge measurement and FEM analysis; Young's modulus and Poisson's ratio of the PDL were determined to be 0.67 MPa and 0.49, respectively. A lower value of 0.07 MPa was also reported, which was determined from autopsy specimens by a similar technique [19]. On the other hand, much larger values, 69 MPa [32] and

50 MPa [18] in the modulus, and different values, 0.45 [32] and 0.25 [18] in Poisson's ratio, have also been reported. These reports showed a wide range of mechanical properties of the PDL. Therefore, we also examined the effect of the material constants on the results of the stress analysis. Changes in Young's modulus of the PDL had little effect on the stress level, because the PDL is a soft tissue situated between hard tissues; the moduli of the hard and soft tissues have quite different values. As for Poisson's ratio, when it was changed from 0.49 to 0.4 the stress level decreased by 50%–75%. Even if a soft tissue is generally treated as incompressible, Poisson's ratio of the PDL under a long period of compression might have to be modified. In addition, most investigations have been performed assuming linear, elastic, and isotropic properties, although it is known that the PDL is nonlinear, orthotropic, nonhomogeneous, and viscoelastic. Further studies should pay more attention to the mechanical properties of the PDL.

Tanne et al. [22] investigated histological changes in the PDL of the second premolar of a dog subjected to experimental tooth movement and compared these findings with the stress distributions obtained by a 3-D FEM analysis. They found that principal stress distribution in the PDL from the apex to cervix coincided with resorption and apposition induced by osteoclasts and osteoblasts, although their comparison was rather qualitative. In our study, the stress level where the osteoclasts appeared was investigated by specimen-specific 2-D FEM models, the discretization of which was fine enough to model the detail structure of tissue sections. Our results also suggest that the presence of osteoclasts highly correlates with the principal stress in the PDL (on the alveolar wall). When another stress such as von Mieses equivalent stress was chosen, we could not find any correlation. The results have clearly demonstrated that osteoclasts appear at a specific site where the principal stress lies within a relatively narrow range.

6 Conclusion

The way in which an orthodontic force is distributed to the tooth root is of fundamental importance in orthodontics. The applications of FEM analysis in this field were briefly reviewed. Quantitative relationships between the orthodontic force and the stress distribution around the tooth root have recently been established by many investigations using 3-D FEM models. However, little information with respect to the quantitative relation of mechanical factors to alveolar bone remodeling is available.

To determine the alveolar resorption rate during orthodontic treatment, we analyzed mechanical stress around the canine tooth using a 3-D FEM model and evaluated the alveolar bone resorption, which was estimated from the 3-D measurement of tooth movement under various clinical treatments. The alveolar resorption rate to a unit stress was found to be $0.6\,\mu m/(kPa\cdot day)$, ranging from 0.4 to $0.8\,\mu m/(kPa\cdot day)$.

Specimen-specific finite-element analysis combined with histological analysis was also performed. The results clearly demonstrated that there is a close correlation between the appearance of osteoclasts and the principal stress distribution in the PDL (on the alveolar wall). The osteoclasts appeared at specific sites where the compressive stress level is 40–50 kPa. However, further investigation is needed to determine whether this magnitude is appropriate for an optimal stress level, in connection with blood perfusion into the PDL.

Recent publications and ongoing research reveal a growing interest in the application of the FEM to biomechanical studies of teeth. Tooth movement during orthodontic treatment is one of the most dynamic processes of bone remodeling. Moreover, the force in orthodontics is well controlled. Computational analysis based on the FEM is a promising technique, not only for finding the optimal stress level in clinical orthodontics but also for understanding bone remodeling.

Acknowledgment. This research was supported in part by the Grant-in-Aid for Scientific Research on Priority Area (No. 04237202, 05221206 and 06213203) and for Scientific Research (No. 07407059) from the Ministry of Education, Science and Culture in Japan.

References

1. Storey E, Smith R (1952) Force in orthodontics and its relation to tooth movement. Aust J Dent 56:11–18
2. Lee BW (1965) Relationship between tooth-movement rate and estimated pressure applied. J Dent Res 44:1053
3. Storey E (1973) The nature of tooth movement. Am J Orthod 63:292–314
4. Nikoli RJ (1975) On optimum orthodontic force theory as applied to canine retraction. Am J Orthod 68:290–302
5. Burstone CJ (1962) The biomechanics of tooth movement. In: Kraus BS, Riedel RA (eds) Vistas in orthodontics. Lea and Febiger, Philadelphia, pp 197–213
6. Burstone CJ (1989) The biophysics of bone remodeling during orthodontics—optimal force considerations. In: Norton LA, Burstone CJ (eds) The biology of tooth movement. CRC Press, Boca Raton, pp 321–333
7. Thresher RW, Saito GE (1973) The stress analysis of human teeth. J Biomech 6:443–449
8. Farah JW, Craig RG, Sikarskie DL (1973) Photoelastic and finite element stress analysis of a restored axisymmetric first molar. J Biomech 6:511–520
9. Nokubi T, Yamaga T, Okuno Y, Tsutsumi S, Ida K (1977) Finite element stress analysis of tooth, periodontal membrane and alveolar bone (part I). Two-dimensional model with nonlinear behavior. J Osaka Univ Dent Sch 17:9–22
10. Yettram AL, Wright KWJ, Houston WJB (1977) Centre of rotation of a maxillary central incisor under orthodontic loading. Br J Orthod 4:23–27
11. Tsutsumi S, Ida K, Nokubi T, Yamaga T, Okuno Y, Tanne K, Sakuda M (1977) Finite element stress analysis of tooth, periodontal membrane and alveolar bone (part II). Three-dimensional elastic model (in Japanese). J Osaka Univ Dent Sch 17:23–34

12. Takahashi N, Kitagami T, Komori T (1980) Behaviour of teeth under various loading conditions with finite element method. J Oral Rehabil 7:453–461
13. Tanne K (1983) Stress induced in the periodontal tissue at the initial phase of the application of various types of orthodontic force: three-dimensional analysis by means of the finite element method (in Japanese). J Osaka Univ Dent Soc 28:209–261
14. Williams KR, Edmundson JT (1984) Orthodontic tooth movement analysed by the finite element method. Biomaterials 5:347–351
15. Tanne K, Sakuda M, Burstone CJ (1987) Three-dimensional finite element analysis for stress in the periodontal tissue by orthodontic forces. Am J Othod Dentofacial Orthop 92:499–505
16. Tanne K, Koenig HA, Burstone CJ (1988) Moment to force ratios and the center of rotation. Am J Orthod Dentofacial Orthop 94:426–431
17. Tanne K, Burstone CJ, Sakuda M (1989) Biomechanical responses of tooth associated with different root lengths and alveolar bone heights: changes of stress distributions in the PDL. J Osaka Univ Dent Sch 29:17–24
18. Middleton J, Jones ML, Wilson AN (1990) Three-dimensional analysis of orthodontic tooth movement. J Biomed Eng 12:319–327
19. Andersen KL, Pedersen EH, Melsen B (1991) Material parameters and stress profiles within the periodontal ligament. Am J Orthod Dentofacial Orthop 99:427–440
20. Andersen KL, Mortensen HT, Pedersen EH, Melsen B (1991) Determination of stress levels and profiles in the periodontal ligament by means of an improved three-dimensional finite element model for various types of orthodontic and natural force systems. J Biomed Eng 13:293–303
21. Tanne K, Nagataki T, Inoue Y, Sakuda M, Burstone CJ (1991) Patterns of initial tooth displacements associated with various root length and alveolar bone heights. Am J Orthod Dentofacial Orthop 100:66–71
22. Tanne K, Shibaguchi T, Terada Y, Kato J, Sakuda M (1992) Stress levels in the PDL and biological tooth movement. In: Davidovitch Z (ed) The biological mechanisms of tooth movement and craniofacial adaptation. Ohio State University, College of Dentistry, Columbus, pp 201–209
23. McGuinness N, Wilson AN, Jones M, Middleton J, Robertson NR (1992) Stress induced by edgewise appliances in the periodontal ligament—a finite element study. Angle Orthod 62:15–22
24. Cobo J, Sicilia A, Argüelles J, Suárez D, Vijande M (1993) Initial stress induced in periodontal tissue with diverse degrees of bone loss by an orthodontic force: tridimensional analysis by means of the finite element method. Am J Orthod Dentofacial Orthop 104:448–454
25. Wilson AN, Middleton J (1994) The finite element analysis of stress in the periodontal ligament when subject to vertical orthodontic forces. Br J Orthod 21:161–167
26. Norton LA, Burstone CJ (1989) The biology of tooth movement. CRC Press, Boca Raton
27. Wedendal PR, Bjelkhagen HI (1974) Dynamics of human teeth in function by means of double pulsed holography—an experimental investigation. Appl Opt 13:2481–2485
28. Burstone CJ, Pryputniewicz RJ, Bowley WW (1978) Holographic measurement of tooth mobility in three dimensions. J Periodontal Res 13:283–294
29. Yamamoto K, Hayashi S, Nishikawa H, Nakamura S, Mikami T (1991) Measurements of dental cast profile and three-dimensional tooth movement during orthodontic treatment. IEEE Trans Biomed Eng 38:360–365

30. Caputo AA, Chaconas SJ, Hayashi RK (1974) Photoelastic visualization of orthodontic forces during canine retraction. Am J Orthod 65:250–259
31. Bench RW, Gugino CF, Hilgers JJ (1978) Bioprogressive therapy. J Clin Orthod 12:123–139
32. Widera GEO, Tesk JA, Privitzer E (1976) Interaction effects among cortical bone, cancellous bone, and periodontal membrane of natural teeth and implants. J Biomed Mater Res Biomed Mater Symp 7:613–623

Circulatory Mechanics

Inelastic Constitutive Modeling of Arterial and Ventricular Walls

Eiichi Tanaka[1], Hiroshi Yamada[2], and Sumio Murakami[1]

Summary. The constitutive laws of arterial and ventricular walls are reviewed and their mechanical modeling is discussed. After a brief review of the constitutive modeling of arterial and ventricular walls, an anisotropic inelastic constitutive model of arteries is developed. The hysteresis loops under cyclic loading are assumed to be caused by the dependence of the behavior on the loading path and the loading rate. The elastic part of the deformation is represented by postulating a transversely isotropic strain energy density function, while the inelastic part is formulated by incorporating the transverse isotropy into the viscoplastic model proposed in a previous paper by the authors. A three-dimensional transversely isotropic constitutive model of ventricular walls is then proposed by dividing the stress into the sum of the passive and active parts. The passive part is represented by a strain energy density function similar to the arterial wall, and the active part is formulated by introducing internal variables describing the activities and the sarcomere length. The applicability of the current models is also discussed by comparing them with the corresponding results of experiments.

Key words: Biomechanics—Constitutive equation—Artery—Ventricular wall—Inelasticity—Modeling

1 Introduction

Noninvasive measurements of blood flow and deformation in the artery and the heart are now possible by means of ultrasonic wave and magnetic resonance imaging. In addition, the techniques of numerical simulations such as finite-element and boundary-element methods are also being developed to give quantitative information on the mechanical variables such as pressure, flowrate, and

[1] Department of Mechanical Engineering, Nagoya University, Furo-cho, Chikusa-ku, Nagoya, Aichi, 464-01 Japan
[2] Department of Micro System Engineering, Nagoya University, Furo-cho, Chikusa-ku, Nagoya, Aichi, 464-01 Japan

deformation that are related to vascular and ventricular motion. By these means, we may understand physiological function and the mechanism of diseases from the mechanical point of view by combining numerical simulations with the image data. However, one of the most crucial factors governing the accuracy of these simulations is the reliability of constitutive models describing the mechanical behavior of arterial and ventricular walls [1]. For this reason, a number of constitutive models of arterial and ventricular walls have been proposed [1,2].

In this chapter, after a brief review of those constitutive models, we first discuss the mechanical modeling of an inelastic constitutive model of arteries. Then, we develop a constitutive model of ventricular walls taking account of excitation–contraction coupling [3]. The validity of the proposed constitutive equations is discussed by comparing them with corresponding experimental results.

2 Brief Review of Constitutive Models of Arterial and Ventricular Walls

2.1 Constitutive Models of Arterial Walls

An arterial wall usually shows the intrinsic properties attributable to its three components: elastic fibers, collagen fibers, and smooth muscles. A smooth muscle is an active component, and its mechanical properties change drastically with contraction. The smooth muscles, either active or passive, give rise to quite different mechanical behavior. Although a number of constitutive models have been proposed for the arteries in the passive state [1,2], adequate constitutive models for arteries in the active state are not available.

Tanaka and Fung [4] proposed a one-dimensional model for various canine arteries under uniaxial loading. The nominal stress T is expressed as a differential equation of the stretch ratio λ by

$$\frac{dT}{d\lambda} = \alpha(T + \beta)$$
(1)

where α and β are material constants. An expression of stress response was also proposed [5]:

$$T(t,\lambda) = G(t) * T^{(e)}(\lambda), \quad G(0) = 1$$
(2)

Where $G(t)$ is a function of time, $T^{(e)}(\lambda)$ is a function of strain, and $(*)$ is a composition product denoting convolution. Because the stress–strain relationship of arteries was found to be insensitive to strain rate over a wide range of values by Fung [6], the relaxation function can be written as

$$G(t) = \frac{1}{A}\left[1 + \int_0^\infty S(\tau)e^{-t/\tau}d\tau\right]$$
(3)

In Eq 3:

$$A = \left[1 + \int_0^\infty s(\tau) d\tau \right] \tag{4}$$

is a normalization factor and the spectrum $s(\tau)$ is proposed as follows:

$$s(\tau) = c/\tau \quad \text{for} \quad \tau_1 < \tau < \tau_2$$
$$= 0 \quad \text{for} \quad \tau < \tau_1, \ \tau > \tau_2 \tag{5}$$

where c, τ_1, τ_2 are constants to be determined by relaxation tests. Equation 2 is quasi-linear, because $T^{(e)}(\lambda(\tau))$ is nonlinear and the convolution operator (*) is linear.

For the description of nonlinear finite deformation, elastic or viscoelastic constitutive equations have been proposed by assuming homogeneity and incompressibility of the material [1,7–22]. Usually material is assumed also to have orthotropy or transverse isotropy. Employment of a strain energy density function to represent the elasticity of the wall facilitates the stress analyses in analytical forms.

A strain energy density function of a hyperelastic material is the most popular model of the arterial walls. The second Piola–Kirchhoff stress tensor S is derived by differentiating the strain energy density function $\rho_0 W$ with respect to Green's strain tensor E as

$$S = \frac{\partial(\rho_0 W)}{\partial E} \tag{6}$$

where ρ_0 is the density in the reference state usually taken in the stress-free state or unloaded state, and $\rho_0 W$ is defined in the reference state. The Cauchy stress tensor τ is related to the second Piola–Kirchhoff stress S as

$$\tau = (\det F)^{-1} FSF^T \tag{7}$$

where F is the deformation gradient. Because of the incompressibility of the arterial wall, we may have the following expression instead of $\rho_0 W$ in Eq. 6:

$$\rho_0 W^* = \rho_0 W + \frac{H}{2} \left[(1 + 2E_\theta)(1 + 2E_z)(1 + 2E_r) - 1 \right] \tag{8}$$

where H is the indeterminate pressure determined by boundary conditions. With the assumption of orthotropy of the material, Chuong and Fung [7] proposed a three-dimensional strain energy density function of exponential type as

$$\rho_0 W = \frac{c}{2} \exp Q \tag{9}$$

$$Q = b_1 E_\theta^2 + b_2 E_z^2 + b_3 E_r^2 + 2b_4 E_\theta E_z + 2b_5 E_z E_r + 2b_6 E_r E_\theta \tag{10}$$

where b_1, b_2, b_3, b_4, b_5, b_6, and c are material constants. By using this model, the stress–strain relationship is expressed in the radial (r), circumferential (θ), and longitudinal (z) directions of the vessel as

$$\tau_r = c\left(1+2E_r\right)\left[b_6 E_\theta + b_5 E_z + b_3 E_r\right]\exp Q + H$$
$$\tau_\theta = c\left(1+2E_\theta\right)\left[b_1 E_\theta + b_4 E_z + b_6 E_r\right]\exp Q + H$$
$$\tau_z = c\left(1+2E_z\right)\left[b_4 E_\theta + b_2 E_z + b_5 E_r\right]\exp Q + H \tag{11}$$

Two-dimensional strain energy density functions are also proposed in polynomial, exponential, and logarithmic forms. Vaishnav et al. [11,12] proposed a function of polynomial form:

$$\rho_0 W^{(2)} = AE_\theta^2 + BE_\theta E_z + CE_z^2 + DE_\theta^3 + EE_\theta^2 E_z + FE_\theta E_z^2 + GE_z^3 \tag{12}$$

where A, B, C, D, E, F, and G are material constants.

Fung et al. [8] proposed an exponential form neglecting a principal strain in the radial direction:

$$\rho_0 W^{(2)} = \frac{C'}{2}\exp\left(a_1 E_\theta^2 + a_2 E_z^2 + 2a_4 E_\theta E_z\right) \tag{13}$$

where C', a_1, a_2, and a_4 are material constants. A strain energy density function including shear stress was proposed [21] as

$$\rho_0 W^{(2)} = P + \frac{C}{2}\exp Q \tag{14}$$

$$P = \frac{1}{2}\left[b_1 E_\theta^2 + b_2 E_z^2 + b_3\left(E_{\theta z}^2 + E_{z\theta}^2\right) + 2b_4 E_\theta E_z\right] \tag{15}$$

$$Q = a_1 E_\theta^2 + a_2 E_z^2 + a_3\left(E_{\theta z}^2 + E_{z\theta}^2\right) + 2a_4 E_\theta E_z \tag{16}$$

where C, a_1, a_2, a_3, a_4, b_1, b_2, b_3, and b_4 are material constants.

Takamizawa and Hayashi [20] also proposed a function of the logarithmic form as

$$W = -C\ln\left(1-\psi\right) \tag{17}$$

$$\psi = \frac{1}{2}\left(a_{\theta\theta} E_\theta^2 + a_{zz} E_z^2 + 2a_{\theta z} E_\theta E_z\right) \tag{18}$$

where C, $a_{\theta\theta}$, a_{zz}, and $a_{\theta z}$ are material constants. Residual stress observed in the arteries [22–29] has been taken into account for stress analyses in the wall using a strain energy density function [20,27,28].

Although the arterial wall shows a hysteresis loop under cyclic loading, an elastic model can only describe either a loading or an unloading branch of the loop. To overcome this limitation, a notion of pseudo-strain energy density function was proposed on the basis of pseudo-elasticity, where two sets of material constants are determined, one for the loading and one for the unloading branches of the hysteresis loop [1,8]. However, the notion can be applicable only for a constant stress range or a constant strain range of a hysteresis loop [30], and thus it is impossible to describe general features of hysteresis loop. It was also reported that nonsteady amplitudes of a hysteresis loop give different tangents on the curve, and can be expressed by neither the elastic nor the pseudo-elastic model [8,29].

Viscoelastic models have been also proposed to express viscous properties disregarded in elastic models [4,31-34]. Some viscoelastic models have been proposed on the basis of Green-Rivlin's theory [35], expressed as a function of strain history for a nonlinear viscoelastic deformation [31-34]. Cauchy stress in an incompressible viscoelastic material is expressed as

$$\sigma_{ij}(t) = -p(\boldsymbol{X},t)\delta_{ij} + \frac{\partial x_i(t)}{\partial X_I} \frac{\partial x_j(t)}{\partial X_J} \left[S_1^{IJ}(t) + S_2^{IJ}(t) + \dots \right] \tag{19}$$

where p is the hydrostatic pressure and δ_{ij} is the Kronecker delta. The symbol x_i ($i = 1, 2, 3$), on the other hand, denotes the position in a deformed state at time t of a particle located at X_I ($I = 1, 2, 3$) at time $t = 0$ in the reference state [34]. The Green-St. Venant strain tensor is expressed as

$$E_{KL} = \frac{1}{2}\left(\frac{\partial x_k}{\partial X_K} \frac{\partial x_k}{\partial X_L} - \delta_{KL} \right) \tag{20}$$

Thus, the terms S_1^{IJ}, S_2^{IJ} in Eq. (19) are expressed as

$$S_1^{IJ} = \int_{-\infty}^{t} K^{IJKL}(t - \tau) \frac{\partial E_{KL}(\tau)}{\partial \tau} d\tau \tag{21}$$

$$S_2^{IJ} = \int_{-\infty}^{t}\int_{-\infty}^{t} K^{IJKLMN}(t - \tau_1, t - \tau_2) \frac{\partial E_{KL}(\tau_1)}{\partial \tau_1} \frac{\partial E_{MN}(\tau_2)}{\partial \tau_2} d\tau_1 d\tau_2 \tag{22}$$

where K^{IJKL} and K^{IJKLMN} are the relaxation functions determined by stress relaxation tests.

Cheung and Hsiao [31] and Sato and Ohshima [34] proposed a form of the relaxation functions:

$$\left. \begin{array}{c} K(t) \\ K(t,t) \end{array} \right\} = K_0 - K_1 t^m \tag{23}$$

where K_0, K_1, and m are parameters determined by stress relaxation tests.

As regards $K(t)$, Young et al. [32] proposed another form as

$$K(t) = K_f + (K_i - K_f) \exp(-\alpha t^\beta) \tag{24}$$

where K_f, K_i, α, and β are parameters determined by stress relaxation tests.

Under cyclic loadings, a hysteresis loop shifts in the first several cycles and becomes stabilized after several cycles [5,8,36]. This occurs because the internal structure of the vessel changes with loading history at first, and the homeostasis is then reestablished depending on the loading history [1]. As mentioned, tangents to the stress–strain curve are different for large and small hysteresis loops at the same point because they show different stress–strain relationships [8]. These inelastic phenomena have not been expressed adequately. Even when the stabilized hysteresis loop only is taken into account, viscoelasticity or time-dependent properties are not the only factor to be considered; time-independent properties could also be included in the model. As a history dependence, loading rate dependence as well as loading path dependence should be considered [30]. A functional such as used in Green–Rivlin's theory is not simple enough to be used easily in stress analyses. A constitutive model based on an internal variable theory may give a better expression.

2.2 Constitutive Models of Ventricular Walls

Several constitutive models have been proposed thus far for ventricular walls of both passive and active states. Pinto et al. [37,38] described the viscoelastic behavior of the heart muscle in the passive state by the one-dimensional model of Eqs. 1 and 2. Humphrey and Yin [39] proposed a constitutive model for noncontracting myocardium by using a pseudo-strain energy function W expressed in terms of matrix and fibrous contribution as

$$W = c\left[\exp\{b(I_1 - 3)\} - 1\right] + A\left[\exp\{a(\alpha - 1)\} - 1\right] \tag{25}$$

where c, b, a, and A are material parameters, and α is the stretch ratio in the direction of a muscle fiber defined as

$$\alpha^2 = N^T \cdot C \cdot N \tag{26}$$

In Eq. 26, N is a unit vector coincident with local muscle fiber directions in an undeformed configuration, and C is the right Cauchy–Green tensor. The symbol $(^T)$ denotes the transpose of a tensor, and the variable I_1 in Eq. 25 is the trace of C. Humphrey et al. [40] improved Eq. 25 and introduced the pseudo-strain energy function of a polynomial expression:

$$W = c_1(\alpha - 1)^2 + c_2(\alpha - 1)^3 + c_3(I_1 - 3) + c_4(I_1 - 3)(\alpha - 1) + c_5(I_1 - 3)^2 \tag{27}$$

where c_1, c_2, c_3, c_4, and c_5 are material constants. Equation 27 is formulated more rigorously than Eq. 25, and contains a coupling term between I_1 and α. The identification of the material constants of Eq. 27 is discussed in Humphrey et al. [41]. This model was also used by Sacks and Chuong [42] to characterize the passive biaxial mechanical properties of the right ventricle free-wall myocardium.

Huyghe et al. [43], on the other hand, proposed a quasi-linear viscoelastic law for passive heart muscle tissue. The myocardinal tissue is represented as a mixture of a fluid and a solid component. The total Cauchy stress in the mixture is the difference between the effective Cauchy stress caused by deformation of the solid and the intramyocardinal pressure. The constitutive law of the solid component is expressed as a relationship between the effective second Piola–Kirchhoff stress S and Green's strain tensor E and time t. The stress S is split into two parts, one resulting from volumetric change of the myocardial tissue S^c, the other from viscoelastic shape change of the myocardial tissue S^s:

$$S = S^c(E) + S^s(E,t)$$ (28)

The elastic part is derived from an isotropic strain energy function C by

$$S^c = \frac{\partial C}{\partial E}$$ (29)

with

$$C = \frac{c^c}{2}(J-1)^2$$ (30)

where c^c is the volumetric modulus of empty solid matrix devoid of coronary blood and J is the Jacobian of deformation gradient. The viscoelastic components S^s is described in a spectral form of quasi-linear viscoelasticity [1].

Pinto and Fung [44], on the other hand, discussed the mechanical properties of stimulated papillary muscle based on Hill's three-element model and Huxley's sliding element theory. To analyze the mechanical behavior of the left ventricle, Chadwick [45] utilized the relationship between tension, fiber strain, and activation. The tension T is represented by

$$T = \left[(1-\beta)E + \beta E^*\right]\varepsilon + \beta T_0$$ (31)

where ε is a fiber strain, and E and E^* are a passive and an active modulus in the tension versus fiber strain curves. The constant T_0 is the maximal isometric tension at zero strain. The activation function $\beta(t)$ is a dimensionless periodic function of time oscillating between zero and unity.

Pinto [46] formulated a constitutive model of contracting papillary muscle by taking account of three well-known features of muscle: (1) the slow onset of contraction, (2) the time-dependent pattern of contraction, and (3) the length–tension behavior. Based on these features, he represented active force of contraction $F_A(t)$ by

$$F_A(\lambda,t) = \left[F_{0min} + s(\lambda-1)\right]\left(\frac{e\delta}{\gamma}\right)^{\gamma} t^{\gamma}\exp(-\delta t) \tag{32}$$

where λ and t are the normalized length of the muscle and the time following stimulus, and γ and δ are the parameters expressing the contraction delay and the inotropic state of the muscle under normal physiological conditions. Furthermore, s is the slope of the ascending limb, and F_{0min} is the intercept on the force axis at $\lambda=1$. The total force is represented by the sum of the active force $F_A(\lambda,t)$ and the passive viscoelastic force $F_p(\lambda,t)$; the expression of latter is given by Pinto and Patitucci [38]:

Guccione and McCulloch [47] developed a constitutive model for active fiber stress in cardiac muscle. In this model, contraction is driven by a length-independent free calcium transient. The number of actin sites available to react with myosin is determined from the total number of actin sites, free calcium, and the length history-dependent association and dissociation rates of Ca^{2+} ions and troponin. The relationship between active tension and the number of available actin sites is then described by a general cross-bridge model. This model is incorporated in a continuum mechanics model of the left ventricle [48].

Finally, van Canpen et al. [49] developed a constitutive model for active heart muscle tissue by extending the model for passive tissue [43]. In this case, the effective second Piola–Kirchhoff stress S in Eq. 28 is written as the sum of a passive stress S^p and an active stress S^a, and the passive part S^p is then divided into the sum of S^c and S^s as the right-hand side of Eq. 28. The active stress generated by the sarcomeres is directed parallel to the fiber orientation, and is expressed in terms of

$$S^a = S^a h \otimes h \tag{33}$$

where h is a unit vector of the fiber orientation at the undeformed configurations. Then, the magnitude S^a is transformed into the first Piola–Kirchhoff stress T^a, and the latter is represented by the relationship:

$$T^a = T^{a0} A^t(t^s) A^\ell(\ell^s) A^v(v^s) \tag{34}$$

where ℓ^s and v^s are the current local sarcomere length and the time constant of the former, respectively. Furthermore, T^{a0} is associated with the load of maximum isometric stress, and the factors $A^t(t^s)$, $A^\ell(\ell^s)$, and $A^v(v^s)$ represent the time dependency, the length dependency, and the velocity dependency, respectively, of the active stress development.

3 Formulation of an Inelastic Constitutive Model of Arteries

Although arterial walls show a hysteresis loop of the stress–strain relationship under cyclic loading [1], elastic models disregard such behavior. To describe the behavior, pseudo-elastic and viscoelastic models have been proposed

[1,7,8,33]. The pseudo-elastic models, however, are applicable only to cyclic loading under fixed strain or stress limits because the material constants are separately identified for the loading and the unloading branch of a hysteresis loop. Although the viscoelastic models, on the other hand, can describe the hysteresis loops, they have a number of material functions to identify, in particular when the material is anisotropic. In such a case the models are far from practical.

Tanaka and Yamada [30] formulated a constitutive model by assuming that the hysteresis loop is caused by the two kinds of history dependence, loading path dependence, typically observed in time-independent plasticity, and loading rate dependence, in viscoelasticity. In this section we further extend the previous model [30] to describe the anisotropic mechanical behavior observed in some regions of arteries. In the numerical calculations to validate the model, residual stress [50] is neglected for simplification of calculation.

3.1 Kinematic Relationships

The configuration of a body at the initial time t_0 is chosen as the reference configuration κ. The position vector of a particle and an infinitesimal line element at that point are described by X and dX, respectively. At time t, the particle X moves to x and the line element dX changes to dx. Then the line elements dX and dx are related by the relationship:

$$dx = FdX \tag{35}$$

where F is the deformation gradient.

In addition to these two configurations, we introduce an unloading configuration χ_I to define the inelastic deformation. The deformation gradient F is decomposed into the product of the elastic deformation gradient F^e and the inelastic deformation gradient F^i:

$$F = F^e F^i \tag{36}$$

Strain tensors G, G^e, and G^i defined with respect to the unloading configuration χ_I by

$$G = G^e + G^i, \quad G^e = \frac{1}{2}\left(\left(F^e\right)^T F^e - I\right), \quad G^i = \frac{1}{2}\left(I - \left(F^i\right)^{-T}\left(F^i\right)^{-1}\right) \tag{37}$$

are the strain measures of the total, elastic, and inelastic deformations, respectively, where I is the identity tensor. Inelastic convected time derivatives $\overset{\Delta}{G}$, $\overset{\Delta}{G^e}$, and $\overset{\Delta}{G^i}$ are defined by

$$\overset{\Delta}{G} = \dot{G} + \left(L^i\right)^T G + G L^i, \quad \overset{\Delta}{G^e} = \dot{G^e} + \left(L^i\right)^T G^e + G^e L^i,$$

and $$\overset{\Delta}{G^i} = \dot{G^i} + \left(L^i\right)^T G^i + G^i L^i \tag{38}$$

which are the measures of time derivatives of the total, elastic, and inelastic strains, respectively. In the foregoing equations the superposed symbols (•) and (Δ) over a variable denote the material time derivative and the inelastic convected time derivative, respectively, and L^i is defined by

$$L^i = \dot{F}^i \left(F^i\right)^{-1} \tag{39}$$

Finally, the incompressibility conditions for the elastic and inelastic parts of the deformation are described, respectively, by

$$\det\left(2G^e + I\right) = 1 \tag{40}$$

$$\operatorname{tr} \overset{\Delta}{G^i} = 0 \tag{41}$$

3.2 Constitutive Modeling for the Elastic Part

Arteries are assumed to be homogeneous and incompressible, and smooth muscles in them are assumed to be in a passive state. We also assume that the materials show the mechanical properties of transverse isotropy about the longitudinal axis of the blood vessels. In this section, by taking account of transverse isotropy, we formulate the constitutive equations for the elastic part.

The stress–strain relationship shows an exponential type of curve. The elastic part of the constitutive model is then formulated by modifying the strain energy density function proposed by Chuong and Fung [7] as follows:

$$\rho^* W = a\left(\exp Q\right) + \left(H/2\right)\left[\det\left(2G^e + I\right) - 1\right] \tag{42}$$

where ρ^* is the density in the unloading configuration, and a and H are a material constant and the Lagrange's multiplier related to the incompressibility condition; the latter is determined by boundary conditions. By noting that transverse isotropy is expressed by a fourth-rank tensor [51], the exponent Q in Eq. 42 is expressed by a quadratic form with respect to the elastic strain components:

$$Q = v \operatorname{tr}^2 G^e + 2\mu \operatorname{tr} G^{e^2} + 2\alpha \operatorname{tr} G^e \operatorname{tr}\left(MG^e\right) + 4\beta \operatorname{tr}\left(MG^{e^2}\right) + \gamma \operatorname{tr}^2\left(MG^e\right) \tag{43}$$

where v, μ, α, β and γ are material constants. In Eq. 43, M is a structural tensor [52] defined by a tensor product of h itself:

$$M = h \otimes h \tag{44}$$

where h is a unit vector in the longitudinal direction of the vessel. The positive definiteness of Q gives the following conditions for the constraints

$$\mu > 0,\, v + \mu > 0,\, \beta + \mu > 0,\, \left(v + \mu\right)\left(v + 2\mu + 2\alpha + 4\beta + \gamma\right) - \left(v + \alpha\right)^2 > 0 \tag{45}$$

In the case of axisymmetrical deformation, the values of β and γ cannot be identified independently, but the combination of $4\beta + \gamma$ has a definite meaning. Thus, Eq. 45 (third part) becomes trivial because the value of β can always be chosen to satisfy Eq. 45 for any value of $4\beta + \gamma$ that satisfies Eq. 45 (fourth part).

The second Piola–Kirchhoff stress tensor T^* defined with respect to the unloading configuration is related to the Cauchy stress tensor σ by the definition

$$T^* = \left(\det F^e\right)\left(F^e\right)^{-1}\sigma\left(F^e\right)^{-T} \tag{46}$$

and is derived from the differentiation of ρ^*W with respect to G^e:

$$T^* = \partial\left(\rho^*W\right)/\partial G^e \tag{47}$$

From Eq. 47, we obtain

$$T^* = 2a\left(\exp Q\right)\left[v\left(\operatorname{tr} G^e\right)I + 2\mu G^e + \alpha\left(\left(\operatorname{tr} G^e\right)M + \left(\operatorname{tr} MG^e\right)I\right)\right.$$
$$\left. + 2\beta\left(MG^e + G^e M\right) + \gamma\left(\operatorname{tr} MG^e\right)M\right] + H\left(I + 2G^e\right)^{-1} \tag{48}$$

3.3 Constitutive Modeling for the Inelastic Part

The inelastic part of the deformation in arteries represents the inelastic properties of smooth muscles. In the previous paper, the inelastic part of the model was formulated by modifying the viscoplastic model proposed by Chaboche and Rousselier [53]. By using an equidissipative potential of the von Mises type together with the assumption of zero yield stress, the inelastic strain $\overset{\Delta}{G}{}^i$ is described by

$$\overset{\Delta}{G}{}^i = \left(\frac{\|S - X\|}{k_H}\right)^n \frac{(S - X)}{\|S - X\|} \tag{49}$$

where S is a deviatoric tensor of T^* given by

$$S = T^* - (1/3)\left(\operatorname{tr} T^*\right)I \tag{50}$$

and X is a kinematic hardening variable (deviatoric tensor). Furthermore, k_H and n are material constants, and the symbol ($\|\ \|$) denotes the norm of a tensor; the norms $\|S\|$ and $\|\overset{\Delta}{G}{}^i\|$ in the stress and strain spaces, for example, are defined by

$$\|S\| = \sqrt{(3/2)\operatorname{tr}\left(SS^T\right)} \tag{51}$$

$$\left\|\overset{\Delta}{G}{}^i\right\| = \sqrt{(2/3)\operatorname{tr}\left(\overset{\Delta}{G}{}^i\,\overset{\Delta}{G}{}^{iT}\right)} \tag{52}$$

Equation 49 describes loading rate dependence because this equation is not a homogeneous function of degree one with respect to time.

In the previous paper [30], the evolution equation of X was formulated as

$$\overset{\circ}{X} = a_k\left[b_k \overset{\vartriangle}{G^i} - (X - Y)\left\| \overset{\vartriangle}{G^i} \right\| \right] \tag{53}$$

where the superposed symbol ($\circ$) denotes the Jaumann time derivative

$$\overset{\circ}{X} = \dot{X} - W^i X + X W^i \tag{54}$$

with respect to an inelastic spin tensor

$$W^i = (1/2)\left(L^i - L^{iT} \right) \tag{55}$$

In Eq. 53, a_k and b_k are material constants. Eq. 53 describes the loading path dependence and dominates the shape of hysteresis loops. The constant a_k determines the width of the hysteresis loop, while b_k determines the size of the translation range of the kinematic hardening variable. These characteristics suggest that one of the simplest ways to express the direction dependence of the hysteresis loop is to change the value of a_k in each direction. Thus, the evolution equation of X is modified as

$$\overset{\circ}{X} = D\left[b_k \overset{\vartriangle}{G^i} - (X - Y)\left\| \overset{\vartriangle}{G^i} \right\| \right] \tag{56}$$

where D is the fourth-rank tensor of transverse isotropy. Defining Z as

$$Z = b_k \overset{\vartriangle}{G^i} - (X - Y)\left\| \overset{\vartriangle}{G^i} \right\| \tag{57}$$

Eq. 56 is described by

$$\overset{\circ}{X} = 2\mu' Z + \alpha'(\operatorname{tr} MZ)I + 2\beta'(MZ + ZM) - (3\alpha' + 4\beta')(\operatorname{tr} MZ)M \tag{58}$$

where μ', α', and β' are material constants. It should be noted that in the case of axisymmetrical deformation, where the principal axes of M and Z are identical, β' does not contribute to the deformation as mentioned earlier.

The internal variable Y in Eq. 56 to specify the center of the translation range of X is described by the same evolution equation as that of the previous paper [30]:

$$\overset{\circ}{Y} = r_Y \langle \dot{R} \rangle \frac{(S - Y)}{\|S - Y\|} \tag{59}$$

where R is a scalar internal variable to govern Y, and its evolution equation is

$$\dot{R} = r_R \left(\|S - Y\| - R \right) \left\| \overset{\triangle}{G^i} \right\| \tag{60}$$

In the foregoing equations, r_Y and r_R and material constants. The symbol $\langle \rangle$ denotes the Macauley bracket defined by

$$\langle x \rangle = x U[x] \tag{61}$$

where $U[x]$ is the unit step function with $U[0] = 0$.

3.4 Numerical Results and Discussion

Numerical calculations were performed to evaluate the proposed constitutive model, Eqs. 48, 49, and 58–60. For comparison of uniaxial loading tests and stress relaxation tests, the experimental results by Azuma and Hasegawa were adopted [54]. In their experiment, seven regions of vascular walls of mongrel dogs from the ascending aorta to the femoral artery were excised to 5-mm-wide strips in the longitudinal and circumferential directions. In this study, we chose the external iliac artery as the typical region to show anisotropic mechanical behavior.

The calculations of the uniaxial cyclic loading/unloading tests were performed by changing the stretch ratio $\lambda = L/L_0$ (L is the length of the specimen after deformation) in the range of $\lambda = 1.0$–1.5 at the rate of $|\dot{\lambda}| = 0.01\,\text{s}^{-1}$. These results were used to identify the material constants in the model. The constants in the elastic part were identified first and then those in the inelastic part. These constants were adjusted by a trial-and-error method. The constants obtained are

$$a = 100\,\text{kPa}, \ v = 0.735, \ \mu = 0.0025, \ \alpha = -0.235, \ 4\beta + \gamma = 0.418,$$
$$k_H = 40\,\text{kPa} \cdot \text{s}^{1/3}, \ n = 3, \ \mu' = 1.25, \ \alpha' = -9.17, \ b_k = 40\,\text{kPa},$$
$$r_R = 2.0, \ r_Y = 50 \tag{62}$$

The calculations shown next were performed using these material constants. The strain rate dependence of hysteresis loops was examined by simulating the cyclic loading/unloading tests for the three cases of stretch rate; $|\dot{\lambda}| = 0.1, 0.01$, and $0.001\,\text{s}^{-1}$. The stress relaxation tests were then simulated. By stretching the specimens from $\lambda = 1.0$ to $\lambda = 1.5$ with $|\dot{\lambda}| = 0.5\,\text{s}^{-1}$ first and then by holding λ constant, we obtained the Cauchy stress versus time relations for 5 min from the beginning of stretching. Finally, we simulated the creep tests: by first stretching the specimens from $\lambda = 1.0$ to $\lambda = 1.5$ at the rate of $|\dot{\lambda}| = 0.01\,\text{s}^{-1}$ and then by holding the stress constant, we obtained the stretch ratio λ versus time t curves for 5 min.

The relations between the Cauchy stress and the stretch ratio under uniaxial cyclic loading/unloading tests are shown in Fig. 1. The solid lines show the stable

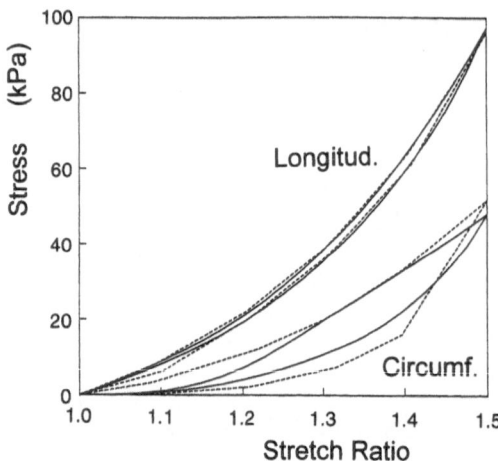

Fig. 1. Stress–stretch ratio relationship under uniaxial cyclic loading/unloading for circumferential (*Circumf.*) and longitudinal (*Longitud.*) strips excised from canine external iliac artery. *Solid line*, calculated; *dashed line*, Azuma and Hasegawa [54]

hysteresis loops at the tenth cycle. The dashed lines, on the other hand, show the corresponding experimental results by Azuma and Hasegawa [54], which are the average of ten experiments. It is found that the current model can describe relatively well the anisotropy of hysteresis loops observed in the experimental results.

Figure 2 shows the strain rate dependence of the hysteresis loops. The small and the positive strain rate dependence in the model agrees well with that of the experimental values for soft tissues such as the canine carotid artery and lung tissue [8,50]. It is also pointed out that the degree of strain rate dependence in the circumferential direction is higher than that in the longitudinal direction, which reflects the fiber orientation of smooth muscles.

The numerical results of the stress relaxation tests are shown in Fig. 3a and 3b. The triangle and circle symbols in the figure denote the averages of eight to ten experiments by Azuma and Hasegawa in the longitudinal and the circumferential direction, respectively. These symbols are plotted for the first 1 min and the last 30 s in the 5-min experiments. The current model well expresses the qualitative tendency of the experimental results: a relatively small stress relaxation and a high stress level after relaxation in the longitudinal direction and a large relaxation and a low stress level after relaxation in the circumferential direction. The relaxations mostly occur just after the strain hold, and a faster initial stretch rate does not raise the level of peak stress much more in this simulation.

The numerical results of the creep tests suggest that no significant creep occurs in either directions. We assume the creep effect is small enough to neglect. However, it is important to clarify the creep phenomena in detail throughout the experiments.

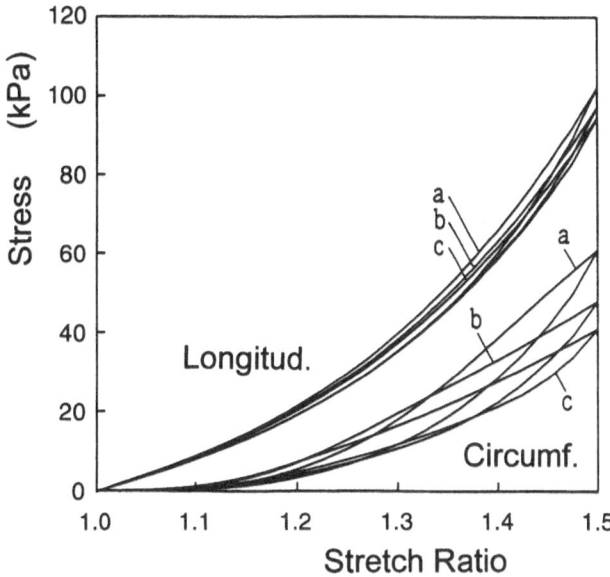

FIG. 2. Strain rate dependence of the hysteresis loops of Fig. 1. a, $|\dot{\lambda}| = 0.1\,\mathrm{s^{-1}}$; b, $|\dot{\lambda}| = 0.01\,\mathrm{s^{-1}}$; c, $|\dot{\lambda}| = 0.001\,\mathrm{s^{-1}}$

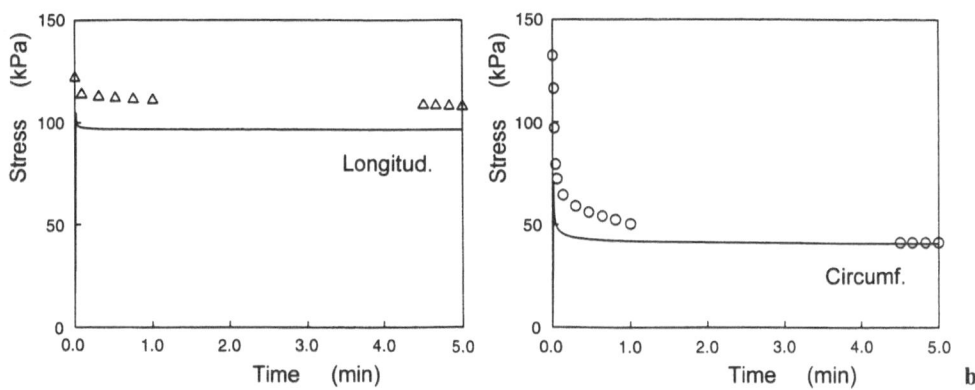

FIG. 3. Stress relaxation curves of longitudinal and circumferential strips excised from canine external iliac artery [54]. **a** Longitudinal strip: *solid line*, calculated; *triangles*, Azuma and Hasegawa. **b** Circumferential strip: *solid line*, calculated; *circles*, Azuma and Hasegawa

4 Mechanical Models of Ventricular Wall Taking Account of Excitation–Contraction Coupling

In this section, a transversely isotropic three-dimensional constitutive model of ventricular walls, which can describe the mechanical behavior of ventricular wall in both passive and active states and the effects of inotropism, is proposed by taking into account the excitation–contraction coupling.

4.1 Excitation–Contraction Coupling

Before developing a constitutive model of ventricular walls, we summarize the following important features of the phenomena of excitation–contraction coupling by examing the literature [55]:

   a. The generation of tension or contraction of the cardiac muscle is controlled by the concentration of Ca^{2+} in the cell.
   b. There are threshold and saturated values in the response for the concentration of Ca^{2+}.
   c. In the process mentioned, the subsequent stage is caused by the preceding one, and time is needed for the reaction in each stage. In other words, a time delay is induced in each stage. Thus we may suppose that the concentration of Ca^{2+} influences the rate, or higher time derivatives of the tension or contraction. Furthermore, the existence of the threshold and the saturated value of Ca^{2+} makes these relationships complicated.

4.2 Basic Assumptions for a Constitutive Model of Ventricular Walls

Ventricular walls show very complicated behavior [38,56,57]. To simplify the formulation, we make the following basic assumptions:

1. Ventricular walls are incompressible.
2. Mechanical properties in the plane perpendicular to the muscle fiber are isotropic; that is, ventricular walls are transversely isotropic.
3. Mechanical properties of ventricular walls are passive in the directions perpendicular to the muscle fiber. In other words, the active properties are observed only in the muscle fiber direction.
4. Viscoelastic properties of ventricular walls can be neglected.
5. The stress acting on the ventricular walls is expressed as the sum of passive stress T^p and active stress T^a; that is, the second Piola–Kirchhoff stress T is expressed as:

$$T = T^a + T^p \tag{63}$$

4.3 Constitutive Relationship for the Passive State

In the passive state, the strain in the ventricular walls is induced by externally applied forces. We describe this response by nonlinear elastic materials. On the basis of the experimental results by Sonnenblick [58], the passive stress T^p may be expressed by

$$T^p = \partial \rho_0 W / \partial E \tag{64}$$

where $\rho_0 W$ is the strain energy density function of exponential type proposed by Chuong and Fung [7]:

$$\rho_0 W = a(\exp Q) + (H/2)\{\det(2E+I) - 1\} \tag{65}$$

where ρ_0 denotes the mass density in the undeformed configuration, a is a material constant, and H is Lagrange's multiplier related to the incompressible condition. The variables E and I are Green's strain tensor and the identity tensor, respectively. Furthermore, Q is the quadratic form with respect to the components of E that represents the transverse isotropy, and is expressed as

$$Q = v\,\mathrm{tr}^2 E + 2\mu\,\mathrm{tr}\,E^2 + 2\gamma\,\mathrm{tr}\,E\,\mathrm{tr}\,ME + 4\eta\,\mathrm{tr}\,ME^2 + \lambda\,\mathrm{tr}^2 ME \tag{66}$$

where v, μ, γ, η, and λ are material constants. In this equation, M is the structural tensor of the transverse isotropy with respect to the unit vector h that represents the direction of cardiac muscle fiber in the undeformed configuration, and thus the tensor M is defined by

$$M = h \otimes h \tag{67}$$

By using the Eqs. 64–66, the passive stress T^p is expressed by the following equation:

$$T^p = 2a(\exp Q)\big[v(\mathrm{tr}\,E)I + 2\mu E + \gamma\{(\mathrm{tr}\,E)M + (\mathrm{tr}\,ME)I\}$$
$$+ 2\eta(ME + EM) + \lambda(\mathrm{tr}\,ME)M\big] + H(I + 2E)^{-1} \tag{68}$$

4.4 Constitutive Relationship for the Active State

The activation of cardiac muscles induces the contraction of muscle fibers or the generation of additional tension. According to the foregoing basic assumption, 3, the active stress T^a can be expressed by

$$T^a = \tau^a M \tag{69}$$

where τ^a is the activated stress caused by the activation. The maximum value of τ^a depends on the length of the cardiac muscle [58] because the maximum number of cross-bridges between myosin and actin filaments, which determines the maximum value of the tension, differs with the length of the muscles. The magnitude of the tension is also governed by the activity that expresses the ratio of bonding of troponin with Ca^{2+}, that is, the ratio of active filaments. In the following, we denote the activity and the strain of muscle fibers by α and E_h, respectively.

Now let us express E_h in terms of Green's strain tensor E. First, we denote an infinitesimal line element in the cardiac muscle fiber direction at the undeformed configuration by dX_h, and the magnitude of dX_h by dS_h. Similarly, the magnitude of the corresponding line element at the current configuration is denoted by ds_h. Then the difference between the square of the length elements can be expressed by

$$\left(ds_h\right)^2 - \left(dS_h\right)^2 = 2EdX_h \cdot dX_h = 2Eh \cdot h\left(dS_h\right)^2 \tag{70}$$

From this equation we may define E_h by

$$E_h \equiv \left\{\left(ds_h\right)^2 - \left(dS_h\right)^2\right\} \Big/ \left\{2\left(dS_h\right)^2\right\} = Eh \cdot h \tag{71}$$

Let us next consider the state in which the cardiac muscle is soaked in Ca^{2+} solution of a constant concentration for a long time under the condition of a constant length. In this situation, the active stress τ^a will approach the asymptotic value τ^{as}. We suppose that the value τ^{as} is determined only by E_h and α, and express the relationship by

$$\tau^{as} = \tau^{as}\left(E_h, \alpha\right) = \tau^{as}_{\max} F\left(E_h\right) A\left(\alpha\right) \tag{72}$$

In this relationship, $F(E_h)$ and $A(\alpha)$ are the normalized functions expressing the dependence of E_h and α on τ^{as}, respectively, and $\tau^{as}_{\max}$ is a constant representing the maximum value of active stress.

As was described in Section 4.1, on the other hand, the generation of contraction and tension is not induced immediately after the change of action potential or the rise of the concentration of Ca^{2+}. In other words, there exists a time delay between these phenomena. In view of this delay, we assume that the rate of the active stress is governed by the difference between the target value τ^{as} and the current value of active stress τ^a:

$$\dot{\tau}^a = b\left(\tau^{as} - \tau^a\right) \tag{73}$$

where b is a material constant specifying the rate of change.

The function $F(E_h)$ was determined on the basis of the relationship between the sarcomere length and tension by Sonnenblick [58]:

$$F\left(E_h\right) = \left\langle\left(1 + F_0\right)\exp\left[-\left\{\left(E_h - E_{h0}\right)/\Delta E_h\right\}^2\right] - F_0\right\rangle \tag{74}$$

Here E_{h0} is the value of E_h at the maximum tension, ΔE_h is the half the range of E_h generating the tension, and F_0 is a material constant. The symbol $\langle \ \rangle$ represents the Macauley bracket defined in Eq. 61. The function $A(\alpha)$ in Eq. 72 is expressed by

$$A(\alpha) = \left\langle 1 - \exp\left[-m\left(\alpha - \alpha_{ths}\right)\right]\right\rangle \tag{75}$$

This relationship was formulated with reference to the relationship between the tension and the concentration of Ca^{2+} at the saturated state by Fabiato [59]. In Eq. 75, m is a material constant and α_{ths} is a value corresponding to the threshold of Ca^{2+} that can generate the tension.

We are now in a position to discuss the relationship between the activity α and the concentration of Ca^{2+}. Because of lack of data, we have to assume a proper form of the relationship. According to our preliminary numerical experiments, the evolution equation

$$\dot{\alpha} = c\left(\beta - \alpha\right) \tag{76}$$

gave satisfactory predictions for the experimental results. In other words, the rate of the activity is governed by the difference between the concentration β of Ca^{2+} and the current activity α, where c is a material constant. Equation 76 is considered as the expression of the phenomena of the diffusion process of Ca^{2+} and the bonding process of troponin. However, further investigation will be required for more elaborate formulation of this phenomenon.

Finally, we need to specify the time variation of the current concentration β. The concentration β is closely related to the release of Ca^{2+} from the sarcoplasmic reticulum in cardiac muscle cells. The trigger and the quantity of the release are governed by the action potential. Accordingly, those mechanisms need to be clarified to specify the time variation of β. However, they have not been sufficiently elucidated [60]. Thus, it is very difficult to formulate the relationship between β and the action potential. Furthermore, such a relationship is not necessarily convenient for the analyses. Thus, we specify β as a function of time t. With reference to the experimental results for cardiac muscles of mice by Cannel et al. [61], we assume the relationship

$$\beta = \beta_0 t^k \exp\left(-\ell t\right) \tag{77}$$

where β_0, k, and ℓ are material constants.

4.5 Experimental Results for Examination and Identification of Material Constants

We performed numerical simulations of the proposed constitutive model to evaluate the accuracy of the description of the mechanical behavior of the ventricular wall. For comparison, we selected the experimental results by

Sonnenblick [58]. He soaked the papillary muscles excised from the right ventricle of a cat in Krebs-Ringer solution at 21°–23°C, and measured the time variation of the tension under isometric contraction and the shortening under isotonic contraction. In the isometric tests, he gave the initial strains of 0.236, 0.191, and 0.094 to specimens, respectively. He then gave electric stimulation to the specimens under the isometric condition to generate the tension. In the isotonic contraction tests, on the other hand, he gave a preload of 3.9 mN to specimens of 11.0 mm in length, and then added the afterloads of 11.4, 17.3, 24.5, and 32.5 mN, respectively. After that, he stimulated each specimen to shorten the cardiac muscles. In the current study, Sonnenblick's data were selected for comparison.

By applying a uniaxial expression of Eq. 68 to the experimental results of Sonnenblick [58], we identified the material constants as follows:

$$v = 34.0, \ \mu = 5.0, \ a = 0.2(\text{kPa}), \ \tau_{\max}^{as} = 107.9(\text{kPa}), \ E_{h0} = 0.322,$$

$$\Delta E_h = 0.205, \ F_0 = 0.032, \ m = 0.16(1/\text{m}M), \ \alpha_{ths} = 0.56(\text{m}M),$$

$$\beta_0 = 0.0326\left(\text{m}M/(\text{ms})^k\right), \ k = 1.0, \ \ell = 0.004(1/\text{ms}), \ b = 0.007(1/\text{ms}),$$

$$c = 0.018(1/\text{ms}) \tag{78}$$

4.6 Examination of the Applicability of the Proposed Model

To examine the validity of the proposed model (Eqs. 63, 66–69, and 71–77) to reproduce or describe the experimental data, we applied the model to the experimental results [58] mentioned earlier. Figure 4 shows the passive stress versus strain relationship (Eq. 68) and the active stress versus strain relationship (Eq. 72) for the case of $A(\alpha) = 1$. In the figure, the various symbols denote the experimental results, while the solid lines are the results calculated by the model. We see that the model can reasonably reproduce the experimental data.

Figure 5 shows the time variation of the tension in the isometric contraction. The values of 0.094, 0.191, and 0.236 are taken as the specified strain E_h of cardiac muscle. In the cases of $E_h = 0.236$ and 0.191, the rising of the tension curves shows some delay in comparison with the experimental data, but the peak times, the peak values, and the relaxation curves can be described well.

Figure 6a and 6b shows the time variation of the strain decrease and the tension for the isotonic contraction experiments. A value of $E_h = 0.217$ (corresponding to 3.9 mN) is chosen as the prestrain for every case. The afterloads are 11.4, 17.3, 24.5, and 32.5 mN, respectively. From Fig. 6a in particular we see that there is a significant difference between the calculations and the experiments. The causes of these discrepancies are discussed elsewhere [62].

The inotropism is defined as the change of contractility of cardiac muscles, and is caused by the change of the time variation curve of the concentration of Ca^{2+} in the cardiac muscles by medication, stimulation, or temperature variation, as

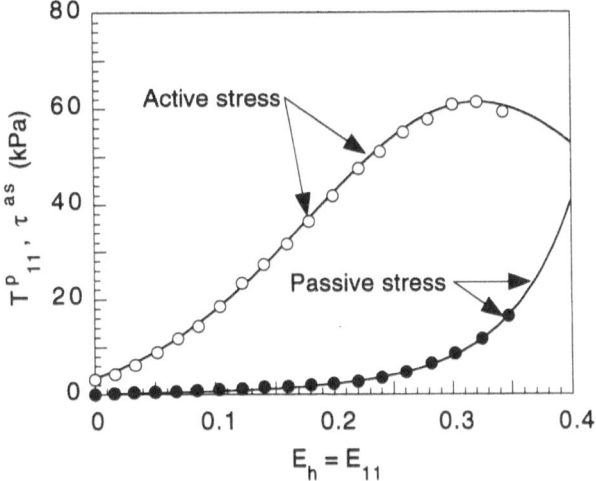

FIG. 4. Passive stress versus cardiac muscle fiber strain relationship (*solid line*, calculated result; *solid circles*, experimental result [58]) and relationship of maximum of the isometric tension versus cardiac muscle fiber strain (*solid line*, calculated result; *open circles*, experimental result [58]) of the papillary muscles of a cat

FIG. 5. Accuracy of the description of isometric contraction. *Solid lines*, calculated results; *symbols*, experimental results [58]

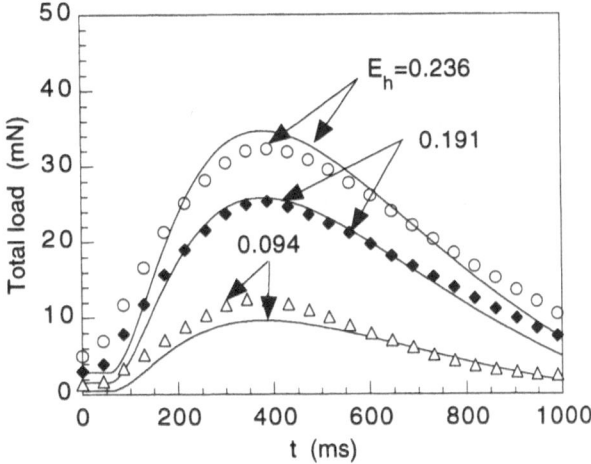

well as the temperature dependence of the actomyosin interaction [63]. In the following, we assume a time variation curve of the Ca^{2+} concentration based on the experimental facts [63–65], and discuss the adequacy of the proposed model by comparing with the literature the typical features of the generated active stress corresponding to the assumed curves of the Ca^{2+} concentration. In the following figures, the various thin lines in the upper half of each figure denote the time variation of the concentration of Ca^{2+}, while the corresponding active stresses are represented by the thick lines in the lower half of the figure.

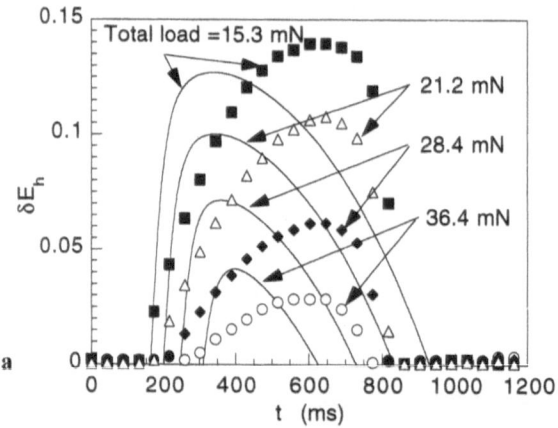

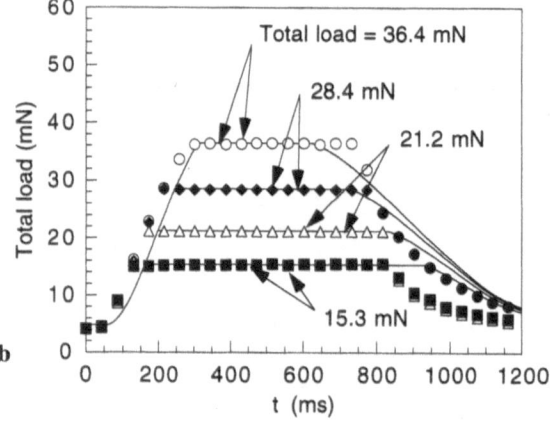

Fɪɢ. 6. Accuracy of the description of isotonic contraction. **a** Time variation of strain decrease. **b** Time variation of tension

The increase of frequency of stimulation to a cardiac muscle cell results in the rise of the maximum value of the concentration of Ca^{2+} [63], and thereby increases the maximum value of the tension [65,66], that is, the Bowditch effect. The results of the simulation are shown in Fig. 7. We see that the model can represent qualitatively the tendency of the variation of the maximum tension.

The peak time of the Ca^{2+} concentration is governed by the inflow rate. Increase in inflow rate is caused by the increase of catecholamines and a drop in temperature [63], and results in increase of the tension rate and decrease of the period generating the tension. Decrease of inflow rate is induced by a dosage of calcium antagonist [63,65], and results in the delay of the peak time of the tension. The corresponding simulation results are shown in Fig. 8. It is found that the later the peak time of the Ca^{2+} curve, the longer the period of generation of tension.

The rate of decreasing of the Ca^{2+} concentration is governed by the discharge of ions from the cell. Reduction of this ion discharge ability is generally induced by dosage of such cardiac drugs as ouabain and digitalis [63]. These medicines

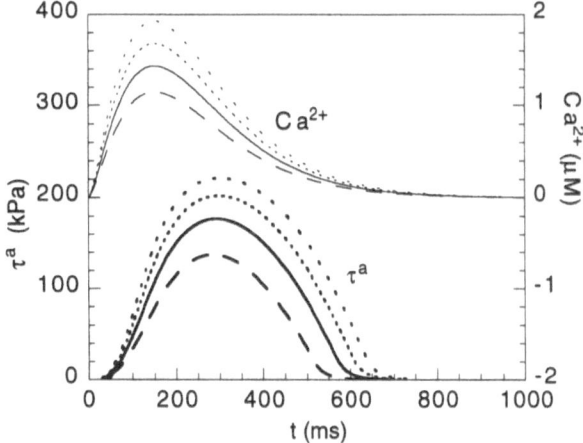

FIG. 7. Effects of maximum values of Ca²⁺ concentration on generated stress. *Fine lines*, Ca²⁺ variations; *bold lines*, corresponding τ^a variations

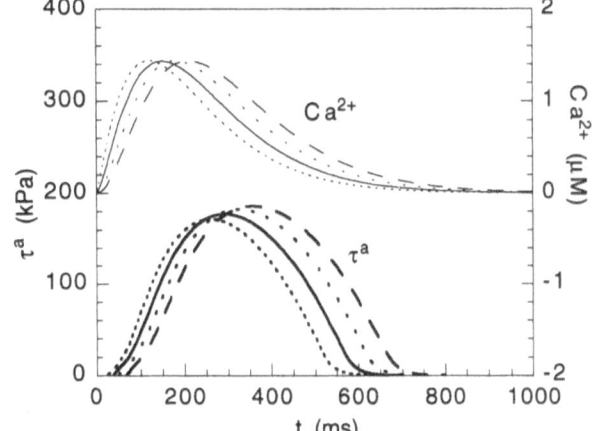

FIG. 8. Effects of arrival time of peak of Ca²⁺ concentration on generated stress

increase the contractibility, and thereby the maximum value of the tension is increased. By assuming a constant temperature and no change of actomyosin interaction, we simulated the decreasing rate of Ca²⁺ concentration (Fig. 9). We see that the magnitude of the tension is increased by the drop.

5 Conclusions

In this study, the constitutive models of arterial and vascular walls were first reviewed. Then, an inelastic constitutive model was formulated to describe the anisotropic mechanical behavior of arteries. To evaluate the proposed model, cyclic loading/unloading and stress relaxation tests were first simulated and then compared with the experimental results.

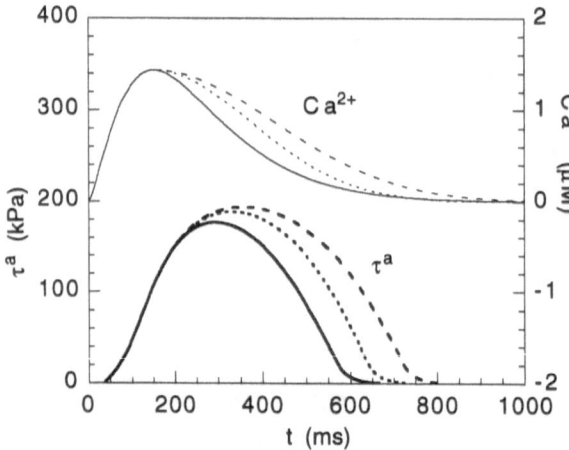

FIG. 9. Effects of the rate of decrease in Ca^{2+} concentration on generated stress

A three-dimensional transversely isotropic constitutive model for ventricular walls was also formulated. Experiments of isometric and isotonic contraction were simulated by this model to evaluate its adequacy.

Acknowledgment. This research was supported by the Ministry of Education, Science and Culture of Japan under a Grant in Aid for Scientific Research on Priority Areas (Biomechanics, No. 04237104) of the fiscal years 1992–1994.

References

1. Fung YC (1981) Biomechanics: mechanical properties of living tissues. Springer, Berlin Heidelberg New York
2. Hayashi K (1993) Experimental approaches on measuring the mechanical properties and constitutive laws of arterial walls. ASME J Biomech Eng 115:481–488
3. Iriki M, Toyama K (eds) (1986) Physiology, vol 2 (in Japanese). Bunkodo, Tokyo, pp 17–21
4. Tanaka TT, Fung YC (1974) Elastic and inelastic properties of the canine aorta and their variation along the aortic tree. J Biomech 7:357–370
5. Goto M, Kimoto Y (1966) Hysteresis and stress-relaxation of the blood vessels studied by a universal tensile testing instrument. Jpn J Physiol 15:169–184
6. Fung YC (1972) Stress-strain history relations of soft tissues in simple elongation. In: Fung YC, Perrone N, Anliker M (eds) Biomechanics: its foundations and objectives. Prentice-Hall, Englewood Cliffs, NJ, pp 181–208
7. Chuong CJ, Fung YC (1983) Three-dimensional stress distribution in arteries. ASME J Biomech Eng 105:268–274
8. Fung YC, Fronek K, Patitucci P (1979) Pseudoelasticity of arteries and the choice of its mathematical expression. Am J Physiol 237:H620–H631
9. Tickner EG, Sacks AH (1967) A theory for the static elastic behavior of blood vessels. Biorheology 4:151–168

10. Vito RP, Hickey J (1980) The mechanical properties of soft tissues. I: The elastic response of arterial segments. J Biomech 13:951–957
11. Vaishnav RN, Young JT, Janicki JS, Patel DJ (1972) Nonlinear anisotropic elastic properties of the canine aorta. Biophys J 12:1008–1027
12. Vaishnav RN, Young JT, Patel DJ (1973) Distribution of stresses and of strain-energy density through the wall thickness in a canine aortic segment. Circ Res 32:577–583
13. Mirsky I (1973) Ventricular and arterial wall stresses based on large deformation analyses. Biophys J 13:1141–1159
14. Simon BR, Kobayashi AS, Strandness DE (1972) Reevaluation of arterial constitutive relations: a finite-deformation approach. Circ Res 30:491–500
15. Sharma MG (1974) Viscoelastic behavior of conduit arteries. Biorheology 11:279–291
16. Demiray H, Weisacker HW, Pascale K, Erbay HA (1988) A stress-strain relation for a rat abdominal aorta. J Biomech 21:369–374
17. von Maltzahn WW, Besdo D, Wiemer W (1981) Elastic properties of arteries: a nonlinear two-layer cylindrical model. J Biomech 14:389–397
18. von Maltzahn WW (1983) Parameter sensitivity analysis and improvement of a two-layer arterial wall model. ASME J Biomech Eng 105:389–392
19. von Maltzahn WW, Warriyar RG, Keizer WF (1984) Experimental measurements of elastic properties of media and adventitia of bovine carotid arteries. J Biomech 17:839–847
20. Takamizawa K, Hayashi K (1987) Strain energy density function and uniform strain hypothesis for arterial mechanics. J Biomech 20:7–17
21. Vaishnav RN, Vossoughi J (1984) Incremental formulations in vascular mechanics. ASME J Biomech Eng 106:105–111
22. Elad D, Foux A, Kivity Y (1988) A model for the nonlinear elastic response of large arteries. ASME J Biomech Eng 110:185–189
23. Fung YC (1993) Biomechanics: mechanical properties of living tissues, 2nd edn. Springer, Berlin Heidelberg New York, pp 342–343
24. Fung YC (1984) Biodynamics: circulation. Springer-Verlag, New York, pp 54–63
25. Vaishnav RN, Vossoughi J (1987) Residual stress and strain in aortic segments. J Biomech 20:235–239
26. Liu SQ, Fung YC (1989) Zero-stress state of arteries. ASME J Biomech Eng 110:82–84
27. Chuong CJ, Fung YC (1986) Residual stress in arteries. In: Schmid-Schoenbein GW, Woo SLY, Zweifach BW (eds) Frontiers in biomechanics. Springer, Berlin Heidelberg New York, pp 117–129
28. Chuong CJ, Fung YC (1986) On residual stresses in arteries. ASME J Biomech Eng 108:189–192
29. Fung YC (1990) Biomechanics: motion, flow, stress, and growth. Springer, Berlin Heidelberg New York, pp 382–394
30. Tanaka E, Yamada H (1990) An inelastic constitutive model of blood vessels. Acta Mech 82:21–30
31. Cheung JB, Hsiao CC (1972) Nonlinear anisotropic viscoelastic stresses in blood vessels. J Biomech 5:607–619
32. Young JT, Vaishnav RN, Patel DJ (1977) Nonlinear anisotropic viscoelastic properties of canine arterial segments. J Biomech 10:549–559
33. Wu SG, Lee GC (1984) On nonlinear viscoelastic properties of arterial tissue. ASME J Biomech Eng 106:42–47

34. Sato M, Ohshima N (1985) Nonlinear viscoelastic behavior of canine arterial walls. Med & Biol Eng & Comput 23:565–571
35. Green AE, Rivlin RS (1957) The mechanics of non-linear materials with memory. I. Arch Rat Anal 1:1–21
36. Remington JW (1955) Hysteresis loop behavior of the aorta and other extensile tissues. Am J Physiol 180:83–95
37. Pinto JG, Fung YC (1973) Mechanical properties of the heart muscle in the passive state. J Biomech 6:597–616
38. Pinto JG, Patitucci PJ (1980) Visco-elasticity of passive cardiac muscle. ASME J Biomech Eng 102:57–61
39. Humphrey JD, Yin FCP (1987) A new constitutive formulation for characterizing the mechanical behavior of soft tissues. Biophys J 52:563–570
40. Humphrey JD, Strumpf RK, Yin FCP (1990) Determination of a constitutive relation for passive myocardium: I. A new functional form. ASME J Biomech Eng 112:333–339
41. Humphrey JD, Strumpf RK, Yin FCP (1990) Determination of a constitutive relation for passive myocardium: II. Parameter estimation. ASME J Biomech Eng 112:340–346
42. Sacks MS, Chuong CJ (1993) A constitutive relation for passive right-ventricular free wall myocardium. J Biomech 26:1341–1345
43. Huyghe JM, van Canpen DH, Arts T, Heethaar RM (1991) The constitutive behavior of passive heart muscle tissue: a quasi-linear viscoelastic formulation. J Biomech 24:841–849
44. Pinto JG, Fung YC (1973) Mechanical properties of the stimulated papillary muscle in quick-release experiment. J Biomech 6:617–630
45. Chadwick RS (1982) Mechanics of the left ventricle. Biophys J 39:279–288
46. Pinto JG (1987) A constitutive description of contracting papillary muscle and its implications to the dynamics of the intact heart. ASME J Biomech Eng 109:181–191
47. Guccione JM, McCulloch AD (1993) Mechanics of active contraction in cardiac muscle: Part I. Constitutive relations for fiber stress that describe deactivation. ASME J Biomech Eng 115:72–81
48. Guccione JM, Waldman LK, McCulloch AD (1993) Mechanics of active contraction in cardiac muscle: Part II. Cylindrical models of the systolic left ventricle. ASME J Biomech Eng 115:82–90
49. van Canpen DH, Huyghe JM, Bovendeerd PHM, Arts T (1994) Biomechanics of the heart muscle. Eur J Mech A/Solids 13(suppl):19–41
50. Fung YC (1984) Structure and stress-strain relationship of soft tissues. Am Zool 24:13–22
51. Jaunzemis W (1967) Continuum mechanics. Macmillan, New York, p 306
52. Boehler JP (1987) Representations for isotropic and anisotropic non-polynomial tensor functions: applications of tensor functions in solid mechanics. In: Boehler JP (ed) CISM Courses and lectures, no. 292. Springer, Berlin Heidelberg New York Vienna, p 31
53. Chaboche JL, Rousselier G (1983) On the plastic and viscoplastic constitutive equations. Part 1: Rules developed with internal variables concept. Trans ASME J Pressure Vessel Technol 105:153–158
54. Azuma T, Hasegawa M (1971) A rheological approach to the architecture of arterial walls. Jpn J Physiol 21:27–47
55. Mashima H (1986) Physiology (in Japanese). Bunkodo, Tokyo, pp 59–61

56. Demer LL, Yin FCP (1983) Passive biaxial mechanical properties of isolated canine myocardium. J Physiol 339:615–630
57. Pinto JG, Pattitucci PJ (1977) Creep in cardiac muscle. Am J Physiol 232(6):H553–H563
58. Sonnenblick EH (1962) Implications of muscle mechanics in the heart. Fed Proc 21:975–990
59. Fabiato A (1985) Time and calcium dependence of activation and inactivation of calcium-induced release of calcium from the sarcoplasmic reticulum of a skinned canine cardiac Purkinje cell. J Gen Physiol 85:247–289
60. Endo M (1977) Calcium release from the sarcoplasmic reticulum. Physiol Rev 57(1):71–108
61. Cannel MB, Berlin JR, Lederer WJ (1987) Effect of membrane potential changes on the calcium transient in single rat cardiac muscle cells. Science 238:1419–1423
62. Tanaka E, Takahashi T, Murakami S (1994) A mechanical model of cardiac muscle taking account of excitation-contraction coupling (in Japanese). Trans Jpn Soc Mech Eng (Series B) 60:3726–3731
63. Mashima H (1986) Physiology (in Japanese). Bunkodo, Tokyo, pp 364–365
64. Endo M, Nishizuka Y, Yagi K, Miyamoto H (eds) (1988) Calcium ion and cell functions (in Japanese). Kyoritsu-shuppan, Tokyo, p 175
65. Iriki M, Toyama K (eds) (1986) Physiology, vol 2 (in Japanese). Bunkodo, Tokyo, pp 45–46
66. Okino H, Sugawara M, Matsuo H (eds) (1980) Mechanics and measurement of cardiovascular systems (in Japanese). Kodansha, Tokyo, pp 13–14

Computational Visualization of Blood Flow

Takami Yamaguchi

Summary. Computational bio-fluid mechanics, in the widest sense, is concerned with all aspects of biological flow, such as blood flow and respiratory flow. In this chapter, a general discussion of studies of blood flow by computational visualization emphasizing physiological relevance and pathological consequences is presented first. Further discussion follows on the extremely complex nature of blood flow, including its susceptibility to the geometrical configuration of blood vessels under unsteady conditions. A concise introduction of the basic governing equations, the methods of numerical computation, and the considerations of various computational conditions, particularly boundary conditions, is also given. Modeling, which is the most important but the most time-consuming part of computational studies, is also briefly discussed. Based on these fundamental discussions, two examples from both extremes of our multilevel computational bio-fluid mechanical studies are shown: realistic modeling and flow computation of the left ventricle, and the cellular-scale flow adjacent to cultured endothelial cells.

Key words: Computational fluid dynamics (CFD)—Blood flow—Visualization—Wall shear stress—Fluid-wall interaction

1 Introduction

Flow phenomena in living systems are not only vital from the point of view of normal physiological conditions but are also significant with respect to various disorders. It is usually difficult to separate the physiological and pathological roles of blood flow because the pathological state begins under normal physiological conditions. In other words, pathological phenomena are part of the continuum of the physiological state [1]. This is particularly true for some vascular diseases, which begin and develop under the strong influence of the flow of blood [2]. Atherosclerosis is a representative of these diseases and is very impor-

Department of Bio-Medical Engineering, School of High-Technology for Human Welfare, Tokai University, 317 Nishino, Numazu, Shizuoka, 410-03 Japan

tant because its progression finally causes diminution and cessation of the blood supply to crucial organs, particularly the brain and the heart [3]. Thus, we need to know the physiological flow conditions and their pathological alterations in a unified point of view to understand the mechanism of various diseases.

In this chapter, we present some general discussion on the studies of blood flow, stressing the computational fluid dynamics (CFD) method and visualization based on the computation. Particular emphasis is placed on computational visualization, which has become available in the field of biological flow studies. Although computational visualization has strong potential, there are some points to be discussed in its application to blood flow with respect to both physiological condition and pathological consequences. Computational bio-fluid mechanics constructed on the basis of these considerations is undoubtedly one of the most promising directions in the field of biological flow studies. Indeed, computational fluid mechanics is proving extremely useful in various fields of engineering where fluid dynamics plays the leading role.

1.1 Pathophysiological Significance of Blood Flow

Vascular diseases such as ischemic heart disease and cerebral stroke are known to be strongly influenced by blood flow in terms of their onset and progression [1–3]. Most of these cardio- and cerebrovascular diseases develop as sequelae of atherosclerosis, which has been postulated to start at vessel locations where the wall shear stress is expected to be low [4]. Although so-called low wall shear stress regions of the artery have not yet been located precisely when the flow field is three dimensional (3-D), there are certainly specific locations that are prone to atherosclerosis, as evidenced by accumulated clinical and pathological observations (Fig. 1) [5].

Because wall shear stress is determined by the flow just adjacent to the wall, it is highly likely that the wall shear stress distribution shows markedly different patterns, particularly when the configuration of the artery varies. From this aspect, the vascular system has in fact a complex structure, including branching, curvature, constriction, and dilatation. Blood flow in the artery itself is, moreover, unsteady with a complex time course. The physics of fluid flow, and consequently its governing equations (Navier–Stokes), is highly nonlinear and sometimes results in a surprising deviation from what would be expected by linear superposition.

1.2 Computational Fluid Dynamics

As we previously reported [6–23], CFD can be a powerful tool for investigating a complex system such as blood flow. This is because computing power is becoming readily available to conduct computations assuming unsteady flow, non-Newtonian viscosity, and other complex characteristics of the blood using an extremely complex model based on the real geometry of the blood vessels. Flow-related phenomena such as heat and mass transfer, and any derived parameters

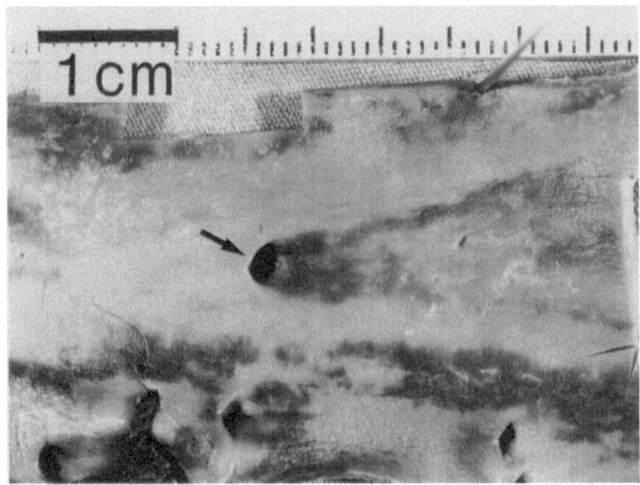

FIG. 1. Spatial distribution of sudanophilic region of the abdominal aorta of an 18-year-old man who died in an accident. *Center*, an opening of the inferior mesenteric artery (*arrow*) supplies blood to the large intestine. The portion of the abdominal aorta shown here is known to be that most prone to early atherosclerosis. A typical fan-shaped sudanophilic region can be seen upstream of the ostium of the inferior vena cava. This pattern is believed to be related to the low wall shear stress zone from the analogy of steady two-dimensional flows

of mechanics, including the wall shear stress exerted by blood flow, are easily computed in CFD. This is particularly noticeable in studies of the role of blood flow in atherogenesis because a combination of spatial as well as temporal variations of these parameters seems to play an influential role in the process. These four-dimensional phenomena (that is, the three spatial dimensions plus time) can be fully analyzed at present only by numerical methods using computers.

1.3 Importance of Geometry

Although the potential of CFD is enormous, its actual applications are still limited mostly to arterial and cardiac flow models based on rather simple idealized geometries. As is frequently pointed out, the most significant factor that affects the flow structure [24] and thus disease [25,26] is the 3-D configuration of the flow field.

Therefore, the degree of realism built into the computational model is crucial for correlating fluid mechanics to physiological and pathophysiological phenomena such as atherogenesis [11,14]. Fortunately, the agreement between the real flow field and the model can be pursued in a flexible way in fluid mechanical studies. We can introduce any arbitrary scaling system so long as it is consistent, so that we can analyze models ranging from the microscopic scale to the very large scale using the same method.

Recent advances in computer technology have enabled us to perform more realistic modeling, and we found vascular casts to be useful in studying complex vascular structures [14,27]. Using the casts as the starting point for realistic modeling, CFD results can be compared to those obtained by blood flow measurement. Three-dimensionally reconstructed images obtained by noninvasive methods such as computed tomography (CT), magnetic resonance imaging (MRI), and ultrasound can also be applied to computational mechanics studies.

1.4 The Significant Role of Visualization

As has been discussed, we need to understand the effect of the 3-D structure of the vasculature. This is essential not only to study fluid motion but eventually to understand the influence of the flow on the wall. It is particularly important for the study of blood flow with respect to vascular disorders. Computational fluid dynamics incorporating computer graphics technology is presently the only method available to allow such an analysis. The 4-D nature of the real flow can be understood by animation techniques in which the changes in the 3-D distribution of computed values with time are displayed using sophisticated rendering techniques with color graphics. Not only velocity components and pressure, but also a variety of derived parameters such as wall shear stress and its spatial derivatives can be displayed from a variety of aspects on the computer screen as well as on video equipment.

2 Computational Method in the Physiological Flow Studies

2.1 Governing Equations

2.1.1 Basic Considerations

As is frequently mentioned, there are several basic problems in applying the Navier–Stokes equations to blood flow. First, it is assumed that the fluid is Newtonian, that is, the viscosity does not vary with the flow condition. This is not strictly true for blood, which is known to show shear-dependent viscosity, particularly when the shear rate is very low [28]. Viscosity becomes relatively constant however if the shear rate exceeds a certain limiting value. Fortunately, the shear rate estimated in larger arteries usually exceeds this threshold and thus we can safely neglect non-Newtonian viscosity when we consider blood flow in large arteries [29].

The next most frequently asked question is related to deformation, particularly that caused by the nonlinear stress–strain relationship of the vessel wall. The walls of arteries and veins deform according to the inside pressure as well as the wall shear stress. The pressure changes mainly due to the pulsatile nature of blood flow, but the fluctuations of the disturbed velocity field such as vortices and turbulence also have an effect. These considerations are unfortunately very difficult to fully incorporate into currently available computational methods; however, intensive studies on this subject have been performed [30,31].

2.1.2 Equations of Motion and Continuity

As was discussed, our usual analysis can be based upon the Navier–Stokes equations of motion and the continuity equation for an incompressible Newtonian fluid as the following [32]:

$$\rho \frac{D\mathbf{v}}{Dt} = -\nabla p + \mu \nabla^2 \mathbf{v} \tag{1}$$

$$\left(\nabla \bullet \mathbf{v} \right) = 0 \tag{2}$$

where ρ is the density, $\mathbf{v}$ is the velocity, $D\mathbf{v}/Dt$ is the substantial velocity time derivative with 3-D partial derivative components of both time and distance in three dimensions, p is the pressure, and μ is the viscosity.

2.1.3 Equations of Transport of Scalar Variables

In the computation, we can integrate the transport equations for heat and mass. Because mass transport in the liquid is particularly convection dependent, the distribution of the solute masses can be computed based on the velocity field obtained by the solution of equations of motion. In heat transfer, natural convection may be important even in a liquid such as blood, and should be modeled as such. Nevertheless, temperature differences have a small range in the living system and heat production within the fluid can be neglected, so that we do not usually have to take the effect of heat on the velocity field into account.

2.1.4 Turbulence

It is well known that turbulence, if it occurs under the same global flow conditions, induces significantly larger wall and intrafluid shear stresses than laminar flow. There is a strong possibility that turbulence in living systems affects various pathophysiological phenomena such as atherosclerosis. Turbulence has been shown to exist in the larger arteries in the cardiovascular system [33–37], particularly when the flow rate is increased, as for example during exercise. Turbulence modeling has been successfully applied to the computation of biological fluid flow and its effect on the wall. In one of these, the so-called κ–ε approach, two averaged properties of turbulent flow are introduced to the equations of motion and are traced in the course of computation [38]. It is noteworthy that the introduction of such parameters is in a sense arbitrary or a priori in terms of recognition of the transition of turbulence. The transition therefore is not predicted by this method, but the average behavior of turbulence can be computed.

2.2 Numerical Method

2.2.1 Pros and Cons of Three Different Methods

In general, currently available techniques in numerical analysis fall into three main classes [39,40], the finite-difference or the finite-volume-type method, the finite-element approach, and the boundary-element method. The finite-difference or finite-volume method was the first method to be developed and has been available for many years. It is established that these methods give stable results with relatively less computation time than that required by other methods. However, model construction is less flexible than with the finite-element method which was developed later. Although the finite-element method allows greater flexibility to build the computational domain, much more time and memory space is necessary for the computation. The boundary-element method is mainly used for a class of flow problems (potential flow) that is not always relevant to blood flow. We have been using a finite-volume method when we compute the fluid flow alone. As pointed out, relatively short computational time is spent to obtain stable results in the finite-volume method, and this point is important because we are using workstation-class computers for their greater flexibility.

It is recognized that the moving-wall-type problem cannot be properly handled by the finite-volume-type approach and indeed may be completely impossible. Most efforts to solve the coupled equations for wall motion and fluid motion reported so far have used the finite-element-type method [30]. In part, this is because mechanics problems in solids have been mostly solved by finite-element methods.

2.2.2 Boundary Conditions

In terms of mathematics, CFD analysis falls into a category of boundary value problems, and so we need three or four sets of boundary conditions: the inlet condition, the wall condition, the outlet condition, and conditions to define the symmetry of the model. The fluid–solid interface, such as that between blood and the arterial wall, is assumed to be a nonslip rigid boundary. In some special cases, the wall may be considered as permeable, allowing a certain flow across it. In an analysis of the coupled motion of the fluid and the wall, the wall moves according to the normal and shear stresses exerted by the fluid. Even in this case, a nonslip condition on the wall is usually assumed.

If the models are like a pipe, the inlet flow boundary is set as if there is an infinitely long inlet before the model starts. This is conducted by assuming some theoretical fluid velocity distribution at the inlet cross section. In unsteady flow cases, however, there are some problems to be considered. When the basic frequency is very low and the flow can be regarded as virtually steady, the flow velocity profile may be parabolic. This is the case when the Wormersley's alpha parameter is very small, and is irrelevant in the larger arteries and airways. In this case, we do not have valid foundations on the inlet boundary condition so that a flat profile is the only choice. Another possibility is to compute appropriate flows to define the inlet boundary condition. This approach is particularly useful when we try to build a general model of the circulatory system. We call this a multilevel CFD model of the flow tracts in the living system (Fig. 2).

A different consideration is necessary for the outlet condition, especially when unsteady flow is calculated. In a unidirectional steady flow case, the outlet condition is rather simple: we just assume zero pressure and zero gradients for all the

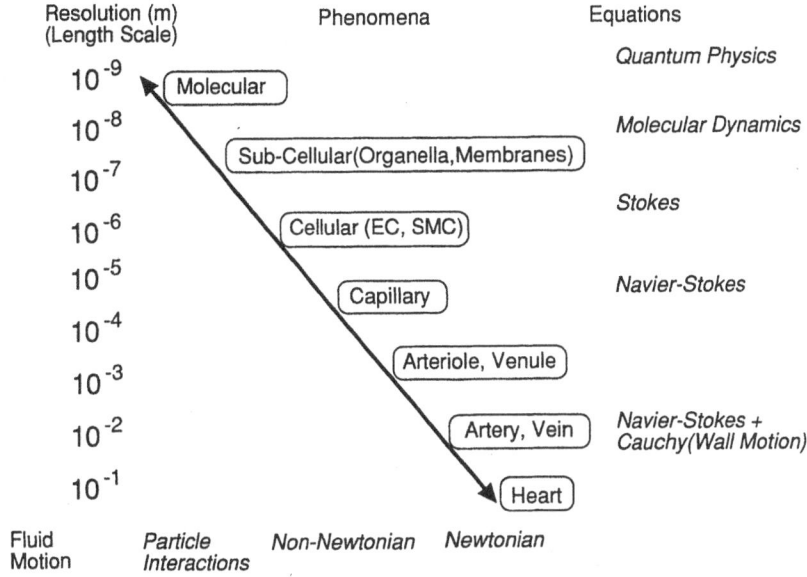

Fig. 2. A scheme of proposed multilevel computational bio-fluid mechanics in blood flow study links various levels of flow-related phenomena. The links are multidimensional: that is, a lower level phenomenon bounds its upper level phenomenon and vice versa. By virtue of the flexibility in the scale conversion of computational method, different scales of phenomena can be united seamlessly. *EC*, endothelial cell; *SMC*, smooth muscle cell

dependent variables such as velocity components and pressure. Nevertheless, for unsteady flow, the pressure gradient can be reversed anywhere in the computing domain, including the outlet cross section. In such a case, we need to know what is happening outside the model.

2.3 Importance of the Pre-Postprocessing [41]

2.3.1 Preprocessor

Because we are trying to tackle the complex configuration of the flow tract, the preprocessor is very important. It is frequently estimated that the preprocessing, that is, the model building, requires more than 90% of the effort of computational analysis. Expertise is still necessary to build a complex model, particularly when it is 3-D, even when using the most advanced computer-aided design-(CAD-) based preprocessor system. There are two types of difficulties in preprocessing. The first is to define the complex surface shape of the model; this aspect has been very much improved by introducing the 3-D CAD software. The second difficulty is defining the computational mesh inside the flow tract. The computational mesh should be carefully located by paying attention to the predicted flow distribution [42,43].

2.3.2 Postprocessor

First, it is important to convert and process the numerical values, because we cannot necessarily be content with the raw output of the computational fluid mechanical simulation. Second, the graphics representation is mandatory for understanding the flow itself and its effect on the vascular wall. Another issue is related to the data compatibility between the CFD system and other systems used for postprocessing, which we will not discuss here.

Three-dimensional velocity and pressure values are usually obtained from the computation. The velocity itself is undoubtedly important to understand the flow field, and is directly calculated in the computational study. The virtue of computational methods is that the data obtained can be easily reprocessed. We always make color graphic mapping of the distribution of the wall shear stress and derived parameters such as plain average and root mean square (rms) values. This is usually difficult to carry out using the experimental data because of the limitations of measurement. Temporal as well as spatial correlation between these derived parameters and other mechanical or physiological parameters can also be processed using the computed results. By doing this, we can search the physiologically significant characteristics with respect to the normal and abnormal state of the living system.

2.4 Visualization Techniques

2.4.1 Computer Graphics

In usual scientific publication, color printing is prohibitively expensive and most graphics are represented as black-and-white drawings or half-tone photos. However, in advanced computer graphics, color representations are easier than graphics of the black-and-white line drawing type, especially in 3-D graphics. This is particularly true if we need to build a specialized graphics system to visualize the CFD results.

As has been repeatedly stressed, we are interested in the true 3-D distribution of a certain class of physical properties, such as the wall shear stress in a complex 3-D configuration. To render these attributes, we need to visualize the geometry of the computational domain and the computed results in the same frame at the same time. Most modern computer graphics tools are based on color graphics, using polygonal drawing with areas of light and shade. This means that the surface of a 3-D object is easily rendered with various effects.

2.4.2 Virtual Reality Technology

The cathode ray tube (CRT) display used for computer graphics is flat and can only show a pseudo-3-D effect by using various techniques of perspective. It is therefore difficult if not impossible to comprehend the true 3-D spatial location of physical objects through a static graphical drawing. To overcome this, virtual reality technology is one of the most promising, but not widely used, modalities. Here, we use the phrase "virtual reality" to mean a technology that gives an interactively controllable or modifiable graphically represented imaginary environment, which gives the user a sense of immersion as if in an imaginary world.

To actualize this, there are three important component technologies, including stereoscopic display (Fig. 3), interactive computer graphics software, and a high-speed graphics computer. Combining these resources, we can produce an imaginary or "virtual" world in which the computational results are displayed and even "touched" by an observer. The technology is thought to be very useful to grasp the complex 3-D structures of the flow field and the fluid–solid interactions in living systems. We can imagine even so-called real-time steering of the computation through such an interface, in which we can control the detail, time course, and what to display in the course of computation of the physical equations.

Although currently available computing systems still lack the required ability to perform this task, we can expect this obstacle to be cleared in the near future because of the rapid advancement of computer technology.

2.4.3 Animation Techniques

Animation techniques are widely use to present physical phenomena of four dimensions, that is, spatial (3-D) plus time (1-D). This is very important in understanding unsteady flow such as that of the cardiovascular system and the respiratory system. It may also be noteworthy that animated figures make it easy to recognize 3-D structures by providing a sense of depth by the differential movement of an object on the view. Animation is therefore a crucial technique nowadays to facilitate the understanding of computational results.

To make an animation video from computer graphics output, there are two major methods. The conventional method we have been using is to convert the graphics output video (RGB) signal into any broadcast format (e.g., NTSC or

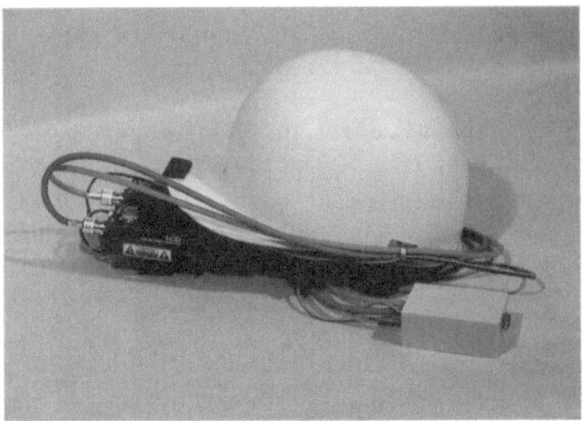

Fig. 3. A stereoscopic (binocular) display system developed to apply virtual reality technology for visualization of the complex 3-D flow field obtained by the computational fluid dynamics (CFD) for blood flow models

PAL) and record it on frame-to-frame video (tape or disk) recording equipment. The relatively new method is to record the graphical output on computer disk in digital format with various data compression technologies (e.g., MPEG).

The graphics output of computers usually has larger scan lines than television format, and thus the video signal is of a higher frequency. Therefore we need to convert the scan rate using special equipment called a scan converter. After this conversion, the video signal is recorded in three separate channels as red, green, and blue (RGB) or in a composite channel according to the broadcasting systems. When recording a frame, we can use a special videotape recorder that can record a single frame, or a disk-type recorder. To use the animation technique for analyzing results, not merely for the purpose of demonstration, a laser disk-type recorder is desirable to decrease the recording time. Using this method, we could compare the minute changes in spatial distribution caused by the combination of the geometrical configuration and the time course of blood flow.

3 Some Results of Computational Visualization of Blood Flow

In the following section, two examples of our computational studies are shown, the intraventricular flow fields of the heart and flow adjacent to cultured endothelial cells. They are shown with the intention of presenting both ends of the spectrum of our computational studies.

3.1 Intraventricular Flow Field

3.1.1 Realistic Modeling of the Left Ventricle

First, we present results from our series of studies on the intraventricular flow fields in the heart. This study is characterized in two ways. First, it is based on an attempt to incorporate uncoupled wall motion into the CFD. Second, the model used in this study is a realistic one based on measurement of the cast of a real heart.

To compute the intracardiac flow field, we made some casts of the left-ventricular chamber of the heart (Fig. 4). This cast was made by injecting a methacrylate resin into the left ventricle of a dog. To reconstruct the true 3-D configuration, it is necessary to obtain the 3-D coordinate values. A coordinate measuring machine was used to measure and digitize the surface of the cast. The measured coordinate positions were digitally sent to a workstation where the values were recorded in a file.

Figure 5 shows the canine left-ventricle representation constructed from the measured surface shape of the cast. The coordinate values of the vascular structure geometric patterns were inserted into the SCRYU (Software Cradle, Osaka, Japan) 3-D flow simulation package, which was used to compute complex flow patterns [11].

Fig. 4. Canine left-ventricle cast made by methacrylate resin in maximally dilatated state. Grids were marked on the surface of the cast to locate the pin sensor of the 3-D coordinate measuring machine measurung its spatial shape

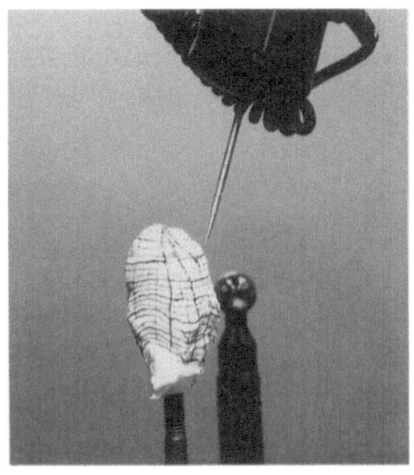

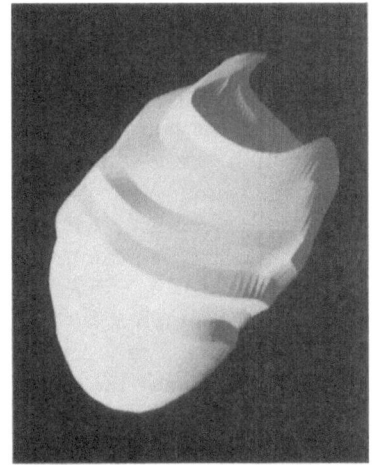

Fig. 5. Smoothed volume representation of the inner cavity of the canine left ventricle in the surface-rendering mode from an animation video in which the normal and the infarcted wall motion were simulated using a specially developed computational method

3.1.2 Computational Modeling of the Ventricular Wall Motion

The software used was the SCRYU flow simulation package by Software Cradle Ltd. This system performs a finite-volume integration of the 3-D Navier–Stokes equations based on the SIMPLE algorithm with a body-fitted coordinate (BFC) system [42,43]. Velocities and pressure values were computed. The computational girds were made using our own user-developed system and the preprocessor system of the SCRYU package, which is able to build BFC grids.

To handle the intraventricular flow as if it were induced by the spontaneous wall motion (i.e., contraction of the heart muscle), we solved the fluid motion and the wall motion in an uncoupled manner assuming the following.

First, the time course of the left-ventricular wall change was assumed to follow a function of time taken from an established cardiac volume measurement without any reaction from the intraventricular fluid. Another important assumption is that the movement of the ventricular wall can be regarded as equivalent to the flow across the wall within a short time period in which the wall does not move significantly. Then, the wall movement can be substituted by a flow across the wall [20].

We assumed that the time scale of the movement of the contracting ventricular wall is much slower than the time scale of the temporal resolution of the computation. In other words, the left-ventricular wall moves much more slowly than nearby fluid particles, and could be assumed to be quasi-steady for the time scale of the velocity development used. By assuming this, we can introduce two different time scales, namely the flow time scale and the cardiac wall time scale. What we assumed is that the cardiac wall time scale is much longer than the flow time scale. If we assume this, we can compute the evolution of the velocity field using a stationary computational grid in each cardiac wall time step. We usually used a flow time scale of an order of magnitude of 10^{-4} s and a cardiac wall time scale of 10^{-2} s.

3.1.3 Results of Systolic and Diastolic Flow Computations

Using the developed model, we simulated various phases of flow in the left ventricle of the heart, including the normal heart [16], the heart with abnormal wall motion because of myocardial infarction, intracardiac systolic blood flow under the condition of aortic stenosis [15], and the interactions of diastolic filling the systolic ejection flow under normal physiological conditions [23] and in heart failure. We show an example of the intraventricular flow pattern in the normal heart at systole (Fig. 6a) and at diastole (Fig. 6b). Cross-sectional velocity vectors were also computed at systole (Fig. 7a) and at diastole (Fig. 7b).

3.1.4 Significance of the Computations of Intraventricular Flow

By introducing different time scales for wall motion and the fluid motion induced by the wall motion, the computation of intraventricular flow fields was shown to be effectively conducted. This was possible because the muscle of the left-ventricular wall exerts much greater power than that needed to give the momentum to the blood before the actual ejection. In this context, the interaction of the blood and the ventricular wall can be regarded as unilateral, and there is very little reaction from the fluid to the muscle. This assumption enabled us to simulate the ventricular wall motion by replacing it by the flow across the wall. This method can be widely applied to different situations in the living system.

It is also noted that the construction of a realistic model whose configuration is based on real vascular structures was established in the studies shown here. This is a necessary technique for correlating fluid mechanics with the atherogenic and other vascular disease processes. This technique, coupled with our computational method, makes it possible to compare simulation results with measurements by various methods such as ultrasound imaging and MRI.

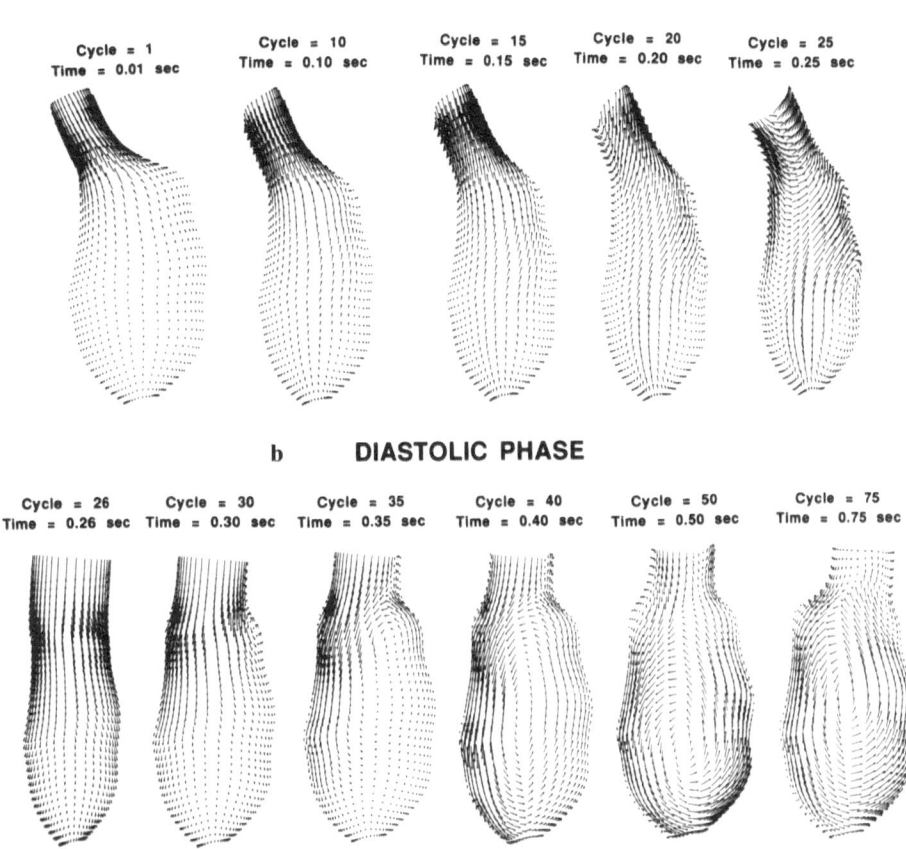

FIG. 6a,b. Intraventricular longitudinal velocity distribution pattern of normal heart; end-systolic ejection fraction is 60%. **a** Systolic flow. **b** Diastolic flow (from [23], with permission)

3.2 Cellular Surface Flow and Wall Shear Stress Distribution

3.2.1 Purpose of the Study

Vascular endothelial cells in situ have long been known to respond to blood flow, and the active role of blood flow in the regulation and remodeling of blood vessels is of the most recent interest [44]. To overcome difficulties in doing experiments using actual blood vessels, investigators have designed in vitro devices for studying the function and morphology of endothelial cells exposed to fluid flow.

When living cultured endothelial cells are examined by a light microscope, their 3-D appearance can be easily appreciated. For example, when cells are cultured on a rigid substrate such as glass or plastic, the center parts of the cells are significantly elevated from the substrate because of the presence of the

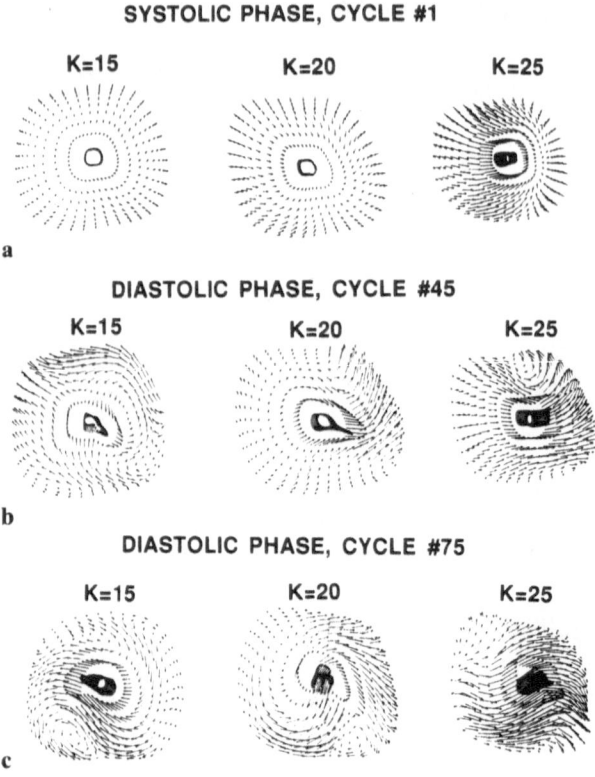

SYSTOLIC PHASE, CYCLE #1

K=15   K=20   K=25

DIASTOLIC PHASE, CYCLE #45

K=15   K=20   K=25

DIASTOLIC PHASE, CYCLE #75

K=15   K=20   K=25

a

b

c

Fig. 7a–c. Intraventricular cross-sectional velocity distribution pattern of normal heart; end-systolic ejection fraction is 60%. **a** Systolic flow. **b,c** Diastolic flow (from [23], with permission)

nucleus; this is the nuclear bulge. We found that the size of the nuclear bulge depended on the nature of the substrate surface, as cells cultured on a collagen gel had smaller nuclear bulges than those cultured on a solid surface. The diameter of the cells ranged from 50 to 70 μm. Thus, the aspect ratio (height/diameter) of these endothelial cells was of the order of 10^{-1}. This aspect ratio should not be overlooked from the fluid mechanical viewpoint, and we decided to investigate the effects of cell shape on the flow pattern over the cell surface and on the consequent wall shear stress exerted by flow on the cell surface by the CFD method [7,13,22].

3.2.2 Modeling of Confluent Endothelial Cells

Two types of confluent cell models were considered: one with cells cultured on type 1 collagen gel substrate, and the other with those cultured on the type 1 collagen-coated glass substrate. Cells on the collagen gel (model 1) express certain features similar to those of the endothelium in vivo.

Optically sliced serial images with a thickness of 0.4 μm for model 1 and 0.9 μm for model 2 were taken under the no-flow condition. The edge of each slice was traced manually to produce a contour drawing, and the contour data were fed into the modeling process developed for the purpose.

3.2.3 Results of Computation and the Wall Shear Stress Distribution

Velocity vectors calculated for confluent cell models are shown in Fig. 8. Figure 8a,b shows vector distributions calculated for model 1 (monolayer formed on a collagen gel substrate) and model 2 (a monolayer on the glass surface coated with

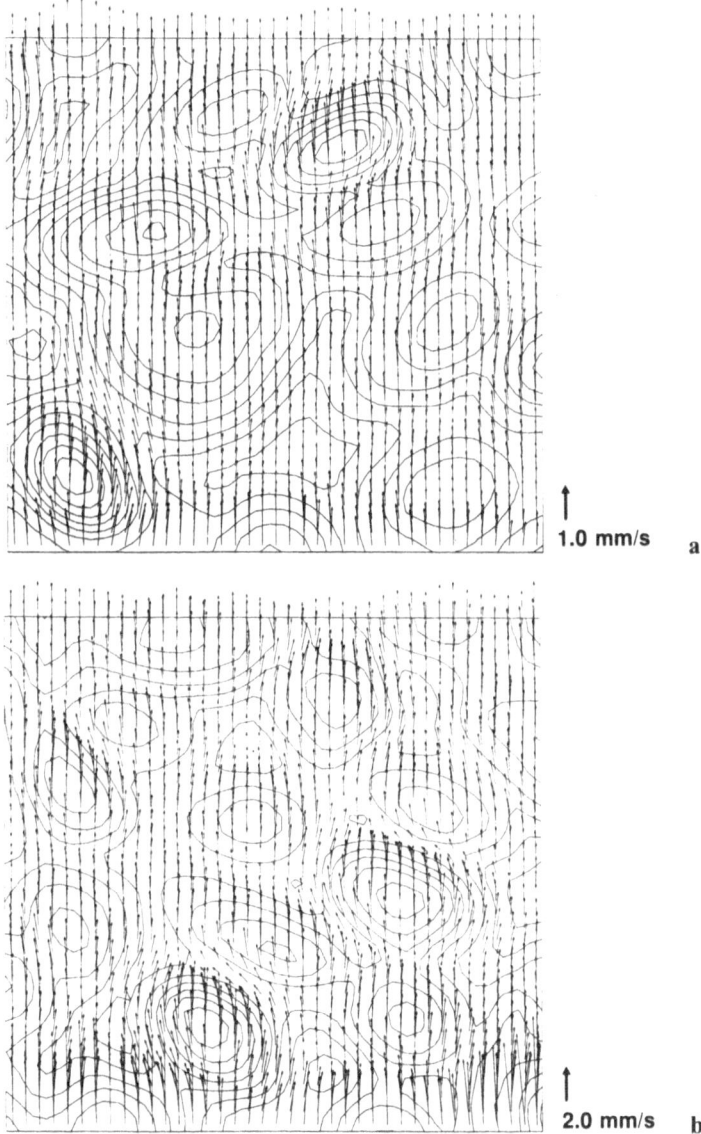

1.0 mm/s   a

2.0 mm/s   b

FIG. 8a,b. Velocity vectors calculated for confluent cell models where substrate shear stress = 1.0 Pa. **a** Cell model 1 (monolayer formed on a collagen gel substrate). **b** Cell model 2 (monolayer formed on a collagen-coated glass substrate)

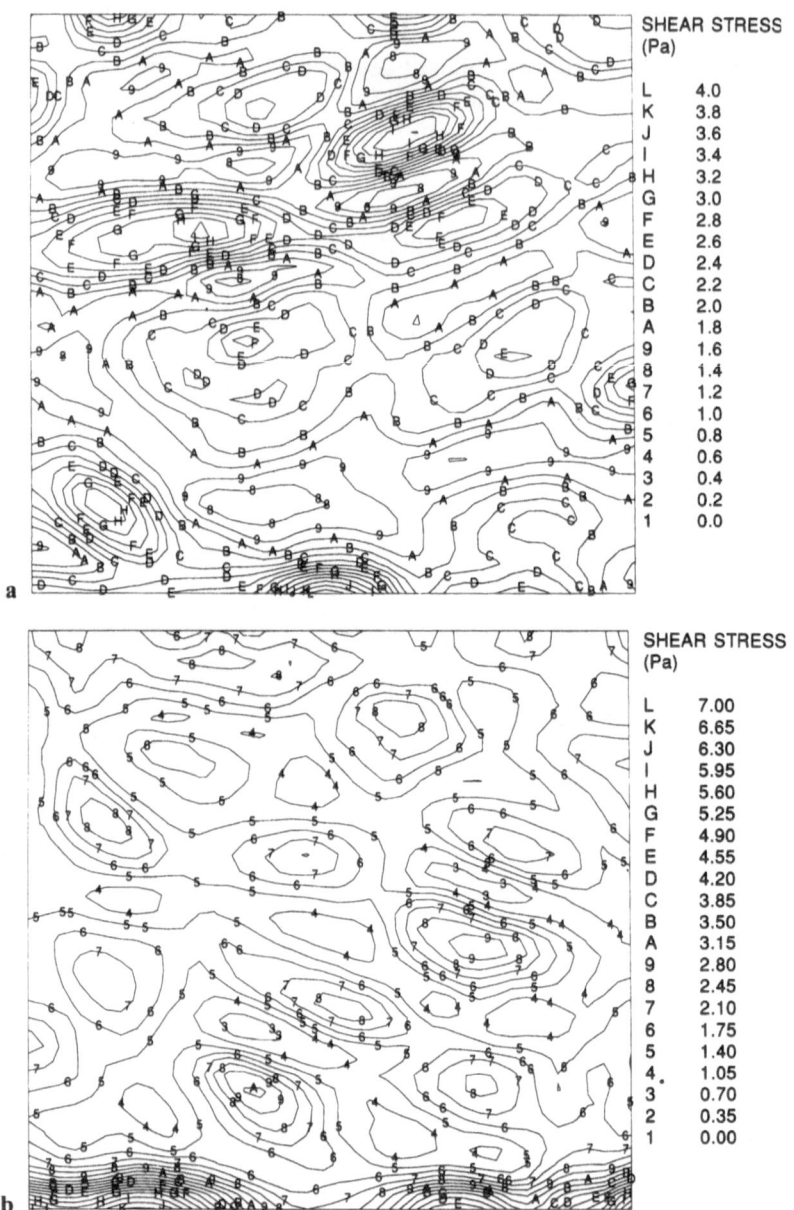

FIG. 9a,b. Wall shear stress distribution where substrate shear stress = 1.0 Pa. **a** Cell model 1 (type 1 collagen gel). **b** Cell model 2 (type 1 collagen-coated glass). Wall shear stress distribution patterns could not be distinguished between low- and high-flow conditions except for values, so the results obtained under the low-flow condition are shown

collagen), respectively. We computed the flow fields under various flow conditions. The main flow that followed the cell surface went around the nuclear bulge. Consequently, fluid that passed over the peak of the nuclear bulge came from higher layers of the flow with higher velocity.

The wall shear stress distribution is shown in Fig. 9; Fig. 9a is model 1 and Fig. 9b is model 2. At the top of the nuclear bulge, shear stress values were two to three times larger than those found on the low areas of the cell surface.

Cell heights were significantly different between the cells cultured on the collagen gel (model 1) and those cultured on the glass surface (model 2). However, the magnitude of shear stress did not differ much between these models. It should be realized that the height of the nuclear bulge was not the only difference between the two models. For example, cell density, configuration, and alignment were clearly different, although we did not quantitatively evaluate them in this study. We have conducted similar computations using more idealistic configurations and reported some preliminary results [45].

4 Concluding Remarks

In this chapter, a general discussion was given on the relevance of the CFD studies of blood flow for correlating physiological state and the pathological consequences. We emphasized that the extremely complex nature of blood flow, including its susceptibility to the geometrical configuration of blood vessels, particularly under unsteady conditions, should be carefully handled. In this sense, the CFD method is the most promising method to reveal the nature of the blood flow and its effects on various physiological and pathological phenomena in the living system.

In a CFD study, modeling is undoubtedly the most important and the most time-consuming part. From our series of attempts to model and to derive the flow field of the cardiovascular system, two examples were shown. The construction of a realistic model whose configuration is based on macro- and microscale vascular structures was shown to be necessary for correlating fluid mechanics to physiological and disease processes. This was thought to allow a finer detail of understanding of the flow than is currently available.

Another aspect that was emphasized was the visualization of the CFD results. We need to know the effect of the 3-D structure of the vasculature. This is necessary not only to understand the fluid motion in blood flow, but finally for understanding the influence of the flow on the wall, particularly for the study of blood flow with respect to the vascular disorders. The four dimensions of the real flow can be understood by animation techniques in which the consecutive changes in the 3-D distribution of computed values are displayed using 3-D rendering with color graphics.

In understanding those graphically presented computational results, we can naturally rely upon the human ability of pattern recognition. The only way in which we are undoubtedly superior to the computing machines is in the intuitive ability of pattern recognition. To fully utilize this ability, we need to visualize the computational results from different aspects, at various thresholds of rendering computed values, and with different time steps. By these rendering techniques, we can depict the subtle changes of spatial parameters and can discuss the underlying physics and physiology. This can be accomplished by the combination of novel hardware, including virtual reality technology, and sophisticated 3-D rendering software.

It should be noted that the available computer power is still unsatisfactory to examine very complicated flow fields in the cardiovascular system. However, the rapid advancement of computer technology has made it possible to compute fairly complicated flow fields, even when using a workstation. Therefore, the use of a realistic model in conjunction with sophisticated visualization of the flow field should become a mandatory part of investigation relating fluid dynamic factors to normal and pathological behavior of vascular tissues and cells.

Acknowledgments. A part of the studies represented in this chapter were supported by the Research Grant for Cardiovascular Diseases (3A-3) from the Ministry of Health and Welfare of Japan, the Grant-in-Aid for Scientific Research on Priority Areas, "Biomechanics of Structure and Function of Living Cells, Tissues, and Organs" (#04237101), and grant #04454537 from the Ministry of Education, Science and Culture of Japan. The author thanks Dr. T.W. Taylor for his help.

References

1. Yoshida Y, Wang S, Yamane T, Okano M, Oyama T, Mitsumata M, Suda K, Yamaguchi T, Ooneda G (1990) Structural differences of arterial walls which are either vulnerable or resistant to atherosclerosis. Acta Med Biol 38:1–19
2. Caro CG, Pedley TJ, Schroter RC, Seed WA (1978) The mechanics of the circulation. Oxford University Press, Oxford, pp 341–346
3. Woolf N (1982) Pathology of atherosclerosis. Butterworth, London pp 187–216
4. Caro CG, Fitz-Gerald JM, Schroter RC (1971) Atheroma and arterial wall shear observation, correlation and proposal of a shear dependent mass transfer mechanism for atherogenesis. Proc R Soc Lond (Biol) 177:109–159
5. Yamaguchi T, Hanai S, Oyama T, Mitsumata M, Yoshida Y (1986) Effect of blood flow on the localization of fibrocellular intimal thickening and atherosclerosis at the young human abdominal aorta-inferior mesenteric artery branching (in Japanese). Recent Adv Cardiovasc Dis 7:97–108
6. Yamaguchi T, Nakano A, Hanai S (1990) Three dimensional shear stress distribution around small atherosclerotic plaques with steady and unsteady flow. In: Mosora F, Caro CG, Krause E, Schmid-Schönbein H, Baquey C, Pelissier R (eds) Biomechanical transport process. Plenum, New York, pp 173–182
7. Sakurai A, Nakano A, Yamaguchi T, Masuda M, Fujiwara K (1991) A computational fluid mechanical study of flow over cultured endothelial cells. Adv Bioeng BED-20:299–302

8. Taylor TW, Yamaguchi T (1992) Three-dimensional simulation of blood flow in an abdominal aortic aneurysm using steady and unsteady computational methods. Adv Bioeng BED-22:229–232

9. Yamaguchi T, Taylor TW (1992) A parametrically defined computational fluid mechanical model for the study of the flow in arterial bifurcations. Adv Bioeng BED-22:237–240

10. Yamaguchi T, Taylor TW (1992) Computational fluid mechanical study of the coronary spasm. Adv Bioeng BED-22:333–340

11. Taylor TW, Yamaguchi T (1992) Three-dimensional graphics and computational model construction of vascular chambers using physiological cast measurements. Adv Bioeng BED-22:469–472

12. Taylor TW, Okino H, Yamaguchi T (1993) Three dimensional analysis of left ventricular ejection using computational fluid dynamics. Bioeng Conf BED-24:136–139

13. Yamaguchi T, Hoshiai K, Okino H, Sakurai A, Hanai S, Masuda M, Fujiwara K (1993) Shear stress distribution over confluently cultured endothelial cells studied by computational fluid mechanics. Bioeng Conf BED-24:167–170

14. Sakurai A, Yamaguchi T, Okino H, Hanai S, Masuda M (1993) A method for formulating realistic mathematical models based on arterial casts for the computational fluid mechanical studies on arterial flow and atherosclerosis. J Phys III 3:1551–1556

15. Taylor TW, Okino H, Yamaguchi T (1993) The effects of supravalvular aortic stenosis on realistic three-dimensional left ventricular blood ejection. Biorheology 30:429–434

16. Taylor TW, Okino H, Yamaguchi T (1993) Realistic three-Dimensional left ventricular ejection determined from computational fluid dynamics. Adv Bioeng BED-26:119–122

17. Yamaguchi T (1993) A computational fluid mechanical study of blood flow in a variety of asymmetric arterial bifurcations. Front Med Biol Eng 5:135–141

18. Yamaguchi T, Taylor TW (1993) Computational fluid mechanical study of the blood flow with moving walls in the cardiovascular system. Theor Appl Mech 42:331–338

19. Taylor TW, Yamaguchi T (1994) Three-dimensional simulation of blood flow in an abdominal aortic aneurysm—steady and unsteady flow cases. J Biomech Eng 116:89–97

20. Taylor TW, Okino H, Yamaguchi T (1994) Three-dimensional analysis of left ventricular ejection using computational fluid mechanics. J Biomech Eng 116:127–130

21. Yamaguchi T, Taylor TW (1994) Some moving boundary problems in computational bio-fluid mechanics. In: Crolet JM, Ohayon R (eds) Computational methods for fluid–structure interaction. Longman, Harlow, UK 306:198–213

22. Yamaguchi T (1994) Maximum wall shear at the nuclear bulge of endothelial cells and their alignment along the blood flow—a computational fluid mechanical study. Adv Bioeng BED-28:347–348

23. Taylor TW, Yamaguchi T (1995) Flow patterns in three-dimensional left ventricular systolic and diastolic flows determined from computational fluid dynamics. Biorheology 32:107–117

24. Friedman MH, Deters OJ, Mark FF, Bargeron CB, Hutchins GM (1983) Arterial geometry affects hemodynamics. A potential risk factor for atherosclerosis. Atherosclerosis 46:225–231

25. Friedman MH, Brinkman AM, Qin JJ, Seed WA (1993) Relation between coronary artery geometry and the distribution of early sudanophilic lesions. Atherosclerosis 98:193–199

26. Masawa N, Glagov S, Zarins CK (1994) Quantitative morphologic study of intimal thickening at the human carotid bifurcation: I. Axial and circumferential distribution of maximum intimal thickening in asymptomatic, uncomplicated plaques. Atherosclerosis 107:137–146
27. Vesely I, Eickmeier B, Campbell G (1991) Automated 3-D reconstruction of vascular structures from high definition casts. IEEE Trans Biomed Eng 38:1123–1129
28. Fung YC (1993) Biomechanics: mechanical properties of living tissues, 2nd edn. Springer, Berlin Heidelberg New York, pp 66–72
29. Perktold K, Resch M, Florian H (1991) Pulsatile non-Newtonian flow characteristics in a three-dimensional human carotid bifurcation model. J Biomech Eng 113:464–475
30. Perktold K, Thurner E, Kenner T (1994) Flow and stress characteristics in rigid walled and compliant carotid artery bifurcation models. Med Biol Eng Comput 32:19–26
31. Reuderink P (1991) Analysis of the flow in a 3D distensible model of the carotid artery bifurcation. Thesis, University of Eindhoven, the Netherlands
32. Bird RB, Stewart WE, Lightfoot EN (1960) Transport phenomena. Wiley, New York, pp 80–81
33. Yamaguchi T, Kikkawa S, Yoshikawa T, Tanishita K, Sugawara M (1983) Measurement of turbulence intensity in the center of the canine ascending aorta with a hot-film anemometer. J Biomech Eng 105:177–187
34. Yamaguchi T, Parker KH (1983) Spatial characteristics of turbulence in the aorta. Ann NY Acad Sci 404:370–373
35. Yamaguchi T, Kikkawa S, Parker KH (1984) Application of Taylor's hypothesis to an unsteady convective field for the spectral analysis of turbulence in the aorta. J Biomech 17:889–895
36. Yamaguchi T, Kikkawa S, Tanishita K, Sugawara M (1988) Spectrum analysis of turbulence in the canine ascending aorta measured with a hot-film anemometer. J Biomech 21:489–495
37. Hanai S, Yamaguchi T, Kikkawa S (1991) Turbulence in the canine ascending aorta and the blood pressure. Biorheology 28:107–116
38. Bradshaw P, Cebeci T, Whitelaw JH (1981) Engineering calculation methods for turbulent flow. Academic Press, London, pp 37–57
39. Peyret R, Taylor TD (1983) Computational methods for fluid flow. Springer-Verlag, New York, pp 18–140
40. Fletcher CAJ (1988) Computational techniques for fluid dynamics, vol 1. Springer, Berlin, pp 98–162
41. Nakahashi K, Fujii K (1995) Grid generation and computer graphics. In: Murakami S (ed) Computational fluid dynamics, series 6 (in Japanese). University of Tokyo Press, Tokyo, pp 1–134
42. Thompson JF, Warsi ZUA, Mastin CW (1982) Boundary-fitted coordinate systems for numerical solutions of partial differential equations—a review. J Comput Physics 47:1–108
43. Thompson JF, Warsi ZUA, Mastin CW (1985) Numerical grid generation foundations and applications. Elsevier, New York
44. Davies PF, Tripathi SC (1993) Mechanical stress mechanisms and the cell: an endothelial paradigm. Circ Res 72:239–245
45. Yamaguchi T (1994) Deformation and alignment of arterial endothelial cells along blood flow (a computational fluid mechanical study) (in Japanese). Trans Jpn Soc Mech Eng B 60:3665–3671

Numerical Analysis of Flow in a Collapsible Vessel Based on Unsteady and Quasi-Steady Flow Theories

Yuji Matsuzaki and Koichiro Seike

Summary. This chapter summarizes the unsteady one-dimensional (1-D) separable flow theory recently proposed by the first author and his co-worker, comparing it to the quasi-steady theory. Numerical analysis was carried out on the self-excited oscillation of the flow in a two-dimensional (2-D) flexible channel to examine the effectiveness of the unsteady flow theory and to compare it with the quasi-steady flow theory. In the unsteady flow theory, the unsteadiness is represented by an additional term in the flow velocity downstream of the flow separation point, whereas this term is not included in the quasi-steady flow theory. The higher frequency components of the flow velocities, the pressures, and the motion of the separation point, therefore, can more accurately be accounted for in the unsteady flow theory. The variances of the velocities and pressures are numerically predicted to be much larger by the unsteady theory than by the quasi-steady theory. On the other hand, the frequency of the higher mode calculated by the latter is about twice that of the former. The introduction of the unsteadiness in the analysis is very important for an accurate prediction of the dynamic features of the flow–channel behavior.

Key words: Unsteady separable flow—One-dimensional flow theory—Flow in a collapsible channel—Flow separation—Self-excited oscillation

1 Introduction

For the past couple of decades, a large number of studies have been performed on theoretical and experimental analyses of self-excited oscillations of flow in a collapsible vessel [1,2]. Flexible tubes and tracts conveying fluid in biological systems show quite complicated oscillatory phenomena that are very significant from both physiological and mechanical aspects. Physiological examples of the tubes and ducts include arteries compressed by a sphygmomanometer cuff,

Department of Aerospace Engineering, Nagoya University, Furo-cho, Chikusa-ku, Nagoya, Aichi, 464-01 Japan

185

intramyocardial coronary blood vessels during systole, pulmonary blood vessels, large intrathoracic airways during forced expiration, the urethra during micturition, and the glottis during phonation. With small positive transmural (external minus internal) pressure, the flexible tube or the duct may collapse into a complex configuration. The configuration of the tube and the tract affects the flow, and vice versa. The flow may easily be separated [3] downstream of the minimum cross section, that is, the throat of the flow channel. At a critical condition, the flow and the channel wall start to be coupled and exhibit self-excited oscillations. Conrad [4] and Katz et al. [5] were the first to demonstrate limit-cycle oscillations by using thin rubber tubes in experiments. Since then, great attention has been attracted to such oscillations because the combination of the flexible channel with the internal flow provides an unexpectedly rich nonlinear system.

The oscillations actually observed and measured were, however, mostly limited to experiments on tubes performed in artificial conditions in laboratories. One of a few actual medical and physiological examples is self-excited oscillation of venae cavae during heart surgery using extracorporeal circulation, for which measured oscillatory blood flow rates are presented in [1]. Voice generation is a very typical example observed in everyday life. The vocal cords and air from the lung are dynamically coupled to produce oscillatory sound sources at the glottis [6]. Although many analyses and experiments have been carried out to reveal the complicated aspects of collapsible channels with internal flow, there remains much to be resolved.

To study the coupled behavior of the channel and the flow, it is important to evalute their three-dimensional (3-D) static and dynamic characteristics. Because 3-D analysis of both the collapsed channel and the separated flow are too complicated, a 1-D or 2-D approach has been taken to understand the basic mechanisms of the complex phenomena observed. The interaction between the flow and the elastic body may really induce very complicated and interesting dynamic phenomena [7]. For a collapsed finite-length tube, Cancelli and Pedley [8] proposed a quasi-steady 1-D separated flow theory, taking into account the flow separation but no flow reattachment downstream. Using the quasi-steady 1-D flow theory, Matsuzaki and his co-workers [9,10] carried out numerical calculations to examine some details of the oscillations of a 2-D collapsible channel conveying fluid.

On evaluating the assumptions introduced in the quasi-steady theory, Matsumoto and Matsuzaki [11] proposed an unsteady 1-D separable flow theory. They introduced a higher order approximation for the flow velocity downstream of the flow separation point, which may account for the unsteadiness in the continuity equations of both the mass and the momentum. The introduction of the quasi-steady assumption into the unsteady flow theory yields the quasi-steady theory. According to their numerical results, the unsteady flow theory predicted that the flow separation point moves mostly together with the throat of the channel, while the quasi-steady theory showed that the former stays far downstream of the latter. As the difference between the numerical results obtained by the unsteady and the quasi-steady theory is substantial, here we exploit more unsteady behavior of a collapsible 2-D channel conveying flow by comparing the unsteady flow theory to the quasi-steady theory.

2 One-Dimensional Unsteady Separable Flow Theory

First, let us summarize the unsteady 1-D flow theory. The X-Z coordinates and a flow in a 2-D channel are shown in Fig. 1, where only the upper half of the channel of breadth $2B(X,T)$ is illustrated because of the assumption of symmetry with respect to the X coordinate. $U^*(X,Z,T)$ and $V^*(X,Z,T)$ are the velocity components in the X- and the Z-direction, respectively. It is assumed that downstream of the flow separation point $X = X_S$, the flow is divided into a parallel jet with uniform profile of the velocity U_S and a pair of stagnant flow zones indicated as a hatched area. One-half of the breadth of the jet is given by $B(X_S,T) = B_S(T)$ independent of X. The static pressure of the flow is assumed uniform over each cross-section of the channel, that is, $P(X,Z,T) = P(X,T)$. Thus, the equations of conservation of mass and momentum governing the flow in the channel are, respectively,

$$\frac{\partial U^*}{\partial X} + \frac{\partial V^*}{\partial Z} = 0 \tag{1}$$

$$\frac{\partial U^*}{\partial T} + U^* \frac{\partial U^*}{\partial X} + V^* \frac{\partial U^*}{\partial Z} = -\frac{1}{\rho} \frac{\partial P}{\partial X} + v \frac{\partial^2 U^*}{\partial Z^2} \tag{2}$$

where ρ and v are the density and the kinematic viscosity of the fluid, respectively. The boundary conditions for the symmetrical flow and the impermeability of the channel wall are, respectively, given by

$$V^* = 0 \quad \text{at} \quad Z = 0, \quad \text{and} \quad V^* = \frac{\partial B}{\partial T} + U^* \frac{\partial B}{\partial X} \quad \text{at} \quad Z = B(X,T) \tag{3}$$

Integrating Eqs. 1 and 2 with respect to Z from 0 to B and applying the Leibniz rule together with the boundary conditions (Eq. 3), we obtain

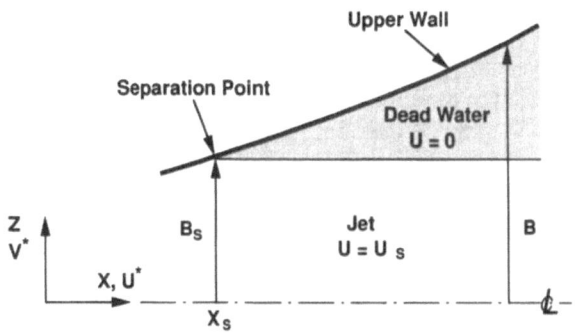

FIG. 1. Flow and channel wall

$$\frac{\partial B}{\partial T} + \frac{\partial Q}{\partial X} = 0 \tag{4}$$

$$\frac{\partial U}{\partial T} + \chi U \frac{\partial U}{\partial X} + 2(1-\chi)\Delta U \frac{\partial U}{\partial X} + (1-\chi)\frac{U}{B}\frac{\partial Q}{\partial X} = -\frac{1}{\rho}\frac{\partial P}{\partial X} - F \tag{5}$$

where we have assumed that

$$U = B_s U_s / B + \Delta U \tag{6}$$

and Q is the flow rate per unit width of the channel and χ is a pressure loss factor [8] set to unity in an unseparated flow region and a value less than unity in a separated flow region, and

$$U(X, T) = \frac{Q}{B} = \frac{1}{B}\int_0^B U^* dZ, \quad \Delta U = \frac{1}{B}\int_{X_s}^X \frac{\partial Q}{\partial X} dX, \quad F = -\frac{v}{B}\frac{\partial U^*}{\partial Z}\bigg|_{Z=B}.$$

When the flow is unseparated, the wall friction per unit width is set to $F = 3vU/B^2$. Otherwise, F is set zero. If the quasi-steady approximation is introduced, that is, $\partial B/\partial T = 0$, then $\partial Q/\partial X = \Delta U = 0$, so that Eq. 5 becomes

$$\frac{\partial U}{\partial T} + \chi U \frac{\partial U}{\partial X} = -\frac{1}{\rho}\frac{\partial P}{\partial X} - F \tag{7}$$

which was originally proposed by Cancelli and Pedley [8] together with the condition on the flow separation:

$$\frac{\partial P}{\partial X} > \gamma_1 \rho U^2 \tag{8.1}$$

$$\frac{\partial P}{\partial X} < \gamma_2 \rho U^2 \tag{8.2}$$

where γ_1 and γ_2 are given constants. If Eq. 8.1 is satisfied at $X = X_1$, then the flow is assumed to be separated downstream of X_1. Therefore, the separation point X_s is the smallest value of X_1. If Eq. 8.2 is satisfied at X_s, the separated flow region is assumed to remain the same. If, however, this is not the case, it is assumed that the separation point retreats downstream so long as Eq. 8.2 is satisfied. In Eq. 8, γ_2 is set to a smaller value than γ_1, so that the hysteresis of the separation–recovery process can be accounted for in the analysis. No condition was proposed in [8] on the flow reattachment, that is, the downstream end of the separated flow region.

To compare to Cancelli–Pedley's theory, Matsumoto and Matsuzaki [11] applied the refined unsteady flow theory based on Eqs. 4 and 5 to an analysis of the self-excited oscillation of a 2-D collapsible channel conveying flow. Next, let us summarize the dynamic analysis of the flow in a 2-D collapsible channel. Figure

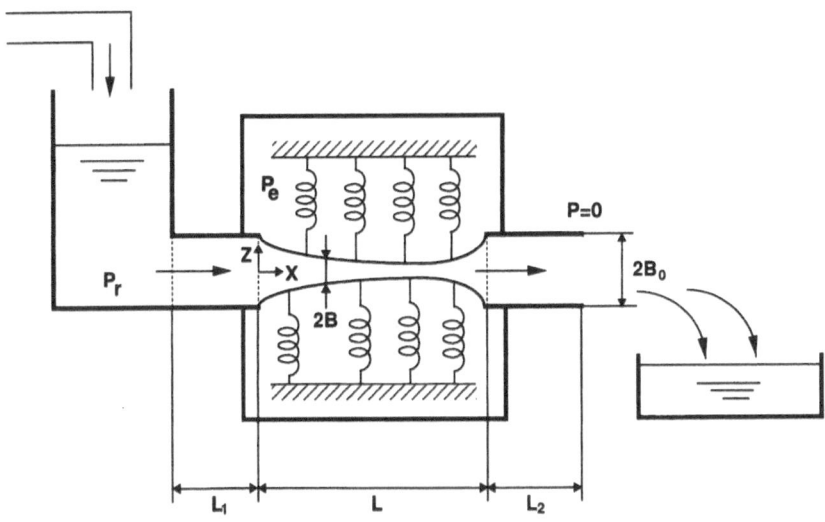

FIG. 2. Two-dimensional (2-D) collapsible channel

2 shows a schematic view of the 2-D channel and the coordinate system. The equilibrium equation of the flexible wall of the 2-D channel is

$$P - P_e + R = 0 \tag{9}$$

where P_e is the external pressure and R is the restoring force per unit area from the wall deflection. The restoring force R is defined by

$$R = K_1 \left[\left(\frac{B}{B_0} \right)^{-1.5} - \left(\frac{B}{B_0} \right)^{20} \right] + K_2 \left[\varepsilon_0 + \frac{1}{2L} \int_0^L \left(\frac{\partial B}{\partial X} \right)^2 dx \right] \kappa \tag{10.1}$$

where K_1 and K_2 are numerical constants relating to the wall stiffness, ε_0 denotes the initial strain of the wall, and κ denotes the longitudinal curvature of the wall, i.e.,

$$\kappa = \frac{\partial^2 B}{\partial X^2} \Bigg/ \left\{ 1 + \left(\frac{\partial B}{\partial X} \right)^2 \right\}^{\frac{3}{2}} \tag{10.2}$$

The boundary conditions of the (upper) wall and the fluid pressures are given at the ends of the collapsible channel:

$$B(0,T) = B(L,T) = B_0 \tag{11.1}$$

$$P(0,T) = P_r - \frac{1}{2}\rho U^2 - \rho L_1 F - \rho L_1 \frac{\partial U}{\partial T} \tag{11.2}$$

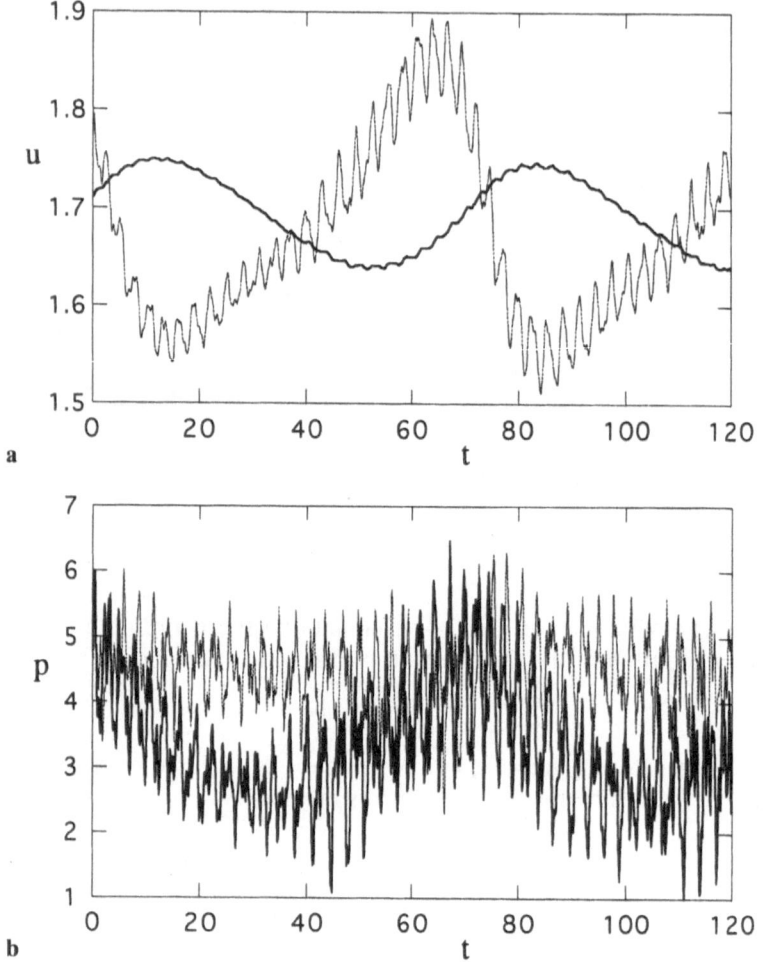

a

b

Fig. 3a–d. Numerical results for $\bar{q} = 1.7$ from the unsteady flow theory. **a** Time courses of velocities (*broken* and *solid curves* denote $u(0)$ and $u(20)$, respectively). **b** Time courses of pressures (*broken* and *solid curves* denote $P(0)$ and $P(20)$, respectively). **c** Time course of $\Delta P = P(0) - P(20)$. **d** Time courses of x_T, x_S, and b_T (*solid*, *broken*, and *thin curves*, respectively)

$$P(L,T) = \rho L_2 F + \rho L_2 \frac{\partial U}{\partial T} \tag{11.3}$$

where the static fluid pressure is zero at the exit of the downstream rigid channel. The separated flow is reattached at the end of the flexible channel. Equations 4, 5, and 9 are solved with the conditions of Eq. 8 under the boundary conditions of Eq. 11. To compare the flow channel oscillations predicted by the unsteady flow theory to those by the quasi-steady theory, Eq. 5 will be replaced by Eq. 7. In addition, the first term will be discarded in Eq. 4.

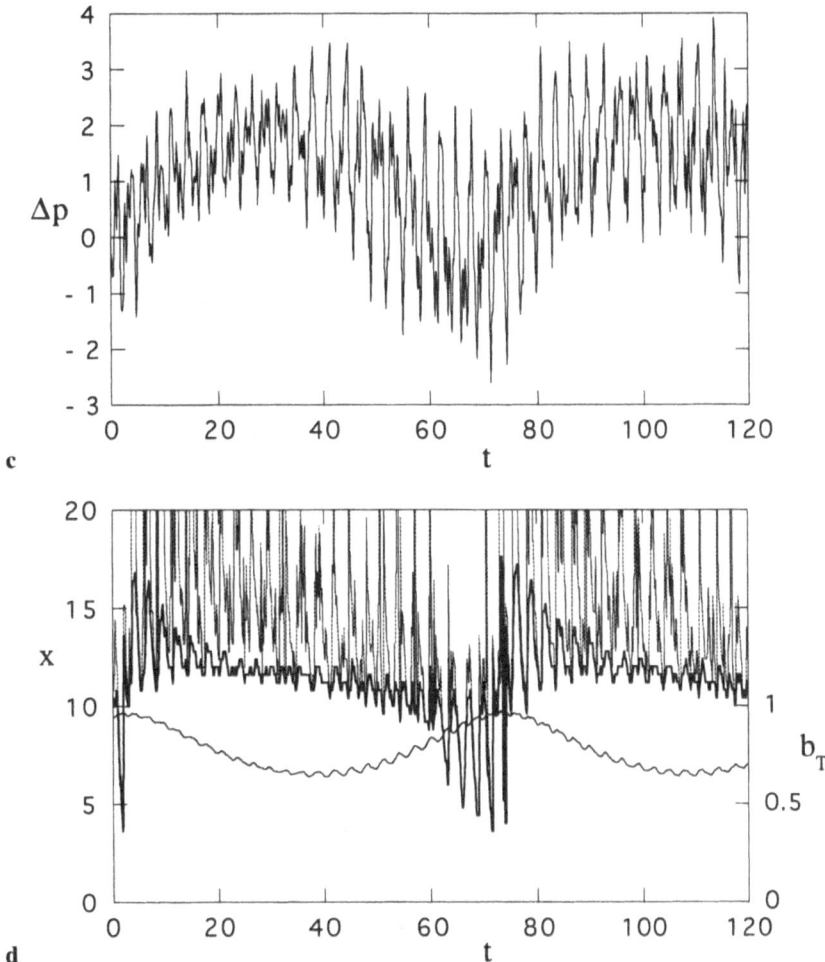

FIG. 3a–d. *Continued*

3 Numerical Analysis and Results

In Matsumoto [12], numerical results showed that the averaged amplitudes of the pressure, the flow velocity, and the motion of the separation point were predicted as much larger by the refined unsteady flow analysis than by the quasi-steady theory. The fundamental frequency of the oscillations calculated by the former was more than double that predicted by the latter. As only a very small number of cases were computed, we will exploit further the coupled oscillatory behavior of the flow and the channel. We solve Eqs. 4, 5, and 9 numerically with the aid of a modified MacCormack explicit finite-difference method, and examine the difference between numerical results calculated by using the unsteady and the

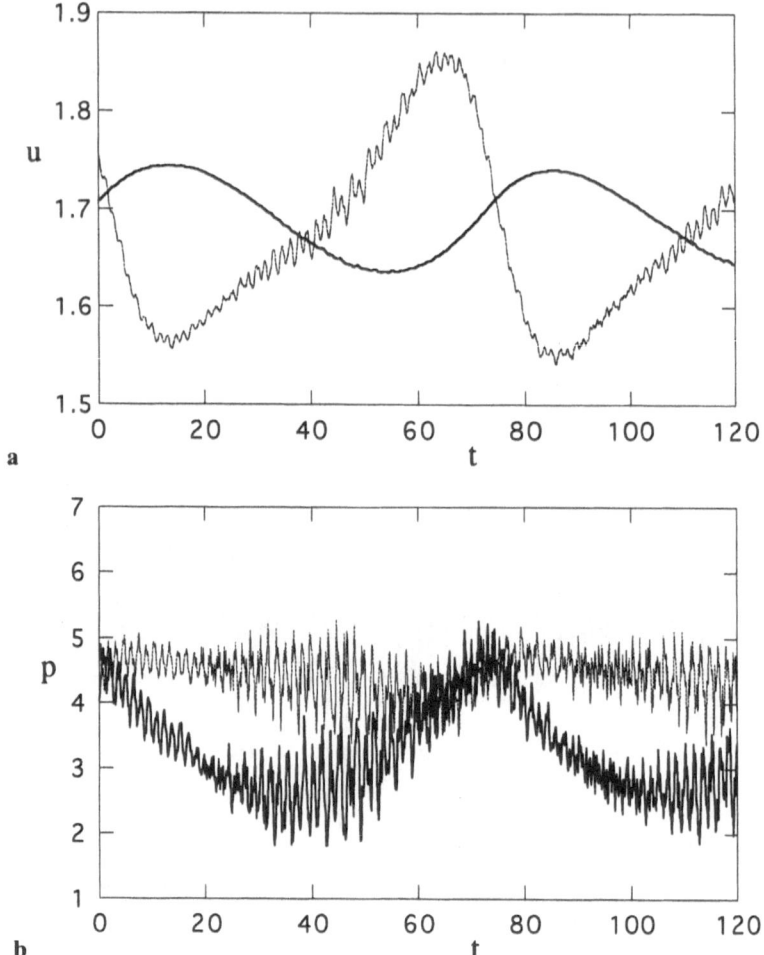

FIG. 4a–d. Numerical results for $\bar{q} = 1.7$ from the quasi-steady flow theory. **a** Time courses of velocities (*broken* and *solid curves* denote $u(0)$ and $u(20)$, respectively). **b** Time courses of pressures (*broken* and *solid curves* denote $P(0)$ and $P(20)$, respectively). **c** Time courses of $\Delta P = P(0) - P(20)$. **d** Time courses of x_T, x_S, and b_T (*solid*, *broken*, and *thin curves*, respectively)

quasi-steady 1-D separable flow theory. The numerical values used in the calculations are mostly the same as in [10], that is, $P_e = 5$, $\ell = 20$, $\ell_1 = 10$, $\ell_2 = 200$, $v_0 = 0.5$, $\varepsilon_0 = 0.25$, $\gamma_1 = 0.05$, $\gamma_2 = 0.02$, $\Delta t = 0.005$, $\Delta t = 0.4$, and $\chi_1 = 1$, and $g_1 = 0.01$ for the unseparated flow, and $\chi_1 = 0.2$ and $g_1 = 0$ for the separated flow. Here, we have introduced nondimensional parameters and variables, which are mostly represented by the corresponding lowercase characters. The lengths, the velocities, the pressures, and the time are referred to B_0, C, ρC^2, and B_0/C, respectively, where

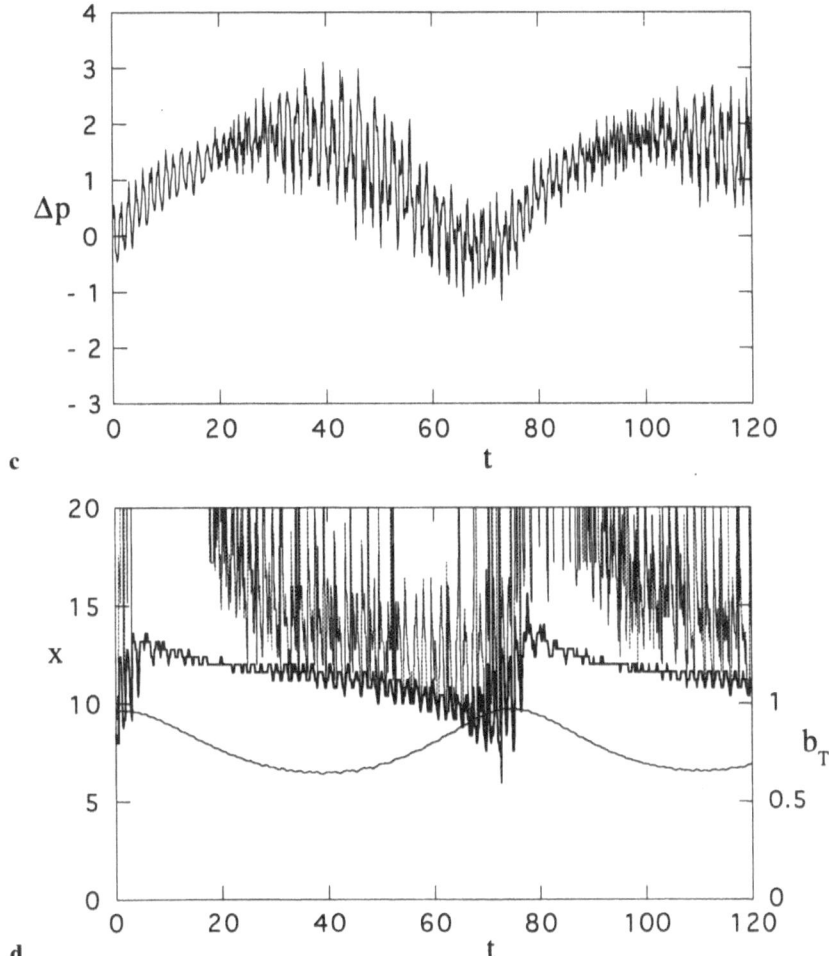

c

d

FIG. 4a–d. *Continued*

C is the propagation velocity of small disturbance. (More detail is available in [10].)

As in Matsuzaki et al. [9,10], the numerical calculations were performed for sufficiently long periods of time, so that the numerical results presented here are not transitional values which were observed in earlier phases from the initial states that were arbitrarily given for the initiation of the computation. Some typical results are presented here. The origin of time will be reassigned in all figures concerning the time course of the responses.

Figures 3 and 4 illustrate numerical results for $\bar{q} = 1.7$ calculated by the unsteady and the quasi-steady theory, respectively, where a bar over q denotes a mean value of q. In Fig. 3a and 3b, $u(0)$ and $p(0)$ and $u(20)$ and $p(20)$ are, respectively, plotted by broken and solid curves. The amplitude of the higher frequency mode seen in $u(20)$ is much smaller than that in $u(0)$ because the inertia force of the fluid in the rigid outlet channel is much larger than that in the inlet channel, as in [10]. Figure 3c illustrates the pressure drop $\Delta p = p(0) - p(20)$. In Fig. 3d, solid, broken, and thin curves denote the locations of the throat, x_T, and the separation point, x_S, and one-half of the breadth of the throat, b_T, respectively.

Figure 4a–d shows the same curves predicted by the quasi-steady theory as Fig. 3a–d. Comparison between the curves of $u(0)$ and $u(20)$ illustrated in Figs. 3a and 4a shows that the mean values of the corresponding velocity agree well with each other. The variance of $u(0)$, that is, the amplitude of the higher frequency component superposed on the fundmental mode observed in Fig. 3a, is several times larger than that in Fig. 4a. This fact is explained as follows: in the unsteady theory, the unsteadiness is introduced by adding Δu to the right-hand side of Eq. 6, while this term is neglected in the quasi-steady theory. This term may more accurately represent additional changes in the amplitude and the frequency of the flow velocity downstream of the separation point. The inclusion of this term also affects the flow and the channel motion upstream of the separation point. The oscillatory characteristic is much strengthened in the responses of $p(0)$ and $p(20)$ illustrated in Figs. 3b and 4b, compared with those of $u(0)$ and $u(20)$. Figures 3c and 4c show that certain aspects of the pressures are magnified in Δp. In Fig. 3d, when b_T approached a peak value, the motion of x_T became very large and x_S moved very closely with x_T. Except for this period, x_S was mostly separated from x_T and stayed far downstream of x_T. The flow was always separated. On the other hand, Fig. 4d shows that the flow was unseparated for a certain period, i.e., from $t = 3$ to $t = 18$, where b_T decreased from a peak value, and that this is not the case for $t = 80$ to $t = 90$ in the same situation. Comparison with Fig. 3d indicates that the motion of x_T was comparatively suppressed and x_S was also mostly far downstream of x_T.

As already pointed out in [10], the higher frequency component in $u(0)$ and $u(20)$ is closely associated with the fundamental frequency of the motion of x_S. The motion of all the variables evaluated by the quasi-steady flow theory was clearly suppressed, but the frequency of the higher mode was almost doubled. As the unsteady flow theory takes into account the higher order approximation, the oscillatory behavior of the higher frequency mode is considered more accurate than those predicted by the quasi-steady theory.

Figure 5 shows the time courses of the pressures at a smaller flow rate $\bar{q} = 1.1$ from the unsteady flow theory. A broken and a solid curve represent $p(0)$ and $p(20)$, respectively. Although the variances of the velocities, the pressures, and the motion of the separation point were much smaller than those observed in Fig. 3 and the fundamental frequency mode disappeared, which is not clearly seen in Fig. 5, the basic features of the oscillations were similar to those presented in Fig. 3.

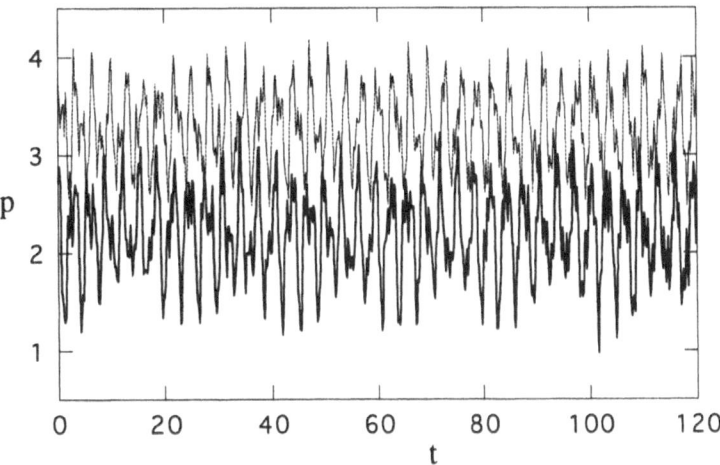

FIG. 5. Time courses of pressures, $\bar{q} = 1.1$ from the unsteady theory (*broken* and *solid* curves denote $P(0)$ and $P(20)$, respectively)

Now, we will examine the "unsteady" dynamic characteristics of the $\Delta p - \bar{q}$ relationship and the breadth of the flexible channel at $x = 10$, which are shown in Figs. 6a and 6b, respectively. A broken and a solid curve denote the mean and the static value, respectively, while a chained curve represents one standard deviation from the mean. Figure 7 shows the oscillatory aspects of the $\Delta p - \bar{q}$ curve for the same parameter values calculated by the quasi-steady flow theory, which is equivalent to Fig. 12a in [10]. Small differences between the corresponding curves of Figs. 7 and 12a are caused by the lengths of the time period used to calculate the means and the standard deviations. As easily anticipated from the comparison between Figs. 3 and 4, the standard deviation of the response predicted by the unsteady flow theory is larger than that by the quasi-steady theory in a flow region between $1.2 < \bar{q} < 2.0$, where the motions of all the variables were large. There was little difference between the standard deviations of $b(10)$ calculated by the unsteady and quasi-steady flow theories, because the motion of the channel wall was in the fundamental low-frequency mode.

The numerical results showed that the variances in the higher mode oscillation of the velocities and the pressures calculated by the unsteady flow theory were much bigger than those by the quasi-steady theory. The frequency of the higher mode was predicted to be approximately double in the latter compared with the former. The dynamic behaviors of the separation point predicted by both theories were quantitatively quite different, although qualitatively similar.

In the current analysis, no flow reattachment was accounted for downstream of the separation point. In other words, the flow was assumed to be reattached at the end of the flexible channel. It is obvious that the flow separation and reattachment influence the dynamic behavior of the flow–channel. Ikeda and Matsuzaki

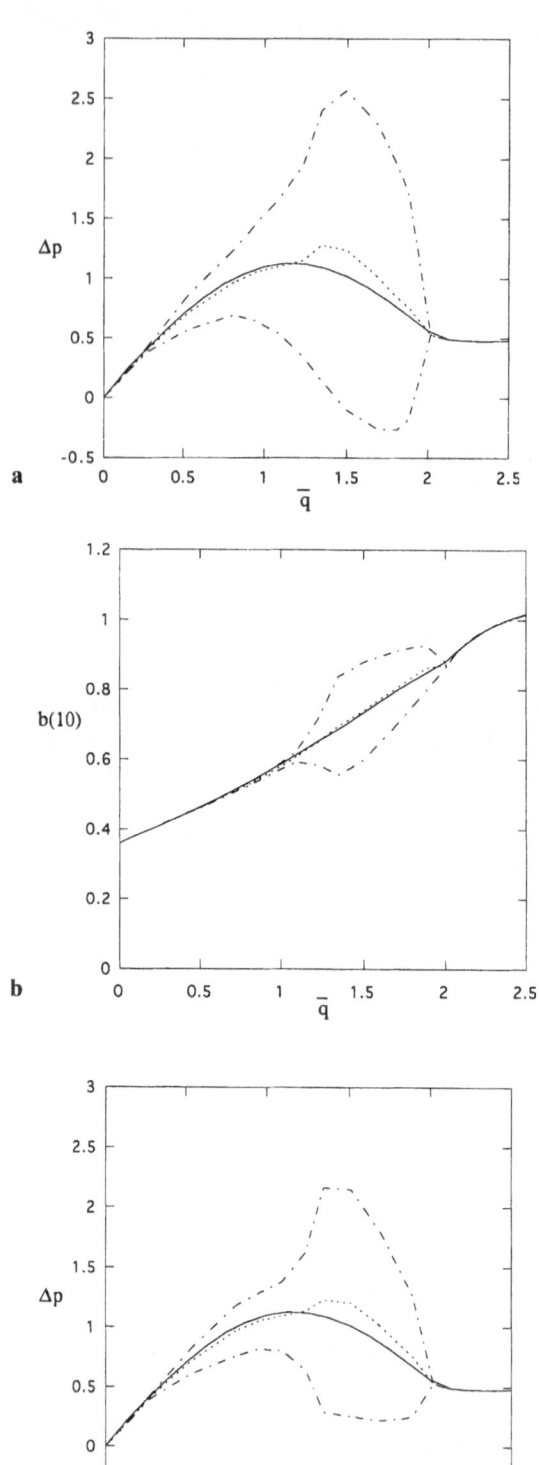

FIG. 6a,b. Oscillatory characterestics of ΔP and $b(10)$ predicted by the unsteady theory (*solid*, *broken*, and *chained curves* denote the static value, the mean value, and the standard deviation, respectively). **a** ΔP versus $\bar{q}$. **b** $b(10)$ versus $\bar{q}$

FIG. 7. Oscillatory characterestics of ΔP versus $\bar{q}$ predicted by the quasi-steady theory (*solid*, *broken*, and *chained curves* denote the static value, the mean value, and the standard deviation, respectively)

[6] have presented an improved 1-D separable flow theory in which the separated flow is reattached downstream of the separation point. If there were accurately observed experimental data on flow separation and the motion of the separation point, such detailed numerical analysis on the flow separation characteristics would be more useful for further improving and establishing a 1-D separable/reattachable flow theory.

4   Conclusions

The self-excited oscillation of the flow in the 2-D collapsible channel was studied numerically by using the unsteady and the quasi-steady 1-D separable flow theories. The oscillatory characteristics of the higher frequency mode of the flow–channel behavior predicted by both theories were different from the quantitative point of view. Because the flow separation, and therefore the flow recovery from the separation, are considered very influential to the dynamic aspects of the self-excited oscillation of the flow–channel, experimental observation and measurement on the motion of the flow separation and reattachment are very important for improvement of the unsteady separable flow theory.

Acknowledgment. This work was partially supported by the Grant-in-Aid for Scientific Research on Priority Area [Biomechanics] (No. 04237103) and for Cooperative Research (A) (No. 04305008) from the Ministry of Education, Science and Culture in Japan.

References

1. Matsuzaki Y (1986) Self-excited oscillation of a collapsible tube conveying fluid. In: Schmid-Schoenbein GW, Woo ALY, Zweifach BW (eds) Frontiers in biomechanics. Springer-Verlag, New York, pp 342–350
2. Kamm RD, Pedley TJ (1989) Flow in collapsible tubes: a brief review. J Biomech Eng 111:177–179
3. Matsuzaki Y, Fung YC (1976) On separation of a divergent flow at moderate Reynolds numbers. J Appl Mech 98:227–231
4. Conrad WA (1969) Pressure-flow relationships in collapsible tubes. IEEE Trans Biomed Eng BME-16:284–295
5. Katz AI, Chen Y, Moreno AH (1969) Flow through a collapsible tube. Experimental analysis and mathematical model. Biophys J 9:1261–1279
6. Ikeda T, Matsuzaki Y (1994) Flow theory for analysis of phonation with a membrane model of vocal cord. In: Proceedings, 1994 international conference on spoken language processing. Acoustical Society of Japan, Yokohama, pp 643–646
7. Matsuzaki Y (1986) Stability of flat plates and cylindrical shells exposed to flows. In: Cheremisinoff NP (ed) Encyclopedia of fluid mechanics. Gulf, Houston, pp 476–509
8. Cancelli C, Pedley TJ (1985) A separated flow model for collapsible-tube oscillations. J Fluid Mech 157:375–404
9. Matsuzaki Y, Matsumoto T (1989) Flow in a two-dimensional collapsible channel with rigid inlet and outlet. J Biomech Eng 111:180–184

10. Matsuzaki Y, Ikeda T, Kitagawa T, Sakata S (1994) Analysis of flow in a two-dimensional collapsible channel using universal "tube" law. J Biomech Eng 116:469–476

11. Matsumoto T, Matsuzaki Y (1994) Mathematical modeling for the unsteady flow separation through a collapsible channel. In: Liepsch D (ed) Proceedings of the 3rd international symposium of biofluid mechanics. VDI, Düsseldorf, pp 261–269

12. Matsumoto T (1991) Flow in a collapsible tube. Ph.D. dissertation. Nagoya University

Numerical Simulator for Left-Ventricular Functions

MASATAKA TOKUDA and YUTAKA SAWAKI[1]

Summary. A numerical simulation system using the three-dimensional finite-element method (FEM) is established to reproduce the performance of the left ventricle during one cardiac cycle, which may ultimately provide useful information for medical diagnoses. The simulation system consists of a 3-D-FEM mechanical model of the left ventricle based on four fundamental models: (1) a mechanical model of myocardial muscle fiber, which produces the active force; (2) a mechanical model of the left ventricle, which is composed of the model muscle fiber; (3) a transmission model of electric stimulus, and (4) a circulatory system model that provides the after- and preloads for the left-ventricular model. In this chapter, the fundamental system of the simulator is explained, and some typical examples of computational results obtained by this system are shown and discussed. The reliability of the simulator is examined by comparing some numerical results on pressure–volume relationships for different peripheral vascular resistances, aortic compliances, and characteristic impedances with the corresponding experimental results obtained from a canine heart.

Key words: Biomechanics—Left ventricle—Numerical simulation—Finite-element analysis—Pressure–volume relationship

1 Introduction

Attempts to apply numerical simulation techniques to evaluations of bionic functions have recently been on the increase; they concern, for example, the functions of the cerebrum, the respiratory system, and so on, including the function of the heart considered here. The background of such activity is as follows: first, the performance of computer hardware has been highly improved from the aspects of calculation speed and memory capacity. Second, in vivo information from a living body, which is necessary for constructing a mathematical model of an organ, can be obtained by several newly developed measuring

---

[1] Department of Mechanical Engineering, Mie University, 1515 Kamihama, Tsu, Mie, 514 Japan

techniques and advanced diagnosis imaging. In particular, magnetic resonance imaging (MRI), X-ray computed tomography (CT), and ultrasonic CT, for example, have been remarkably developed, and they make it possible to observe the in vivo performance of living organs without damaging the living tissues.

The living body can be considered as a quite complex system with many functions, and controlled in a multiplex way to cope with severe, continuous external excitement with optimum efficiency through a complex nerve network (stimulus conduction system). The elegant but complex characteristics of the living body, such as, multiple functions, acclimation, and self-restoration, make it quite difficult to solve intrinsically the problems with respect to the living body [1]. Considering this situation, a numerical simulation technique is expected to be best suited for elucidating this complex system.

In their previous work [2], the authors proposed a fundamental numerical simulation system on the basis of a two-dimensional, finite-element, left-ventricular model closely linked with both a circulatory system of blood and a transmission system of electric stimuli. There are, however, several limitations in the two-dimensional model when we try to analyze several interesting and important features of left ventricle, e.g., the effect of electric stimulus transmission along the three-dimensional nerve network; the effect of myocardial muscle fiber orientation, which is three-dimensionally distributed in some complex manner; and the realistic stress and strain distributions in the ventricular wall for the normal as well as the diseased heart.

In this chapter, we attempt to construct a numerical simulation system on the basis of a three-dimensional finite-element model to estimate the three-dimensional features of the left ventricle [3]. The system proposed here is composed of the following four fundamental and physically supported mathematical model elements: (1) a mechanical model of myocardial muscle fiber [4], (2) a mechanical model of the left ventricle that is constructed by a three-dimensionally distributed muscle fiber model, (3) a three-dimensional transmission model of electric stimuli, and (4) a circulatory system model, including the effect of the vasculature network. The numerical simulation system may be expected to improve heart disease diagnoses [5] from being empirical, subjective, and qualitative to being scientific, objective, and quantitative. The reliability of the present simulation system of the left ventricle is examined by comparing some numerical results and the corresponding canine experimental results on pressure–volume relationships for different peripheral vascular resistances, aortic compliances, and characteristic impedances. Additionally, the effect of three-dimensional muscle fiber orientation on the performances of the left ventricle in one cardiac cycle is discussed through some numerical results obtained by using the simulator constructed here.

2 Mathematical Model of the Left Ventricle

The contraction and relaxation of the left ventricle are cyclically continued by the harmonic and systematic cooperation of the mechanical behavior of numerous muscle fibers excited by the synchronized electric stimulus in the wall of the left ventricle, which interacts with the connected circulatory system. A mathematical model of the left ventricle that can reproduce such elegant cyclic performances is described here.

2.1 Mechanical Model of Myocardial Muscle Fiber

To reproduce the movement of the left ventricle, we first study the active force induced in the myocardium, which is a quite different aspect from the point of view of conventional engineering materials. The myocardium consists of numerous contractile muscle fiber elements called sarcomeres, which produce an active tensile force and contract by themselves after receiving the electric stimulus sent from the so-called pacemaker of the heart (nodus sinuatrialis) [6].

The magnitude of the active tensile force produced by the sarcomeres may be approximated through a set of simple relations proposed by Beyar and Sideman [7] as follows:

$$\sigma_f = \sigma_{max} \sin(\pi t/T_0) \quad (0 \leq t < T_0) \tag{1}$$

$$\sigma_f = 0 \quad (T_0 \leq t) \tag{2}$$

where σ_f is a nominal active tensile stress, that is, the active force divided by the original cross-sectional area of the myocardium, T_0 is the activation time of the myocardium, and t is the time measured from the instance at which the electric stimulus arrives at the myocardium. The maximum active stress σ_{max} induced in the myocardium depends on the length of the sarcomere fiber L, and may be represented in the following manner:

$$\sigma_{max} = 0 \quad (L < 1.65\,\mu m) \tag{3}$$

$$\sigma_{max} = \{(L - 1.65)/0.55\}\sigma_0$$
$$(1.65\,\mu m \leq L < 2.20\,\mu m) \tag{4}$$

$$\sigma_{max} = \sigma_0 \quad (2.20\,\mu m \leq L < 2.40\,\mu m) \tag{5}$$

$$\sigma_{max} = \{(2.40 - L)/0.55\}\,\sigma_0 + \sigma_0$$
$$(2.40\,\mu m \leq L < 2.95\,\mu m) \tag{6}$$

$$\sigma_{max} = 0 \quad (L \geq 2.95\,\mu m) \tag{7}$$

where σ_0 is a material constant.

The following must be taken into consideration when we employ this model for the deformation/stress analysis of the left ventricle; the magnitude of active force induced in the myocardium is proportional to the number of fibers of which the muscle body is composed, rather than the cross-sectional area, because the myocardium fiber element (sarcomere) is a contractile unit. In this work, while the actual stress diminishes with the increase of the cross-sectional area of the muscle owing to its contraction, the magnitude of the resultant force induced in the muscle is independent of cross-sectional area. To incorporate this mechanism, the following stress $\bar{\sigma}_f$, called the normalized active fiber stress, is introduced.

$$dT = \bar{\sigma}_f \, dA_0 = \sigma_f \, dA \tag{8}$$

and thus

$$\bar{\sigma}_f = \sigma_f \, dA_0/dA \tag{9}$$

where T is the active tensile force induced in the muscle body, and A_0 and A are the original and current cross-sectional areas of the muscle body, respectively. This normalized active stress is employed for our analyses.

2.2 Three-Dimensional Transmission Model of Electric Stimulus

The electric stimulus launched from the pacemaker (sinoatrial node) is transmitted first to the apex through a ventricular septum and second to the basis through Purkinje's fibers, which are distributed on the endocardium surface, at a relatively high speed in the meridian direction; last, the stimulus is transmitted in the thickness direction radially from the activated portion of the endocardium to the epicardium.

Considering this transmission pathway, in the present mathematical model it is appropriate to assume that the electric stimulus is launched from the apex in the endocardium (point A in Fig. 1), and transmitted first along the meridian direction on the endocardium (arrow 1 in Fig. 1) and second in the thickness direction (arrow 2 in Fig. 1) from an activated portion (for example, point Q in Fig. 1) to the epicardium. Then the active stress induced at a point P in the muscle fiber in Fig. 1 can be expressed as follows:

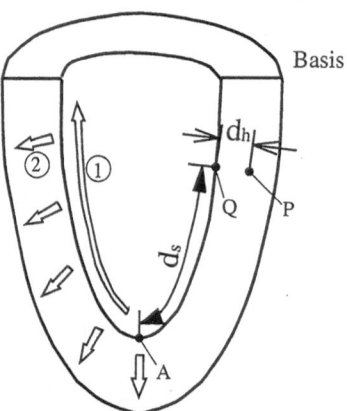

FIG. 1. Pathway of electric stimulus transmission, first along the meridian of the endocardium (*arrow 1*) and then across the ventricle wall (*arrows 2*)

$$\sigma_f = \sigma_{\max} \sin\left[\pi(t - \tau_s - \tau_h)/T_0\right] \qquad (0 \leqq t < T_0) \tag{10}$$

$$\tau_s = d_s/v_s \tag{11}$$

$$\tau_h = d_h/v_h \tag{12}$$

where t is the time counted from the arrival of the electric stimulus at the apex, τ_s and τ_h are the time-lag parameters of the electric stimulus transmission in the meridian and thickness directions, respectively, v_s and v_h are the transmission velocities in each direction, d_s is the distance measured from the apex in the meridian, and d_h is measured from an activated portion Q in the thickness direction.

2.3 Three-Dimensional Finite-Element Model of the Left Ventricle and Installation of Muscle Fiber Orientation

Although the real structure and geometry of the left ventricle are quite complex (particularly the fiber orientation of the myocardium) [8–10], we adopt structure and geometry as simple as possible because our present interest is to construct a basic simulation system as the preliminary step of this project. Several simplified analyses [7,11,12] employing the thin (or thick) spherical (or oval) shell model of the left ventricle, however, are not selected here. To retain the possibility of properly taking into account the realistic complex structure and geometry, a three-dimensional finite-element model [13,14] is constructed in this project. The initial geometry of the left ventricle is assumed to be a prolate spheroid for simplicity in the first construction stage of the finite-element model to make it easy to estimate the complex results obtained.

The three-dimensional finite-element model of the left ventricle constructed here is as follows: the geometry of the left ventricle is selected as a prolate spheroid. The ventricular wall is assumed to be an isotropically elastic material with myocardial muscle fibers whose orientations alter continuously from endocardium to epicardium (Fig. 2). The myocardial fiber angle is installed to the finite-element model by the following manner. First, taking a standard cubic finite-element $A–H$ under the local coordinate system xyz as shown in Fig. 3a, the

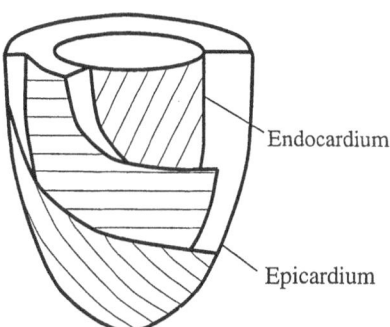

Endocardium

Epicardium

FIG. 2. Schematic structure of myocardial muscle fiber direction in the ventricular wall

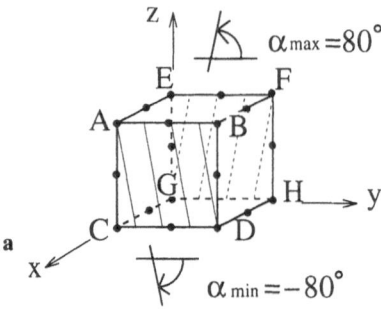

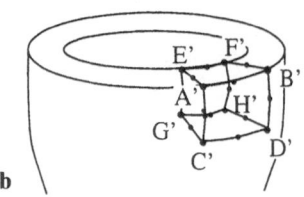

FIG. 3a,b. Modeling of myocardial muscle fiber orientation. **a** Local coordinate system *xyz*. **b** Global coordinate system. *ABCD* (*A'B'C'D'*), epicardium; *EFGH* (*E'F'G'H'*), endocardium; *black circles*, nodal points

fiber angle in the element is assumed to be $\alpha_{max} = +80°$ on the endocardium surface and $\alpha_{min} = -80°$ on the epicardium surface, and interpolated linearly through the cubic element. As a four-point Gauss quadrature is employed in the present analysis, there exist 64 Gaussian points in one finite element. The fiber angle is assigned at each Gaussian point according to the fiber orientation scheme just described. The final fiber orientation in the left-ventricular wall is realized by transforming the standard element *A–H* in the local coordinate system to the element *A'–H'* in the global coordinate system (Fig. 3b).

In the present numerical scheme, the isoparametric parallelepiped finite element with 16 nodes is employed to make it easy to handle the active tensile force induced by the distributed muscle fibers. Such elements, 128 in total, are arranged along the ventricular wall (see Fig. 11 later in this chapter for an example). The active stress in each element is treated as the internal stress induced along a three-dimensionally distributed muscle fiber. Such active stresses are realized by considering them as the time-dependent internal stresses on 64 Gaussian points in each element. In this chapter, the myocardial fiber is considered to be the force-induced element, as described by Eqs. 3–7. On the other hand, it is sometimes considered to be the displacement-induced element. In this case, the internal strain, such as thermal strain, must be considered instead of the internal stress. Real muscle fibers may be between these two models. A more elaborate mechanical model of muscle fiber may be necessary when an attempt to construct a more accurate simulation system of the left ventricle is made at the next stage.

Assuming that the myocardium is the elastic material that produces the internal (active) stress, the relation between the stress vector $\{\sigma\}$ and the strain vector $\{\varepsilon\}$ is

$$\{\sigma\} = [D]\{\varepsilon\} + \{\bar{\sigma}_a\} \tag{13}$$

where $[D]$ is the elastic constant matrix and $\{\bar{\sigma}_a\}$ is the normalized active stress vector. When the cylindrical coordinate system $(x_1, x_2, x_3) = (r, \theta, z)$ is introduced and the orientation of the sarcomere is taken in the $x_2 = \theta$ direction

$$\{\bar{\sigma}_a\} = \{\bar{\sigma}_1, \bar{\sigma}_2, \bar{\sigma}_3, \bar{\sigma}_4, \bar{\sigma}_5, \bar{\sigma}_6\}^T$$
$$= \{0, \bar{\sigma}_f, 0, 0, 0, 0\}^T \qquad (14)$$

where $\bar{\sigma}_f$ is the normalized active stress described in the preceding section.

For each element $\{e\}$, the following identity may be derived by virtue of the so-called principle of virtual work [15]:

$$\{F\}^e = \left(\int_v [B]^T [D][B] dV\right)\{d\}^e + \int_v [B]^T \{\bar{\sigma}_a\} dV - \int_s [N]^T \{p\} dS \qquad (15)$$

where $\{F\}^e$, $\{d\}$, and $\{p\}$ are the equivalent nodal force vector, the displacement vector, and the distributed load applied on the element surface under consideration, respectively; $[B]$, $[D]$, and $[N]$ are the strain displacement matrix, the elastic constant matrix, and the shape function, respectively; and V and S are respectively the element volume and the area of the element on which the distributed load $\{p\}$ acts. In this identity, the stiffness matrix of the element is

$$[K] = \int_v [B]^T [D][B] dV \qquad (16)$$

the nodal force equivalent to the active contractile force is

$$\{F_a\}^e = \int_v [B]^T \{\bar{\sigma}_a\} dV \qquad (17)$$

and the nodal force equivalent to the distributed load is

$$\{F_p\}^e = \int_s [N]^T \{p\} dS \qquad (18)$$

3 Circulatory System Model of the Blood

The left ventricle supplies arterial blood to our body through the vascular network. The barrier that the left ventricle must overcome to eject a sufficient amount of blood, that is, the aorta pressure at the aortic valve, is called the afterload. The afterload depends on the elastic properties of the aorta, the peripheral vascular resistance, and so on. The blood that returns from the lung is reserved temporarily in the left atrium, and after that it flows into the left ventricle. The left ventricle is distended with the blood inflow, whose amount is called the preload. The preload depends on not only the mechanical properties of the left ventricle but also on the mechanical properties of the vasculature, including the left atrium and the pulmonary vein, which belong to the entrance side of the left ventricle.

To concentrate on the estimation of mechanical properties and functions of the left ventricle, we employ the simplified electric circuit analogy model, which provides the proper pre- and afterloads to the left ventricle. Among several proposed models, we select here the electric circuit model constructed by Sekioka [16] (Fig. 4). The left-hand side of the circuit corresponds to the circulatory system model, which produces the preload at the input side, including the effects of the left pulmonary vein, the left atrium, and so on. The right-hand side corresponds to the circulatory system, which produces the afterload at the output side, including the effects of the aortic compliance, the peripheral vasculature, and so on.

In this electric circuit analogy model, the voltage and electric current correspond to the blood pressure and the blood flux, respectively, the resistances correspond to the vascular and valvular resistances for the blood flow, and the condensers correspond to the elastic properties of the vasculature (the amount of blood preserved in the vasculature depends strongly on the elastic property of the vessel). The battery indicates the averaged blood pressure to which the pre- and afterloads are subjects stationarily. In this circuit, the left ventricle is regarded as a kind of generator producing the fluctuating voltage (blood pressure) or fluctuating electric current (the blood flux). The following relations hold among the blood flux (Q, electric current), the blood pressure (P, voltage), the flow resistance (R, electric resistance), and the deformability of the blood vessel (C, electric capacitance).

For the preload system:

$$Q_1(t) = \{P_v - P_{vl}(t)\}/R_{vl} \tag{19}$$

$$Q_2(t) = \{P_{vl}(t) - P_h(t)\}/R_{v2} \tag{20}$$

$$dP_{vl}(t)/dt = \{Q_1(t) - Q_2(t)\}/C_v \tag{21}$$

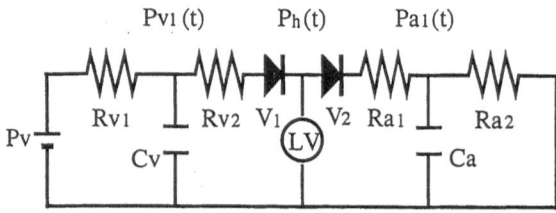

FIG. 4. Circulatory system model. LV, Left ventricle; P_v, mean pulmonary arterial pressure; R_{vl}, pulmonary venous vascular resistance; R_{v2}, mitral valvular resistance; V_1, mitral valve; C_v, pulmonary vein and left atrial compliances; P_a, mean peripheral arterial pressure; R_{a1}, characteristic impedance; P_{a1}, peripheral vascular resistance; V_2, aortic valve; C_a, aortic compliance; $P_h(t)$, left ventricular pressure; $P_{a1}(t)$, aortic pressure; $P_{vl}(t)$, left atrial pressure

The role of the mitral valve preventing a backward flow of blood may be realized by taking

$$Q_2(t) = 0 \qquad (22)$$

when $P_h(t) \geq P_{v1}(t)$. For the afterload system:

$$Q_3(t) = \{P_h(t) - P_{al}(t)\}/R_{al} \qquad (23)$$

$$Q_4(t) = \{P_{al}(t) - P_a\}/R_{a2} \qquad (24)$$

$$dP_{al}(t)/dt = \{Q_3(t) - Q_4(t)\}/C_a \qquad (25)$$

The role of the aortic valve preventing a backward flow of blood also can be realized by taking

$$Q_3(t) = 0 \qquad (26)$$

when $P_h(t) \leq P_{al}(t)$. In Eqs. 20 and 23, $Q_2(t)$ and $Q_3(t)$ are the input and output of the left ventricle, respectively, and they correspond to the variation of the left-ventricular volume. That is, when the aortic valve is open (the ejection period), for the afterload system

$$V(t + dt) = V(t) - Q_3(t)dt \qquad (27)$$

and when the mitral valve is open (the diastolic period), for the preload system

$$V(t + dt) = V(t) + Q_2(t)dt \qquad (28)$$

where $V(t)$ is the volume of the left ventricle at time t.

4 Computational Process for the Proposed Model

The performance of the left ventricle is analyzed by using the mechanical model system just described, composed of four simple and fundamental models: a mechanical model of myocardial muscle fiber, a mechanical model of the left ventricle, a circulatory system model expressed by the electric circuit analogy, and a transmission model of electric stimulus. The phases (period) in a cardiac cycle are judged by comparing the magnitude of ventricular, aortic, and pulmonary pressures: P_h, P_{al}, and P_{v1}. The simulation proceeds with computing the values at time $t + dt$ by using the known values at time t.

4.1 Isovolumetric Contraction period: $P_h(t) \leq P_{al}(t)$ and $P_h(t) \geq P_{v1}(t)$

In this period, both the mitral and aortic valves are closed, and thus $Q_2(t) = Q_3(t) = 0$, as expressed in Eqs. 22 and 26. The values of dP_{v1}/dt and dP_{al}/dt are evaluated from Eqs. 21 and 25 using $Q_1(t)$ and $Q_4(t)$ calculated from Eqs. 19 and 24. At the next time step, $t + dt$,

$$P_{al}(t+dt) = P_{al}(t) + (dP_{al}/dt)dt \tag{29}$$

$$P_{vl}(t+dt) = P_{vl}(t) + (dP_{vl}/dt)dt \tag{30}$$

Independently of this pressure, the magnitude of the active stress $\sigma_f(t)$ in the ventricular wall increases in the current period, and thus the ventricular pressure $P_h(t)$ heightens according to the increase of the active force. Then the active stress $\sigma_f(t + dt)$ at the time $t + dt$ is evaluated by using Eqs. 10–12. The increment of the ventricular pressure $(dP_h/dt)dt$, which keeps the volume of the left ventricle constant against the increase of active stress $(d\sigma_f/dt)dt = \sigma_f(t + dt) - \sigma_f(t)$ is determined through the finite-element analysis described by Eqs. 13–18. Consequently, the ventricular pressure at the next time step can be evaluated in the same form as Eq. 29 or 30, as follows:

$$P_h(t+dt) = P_h(t) + (dP_h/dt)dt \tag{31}$$

In this period, $(dP_{al}/dt)dt < 0$ and $(dP_h/dt)dt > 0$, and thus the aortic pressure P_{al} decreases while the ventricular pressure P_h increases. When $P_{al}(t) = P_h(t)$ is achieved by repeating this numerical procedure, the aortic value is opened, and the ejection period begins.

4.2 Ejection Period: $P_h(t) \geqq P_{al}(t)$ and $P_h(t) \geqq P_{vl}(t)$

In this period, the aortic valve is open and the blood is ejected from the left ventricle with its volume change. The simulation process in this period can be described as follows. As seen in Eq. 22, when $P_h(t) \geqq P_{vl}(t)$, the mitral valve is closed and the blood flux to the left ventricle $Q_2(t)$ vanishes. In this case, the output blood flux $Q_3(t)$ is calculated by Eq. 23. The pressure changes dP_{vl}/dt and dP_{al}/dt are evaluated by Eqs. 21 and 25 with the value of $Q_1(t)$ and $Q_4(t)$ calculated from Eqs. 19 and 24. Therefore, the next time step pressures $P_{al}(t + dt)$ and $P_{vl}(t + dt)$ are determined through Eqs. 29 and 30.

On the other hand, the variation of the ventricular pressure $(dP_h/dt)dt$, in keeping with both the variation of the active stress $(d\bar{\sigma}_f/dt)dt$ and the change of ventricular volume equivalent to the output blood flux $Q_3(t)$, is determined through the present finite-element analysis, and thus the ventricular pressure $P_h(t + dt)$ at the next time step is obtained. In the first half of this period, even if the output blood flux $Q_3(t)$ occurs, the ventricular pressure $P_h(t)$ continues to increase with the increase of active force, and $P_h(t) \geqq P_{al}(t)$ holds. In the latter half of this period, the ventricular pressure $P_h(t)$ decreases according to the decrease of the active stress, and finally $P_h(t) = P_{al}(t)$ occurs. When $P_h(t) = P_{al}(t)$ is fulfilled, the aortic valve is closed immediately to prevent the backflow of blood from the aorta to the left ventricle. And thus, the next phase, named the isovolumetric relaxation period, arises.

4.3 Isovolumetric Relaxation Period: $P_h(t) \leq P_{a1}(t)$ and $P_h(t) \geq P_{v1}(t)$

In this period, both the aortic and mitral valves are closed, and again $Q_2(t) = Q_3(t) = 0$ holds. The simulation procedure is almost the same as that in the isovolumetric contraction period except that the ventricular pressure $P_h(t)$ decreases quickly according to the decrease of the active stress. When $P_h(t) = P_{v1}(t)$ is fulfilled, the mitral valve opens, and the diastolic period, in which the blood flows into the left ventricle from the left atrium, commences.

4.4 Diastolic Period: $P_h(t) \leq P_{a1}(t)$ and $P_h(t) \leq P_{v1}(t)$

In this period, the ventricular volume increases because of input blood flux $Q_2(t)$ from the left atrium. Explanation of the simulation procedure in this period is omitted because there is no essential difference between the diastolic and ejection period except that $Q_2(t) \neq 0$ and $Q_3(t) = 0$ in the diastolic period while $Q_2(t) = 0$ and $Q_3(t) \neq 0$ in the ejection period.

5 Numerical Results and Discussion

When applying the numerical method to the mathematical models of the left ventricle, the mechanical properties of the myocardial muscle fiber, such as Young's modulus, Poisson ratio, maximum active force, and the characteristics of circulation system models must be selected in advance. The former is not determined for a specific individual, but is chosen on the basis of work by others [3,14,17,18] as well as the experience and knowledge of some medical doctors. Furthermore, these material constants are corrected slightly by the trial-and-error technique to adjust some obtained computational results to the corresponding available experimental results (e.g., the pressure–volume relation of left ventricle) [16]. On the other hand, as for the latter, the same parameters as employed in the corresponding canine experiment [16] are selected. Several parameters employed in the simulation are presented in Table 1.

The characteristics of left-ventricular structure may be divided into three main elements: the three-dimensional geometry (shape), the orientation of muscle fibers, and the transmission system of electric stimulus. From the point of view of biomechanics or biomedical mechanics, the relations among these elements related to the structure and the mechanical functions of the left ventricle are quite interesting. In this chapter, the adequacy of the numerical simulator is examined, first by comparing the pressure–volume relations of the left ventricle obtained by experiment with those computed by the current simulator, and then the effect of muscle fiber orientation on the performances of left ventricle for one cardiac cycle is estimated by using the developed numerical simulator.

5.1 Pressure–Volume Relation

The typical pressure-volume relation of the left ventricle computed by using the proposed simulation system assisted by the finite-element technique are shown in Figs. 5–7 for different peripheral vascular resistances (R_{a2}), aortic compliances

TABLE 1. Parameters used in numerical simulation.

Parameter	Value
Young's modulus of left-ventricular wall, E	53.3 (kPa)
Poisson's ratio, left-ventricular wall, v	0.49
Maximum active stress, σ_0	53.3 (kPa)
Activation time, T_0	0.26 (s)
Initial sarcomere length, L	2.00 (μm)
Transmission velocity of electric stimulus (meridian direction), v_s	5.00 m/s
Transmission velocity of electric stimulus (tickness direction), v_h	0.50 m/s
Mean pulmonary arterial pressure, P_v	18.00 (mmHg)
Pulmonary venous vascular resistance, R_{v1}	0.03 (mmHg·s/ml)
Mitral valvular resistance, R_{v2}	0.05 (mmHg·s/ml)
Pulmonary vein and left atrial compliances, C_v	1.00 (ml/mmHg)
Characteristic impedance, R_{a1}	0.10–0.80 (mmHg·s/ml)
Peripheral vascular resistance, R_{a2}	1.00–12.00 (mmHg·s/ml)
Aortic compliance, C_a	0.07–0.80 (ml/mmHg)

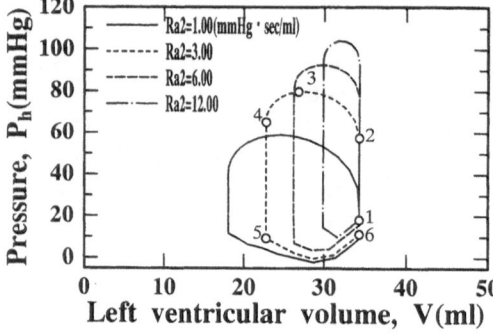

FIG. 5. Pressure–volume relations for different peripheral vascular resistances, R_{a2} (simulation)

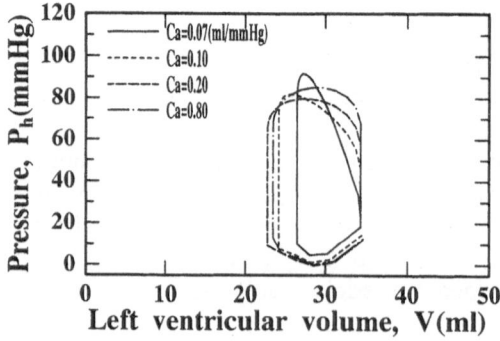

FIG. 6. Pressure–volume relations for different aortic compliance, C_a (simulation)

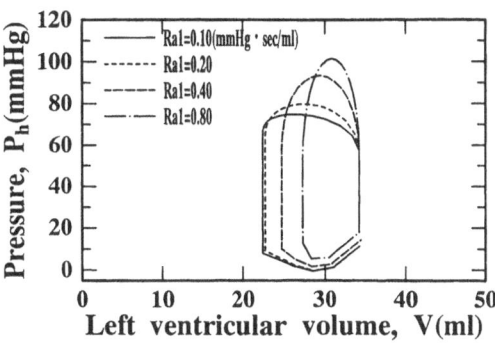

FIG. 7. Pressure–volume relations for different characteristic impedance, R_{a1} (simulation)

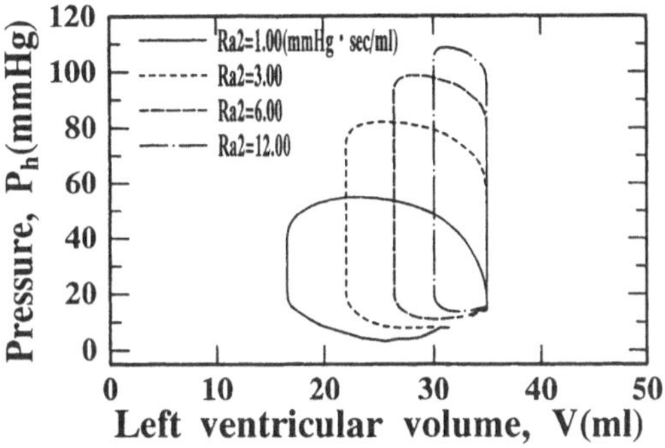

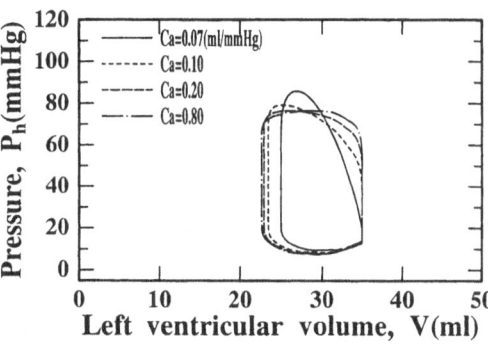

FIG. 8. Pressure–volume relations for different peripheral vascular resistances, R_{a2} (experiments)

FIG. 9. Pressure–volume relations for different aortic compliance, C_a (experiments)

FIG. 10. Pressure–volume relations for different characteristic impedance, R_{a1} (experiments)

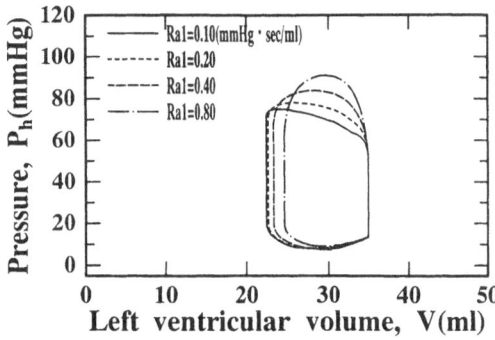

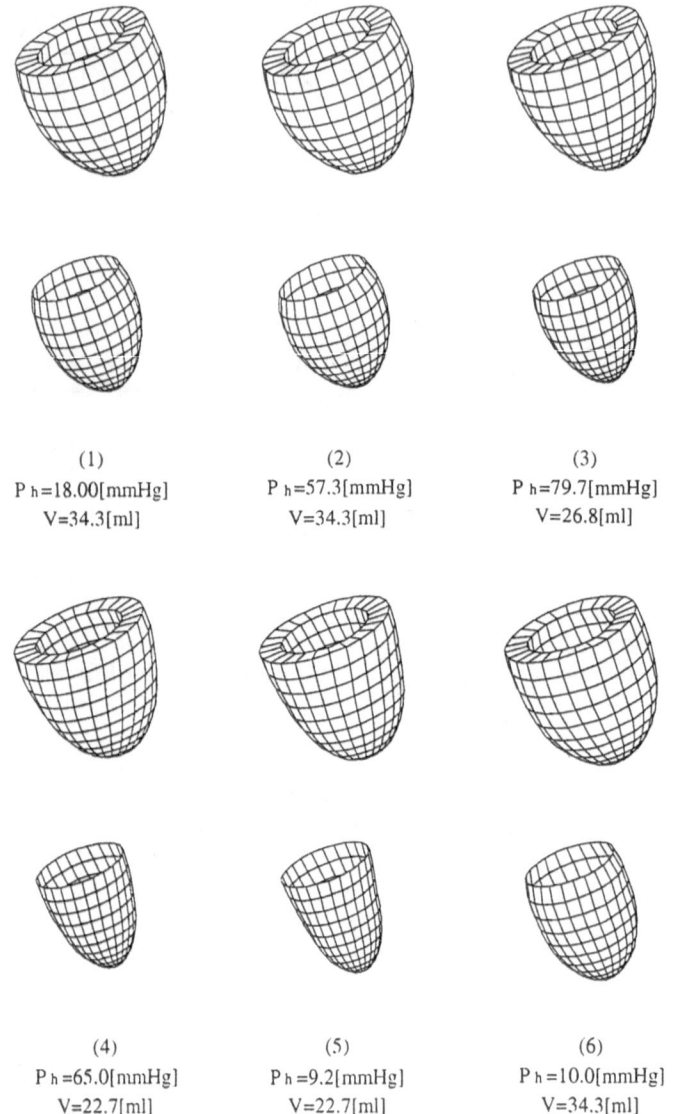

(1)
P h=18.00[mmHg]
V=34.3[ml]

(2)
P h=57.3[mmHg]
V=34.3[ml]

(3)
P h=79.7[mmHg]
V=26.8[ml]

(4)
P h=65.0[mmHg]
V=22.7[ml]

(5)
P h=9.2[mmHg]
V=22.7[ml]

(6)
P h=10.0[mmHg]
V=34.3[ml]

FIG. 11. Simulated performance of left ventricle (R_{a2} = 3.00 mmHg·s/ml)

(C_a), and characteristic impedances (R_{a1}), and the corresponding experimental results are presented in Figs. 8–10. As recognized from these figures, the present simulator may reproduce well the corresponding experimental results. Comparing the computational results for different peripheral vascular resistances R_{a2} (Fig. 5) with the corresponding experimental results (Fig. 8), for example, the following features of the pressure–volume relation are detected: the internal pressure of the left ventricle heightens and the ejection volume per cardiac cycle decreases according to the increase of peripheral vascular resistance value.

Figure 11 depicts the performance of the left ventricle ($R_{a2} = 3.00\,\mathrm{mmHg \cdot s/ml}$) obtained by the numerical simulation. In this figure, the upper side of each figure shows the overall behavior of left ventricle and the lower one illustrates the behavior of the epicardial surface. The numbers (1)–(6) indicated in each figure correspond to circle symbols 1–6 attached on the pressure–volume loop in Fig. 5. From this figure, it can be recognized that the behavior of the left ventricle simulated here reproduces the circumferential torsion phenomenon of the ventricular wall generally seen when the left ventricle is in the ejection period.

5.2 Effect of Muscle Fiber Orientation

The distributions of orientation angle are assumed to be linear through the thickness of ventricular wall as employed here. To examine the effect of myocardial muscle fiber orientation, four kinds of angle ranges, $\alpha_{max}-\alpha_{min} = +80°$ to $-80°$, $+60°$ to $-60°$, $+40°$ to $-40°$, and $+20°$ to $-20°$, are selected in this simulation.

Figure 12 shows the pressure–volume relationship corresponding to the selected muscle fiber orientations obtained by the computations. As seen here, the attained maximum pressure and the ejection volume per cardiac cycle (the stroke volume) are increased with the decrease of the orientation angle range from $\pm80°$ to $\pm20°$; that is, the mechanical pumping function of the left ventricle is rather better when the range of orientation angle is smaller. On the other hand, the realistic range of orientation angle in the left-ventricular wall, $\alpha_{max}-\alpha_{min}$, is reported to be about $+60°$ to $-60°$ [1]. It may be stated that the realistic orientation of the myocardial fiber is not the best from the aspect of pumping functions.

The maximum torsional angle of the left ventricle calculated at the side of the endocardium is presented in Fig. 13; Fig. 14 depicts the geometric variations of the left ventricle at the end-diastole and the end-systole for selected distributions of muscle fiber orientations. As seen from these two figures, the deformation

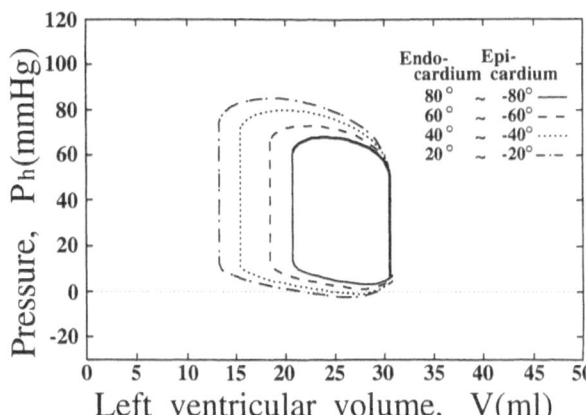

FIG. 12. Effect of muscle fiber orientation on pressure–volume relation

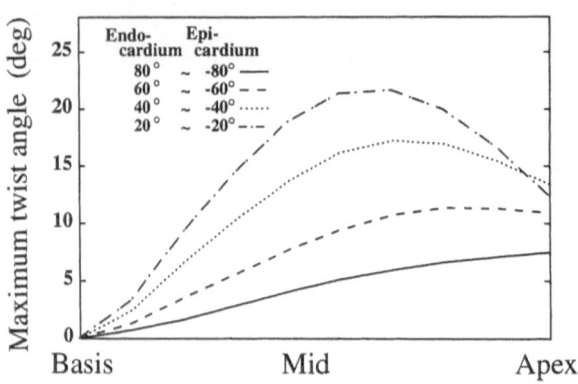

FIG. 13. Effect of muscle fiber orientation on maximum torsional angle on epicardium

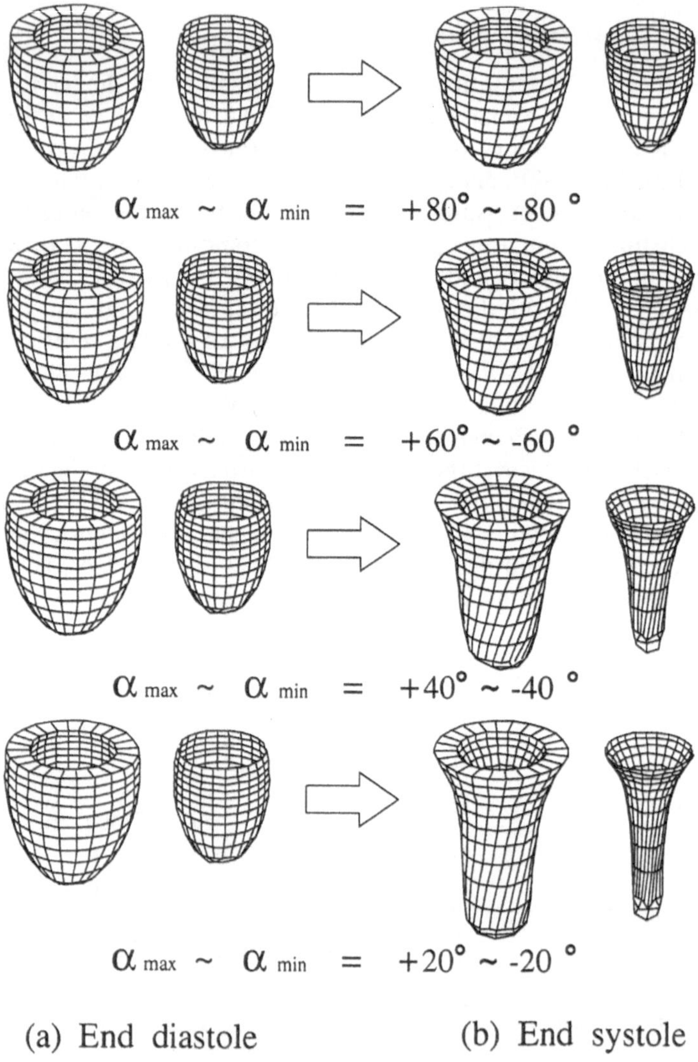

$\alpha_{max} \sim \alpha_{min} = +80° \sim -80°$

$\alpha_{max} \sim \alpha_{min} = +60° \sim -60°$

$\alpha_{max} \sim \alpha_{min} = +40° \sim -40°$

$\alpha_{max} \sim \alpha_{min} = +20° \sim -20°$

(a) End diastole   (b) End systole

FIG. 14a,b. Effect of muscle fiber orientation on variation of ventricular geometry. **a** End-diastole (*left side*). **b** End-systole (*right side*) [change of axial shape (geometry) and torsion] of the left ventricle becomes larger according to the decrease of distribution range of muscle fiber orientation. Large changes in the geometry of the left ventricle may not be compatible with the other organs around the left ventricle in the body. That is, the decrease of the muscle fiber orientation range is acceptable for the mechanical (pump) functions of the left ventricle, although it is not as good from the aspect of interaction of other organs. It is remarked that the realistic distribution range of muscle fiber orientation, $\alpha_{max}-\alpha_{min} = +60°$ to $-60°$ is determined by the compromise of these two aspects in our human body.

6 Concluding Remarks

The basic numerical system for simulating the mechanical properties and functions of the left ventricle has been constructed by combining the mechanical model of the left ventricle with the circulatory system model. The proposed simulation system can reproduce the generally well-accepted properties and functions of the left ventricle, and also makes it possible to estimate, for example, the stress distributions, which are quite difficult to measure, while all the basic elements of the system are very simple and fundamental. By substituting higher grade models for the present basic models, the more complicated performance of the left ventricle could be reproduced in a more precise and reliable manner. Thus, in the future we can expect objective and quantitative diagnoses for heart diseases by improving the present numerical system.

There are still many problems to solve before we can realize the ideal simulation system. One of them is that there is a shortage of reliable in vivo information about the mechanical properties of the biological tissues and organs. Even if we could obtain such information, the characteristic complexity, the time dependence, and the individual differences of organisms become considerable barriers for the numerical simulation. However, it is expected that numerical simulators like the one presented here will play a major role in overcoming these difficulties. In the authors' opinion, both the biomeasurement technique and numerical simulation will be developed by compensating for each other in this research field.

Acknowledgments. The authors express their gratitude to both Professor K. Sekioka and Professor K. Yagi of Mie University for many fruitful discussions and the offering of useful experimental results.

References

1. Fung Y, Seguchi Y (1985) Mechanics applied to living systems (in Japanese). Trans Jpn Soc Mech Eng 88:52–58
2. Tokuda M, Sekioka K, Veno T, Hayashi T, Havlicek F, Sawaki Y (1994) Numerical simulator for estimation of mechanical functions of human left ventricle (study of basic system). Jpn Soc Mech Eng Int J (Series A) 37:64–70

3. Sinoyama S (1988) Cardiac function (in Japanese). Chugai Igaku Sha, Tokyo, pp 70–108
4. Nakamura T, Abe H, Imai J (1978) Bioengineering assessment of cardiac mechanical function (analysis of left ventricular wall stress and strain) (in Japanese). Jpn J Med Electron Biol Eng 16:462–471
5. Furuya K, Tanabe A, Kanemoto M (1978) Various heart diseases (in Japanese). Jpn J Med Electron Biol Eng 16:456–461
6. Huxle HERS (1971) The structural basis of muscular contraction. Proc R Soc Lond Ser B Biol Sci 178:131–149
7. Beyar R, Sideman S (1984) A computer study of the left ventricular performance based on fiber structure, sarcomere dynamics and transmural electrical propagation velocity. Circ Res 55:358–375
8. Greenbaum RA (1981) Left ventricular fiber architecture in man. Br Heart J 45:248–263
9. Streeter DD Jr, Hanna WT (1973) Engineering mechanics for successive states in canine left ventricular myocardium. Circ Res 33:565–664
10. Freeman GL, LeWinter MM, Engler RI, Covell JW (1985) Relationship between myocardial fiber direction and segment shortening in the midwall of the canine left ventricle. Circ Res 56:31–38
11. Chadwick RS (1982) Mechanics of the left ventricle. Biophys J 39:279–288
12. Torezen A (1983) Static analysis of the left ventricle. Trans ASME J Biomech Eng 105:39–46
13. Perl M, Horowitz A, Sideman S (1986) Comprehensive model for the simulation of left ventricle mechanics. Part 1: Model description and simulation procedure. Med Biol Eng Comput 3:145–149
14. Pao YC (1982) Finite elements in stress analysis and estimation of mechanical properties of the working heart. In: Gallagher RH, Simon BR, Johnson PC, Gross JF (eds) Finite element in biomechanics. Wiley, New York, p 127
15. Zienkiewicz OC (1971) The finite element method in engineering science. McGraw-Hill, New York
16. Sekioka S (1988) A digital control system for ventricular loading (in Japanese). Jpn J Med Electron Biol Eng 25:21–28
17. Tokuda M (1991) Research report (in Japanese). Grant-In-Aid for Scientific Research, Japanese Ministry of Education, Tokyo, pp 38–126
18. Nevo E, Lanir Y (1989) Structural finite deformation model of the left ventricle during diastole and systole. Trans ASME J Biomech Eng 111:342–349

Biological and Living Systems

Dynamic Control of the Musculoskeletal System

Koji Ito[1,2]

Summary. Impedance adjustment and dynamic control of the musculoskeletal system are considered. The dynamic characteristics of this system are described by using a bilinear model. Next, the coordinated action of two hands are considered, and it is shown by experiment and a bilinear control model that the impedance adjustment at the joint and muscular levels plays an important role in motor control. Finally, we discuss the neuroscientific standpoints of the precise and flexible motor control mechanisms.

Key words: Musculoskeletal system—Motor impedance—Bilinear model—Motor dynamics—Motor control system

1 Introduction

We perform various movements on a daily basis, such as upright posture control, locomotion such as walking and running, limb movements such as reaching and manipulation, and sports movements like tennis and basketball. All of these are characterized by the fact that a multiple-degrees-of-freedom system of the musculoskeletal system is controlled. Moreover, our body is a very redundant system having more than 100 joint-degrees of freedom and a complex nonlinear dynamic system. As a consequence, to achieve smooth and dexterous movements, these redundant degrees of freedom must be constrained in one form or another [1].

In general, three types of variables are involved in the control of human movement: positional variables (displacement, velocity, acceleration), force-related variables (force, torque), and motor impedance variables (stiffness, viscosity, inertia). The essence of movement control lies in the complex interactions

[1] Department of Information and Computer Sciences, Toyohashi University of Technology, 1-1 Hibarigaoka, Tempaku, Toyohashi, Aichi, 441 Japan
[2] Bio-Mimetic Control Research Center, RIKEN (The Institute of Physical and Chemical Research), 3-8-31 Rokuban, Asuta, Nagoya, Aichi, 456 Japan

between the environment and human movements. For example, when rotating, pinching, or grasping an object, we must control not only the positional variables but also the force variables according to the constraints imposed by the object. Therefore, smooth manipulation requires proper control of the motor impedance connecting these two variables.

In the control mechanism of the brain that has made these movements, a large number of neural circuits are combined in a complicated way and numerous functional modules are formed. In spite of the fact that each module receives different input information, the very act of information processing is localized and autonomous. In addition, spatiotemporal mapping of the information is taking place in parallel between the modules, and a coherent function as a whole is thus created in a self-organizing manner. The system structure is extremely flexible, and there are a variety of information transformations such as the fusion of information of multiple sensors, the generation of symbol-processing information like the motor program, and, moreover, the conversion of such information into the spatiotemporal motor pattern.

First, this chapter tackles the impedance adjustment and the dynamic control of the musculoskeletal system. It is shown that the system's dynamic characteristics can be described using a bilinear model. Next, the coordinated action of two hands will be taken up, and it will be shown by experiment and a bilinear control model that the impedance adjustment at the joint and muscular levels plays an important role in motor control. Finally, we discuss the neuroscientific standpoints of precise and flexible motor control mechanisms.

2 Motor Impedance

Motor impedance is a general term signifying stiffness, compliance, viscosity, and inertia and is a set of parameters for transforming the variables representing motion (displacement, velocity, acceleration) into force and torque.

$$
\begin{array}{llll}
\text{(1) Stiffness:} & \text{Displacement} \to \text{Force} & F = KdX & (1) \\
\text{Compliance:} & \text{Force} \to \text{Displacement} & dX = CF & (2) \\
\text{(2) Viscosity:} & \text{Velocity} \to \text{Force} & F = Bd\dot{X} & (3) \\
\text{(3) Inertia:} & \text{Acceleration} \to \text{Force} & F = Md\ddot{X} & (4)
\end{array}
$$

Here, $dX = X_e - X$, and represents a vector showing the amount of displacement from the equilibrium point X_e. In addition, K, C, B, and M are matrices.

The dynamic characteristics of stiffness can be described as follows. When the end-effecter of the arm is displaced, the reactive force generated at the end-effecter is determined by the stiffness and the amount of displacement (Fig. 1). Now, if the displacement is assumed to be constant, then the larger the stiffness, the bigger is the reaction force, constituting a stiff arm. Inversely, the smaller the stiffness, the smaller the reaction force, constituting a compliant arm. Moreover,

FIG. 1. Relationship among stiffness, amount of displacement, and reaction force

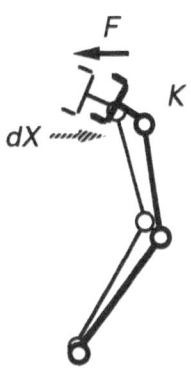

as can be seen from Eq. 1, once the stiffness K is determined, the force F and the displacement dX are no longer independent. It therefore follows that it is not possible to control the force and displacement in the same direction independently.

In addition, viscosity regulates the generated reaction force by a change in velocity, while inertia regulates the generated reaction force by a change in acceleration.

3 Impedance Adjustment Mechanisms

In the musculoskeletal system, the joint becomes compliant if both the flexor and extensor muscles are relaxed, so that they can be easily moved by the external force. Conversely, if they are contracted strongly, the joint becomes very stiff and is in a state of being locked. This implies that the stiffness or viscosity of the joint can be altered by changing the contraction level of the muscles. The degree of freedom about the joint is constrained not only on the basis of variable dynamic characteristics of the muscles but also by positively adjusting various forms of feedback at the spinal cord level, such as the stretch reflex or feedback coupling between the joints.

The relationship between the impulse input from the central nervous system to the muscles and the resulting muscular force depends on the length of the muscles, the contraction velocity, the type of muscles, and the degree of fatigue. However, it is well known that at the macro level the dynamic nature of muscles is represented in terms of the two fundamental functions of length–tension curves and force–velocity curves [2].

Figure 2 shows the tensile force generated when muscles of various lengths are activated with the resting length being set at 100%. These results provide the dynamic characteristics that the longer the muscle is, the greater the tensile force. In addition, as indicated by the broken curves in the diagram, the tensile force becomes larger as the level of muscular activity increases.

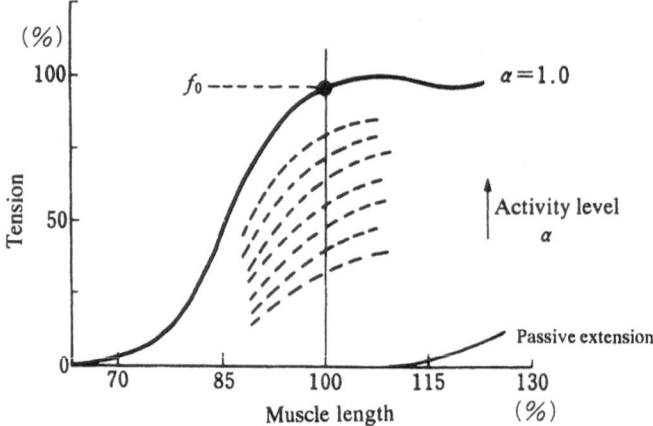

Fig. 2. Length–tension curves

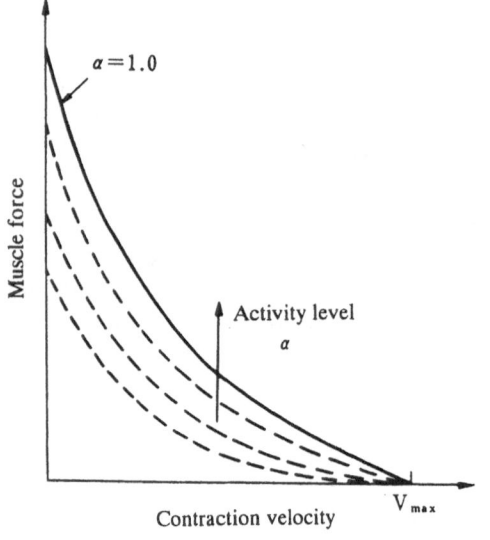

Fig. 3. Force–velocity curves

Figure 3 shows force-versus-velocity relations at various levels of muscular activity. The muscular force decreases in inverse proportion to the contraction velocity of the muscles, thereby indicating the muscle viscosity characteristics. In addition, the muscular force increases with the level of muscular activity.

Now, let us assume here that the muscular force f is proportional to the level of activation α ($0 \leqq \alpha \leqq 1$, normalized at the maximum value). Then the following expression can be obtained:

$$f = a \cdot g(L, V) \qquad (5)$$

where $g(L,V)$ is a nonlinear function that represents the relation at the maximum activity level ($\alpha = 1$), while L and V are the length and the contraction velocity of the muscle, respectively. When $g(L,V)$ is linearly approximated at the point of equilibrium of the muscle and in the neighborhood of the contraction velocity $V = 0$, and the variables are rewritten, the following equation

$$f = u - kux - bu\dot{x} \tag{6}$$

is obtained [3,4]. Here, u is the contraction force of the force-generating element, f is the muscular force, $x = x_e - L$ is the change of the length of the muscle from the point of equilibrium, and k and b are constants. Eq. 26 is a model of the dynamic characteristics of the muscle, and has the characteristics that the elastic and viscous coefficients are not constant but in proportion to the contraction force u.

If the foregoing equation is applied to the horizontal rotational motion of a forearm having a flexor muscle (u_f) and an extensor muscle (u_e), then the equation of motion is given as

$$M/d \cdot \ddot{\theta} = u_f - u_e - (u_f + u_e)(k\theta + b\dot{\theta}) \tag{7}$$

where θ is joint angle, M is inertial moment of the forearm, d is the moment arm (Fig. 4). The foregoing equation forms a bilinear system in which the difference $u_f - u_e$ of the flexor and extensor muscles adjusts the driving force of the joint, and the sum of the contraction forces, $u_f + u_e$, adjusts the parameters (elasticity and viscosity).

In addition to the variable elastic and viscous characteristics of the muscle, the motor impedance is also controlled by the parameter adjustment mechanism at the spinal cord level and the posture selection of the limb utilizing the redundant degrees of freedom.

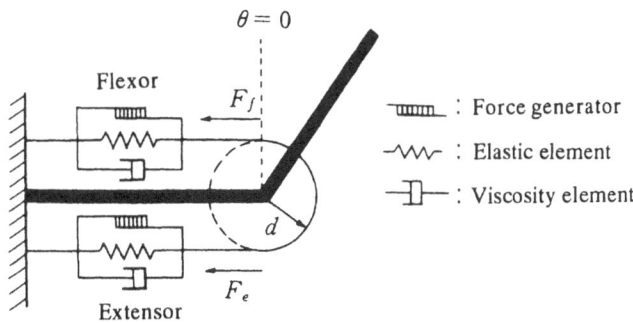

FIG. 4. Musculoskeletal system of the forearm

4 Coordinated Actions of Two Hands and Impedance Adjustment

4.1 Experiment on Coordinated Actions

In the case of holding a ball or a box with two hands, it is necessary to control not only the position and posture of the object but also the internal forces applied to it at the same time. In the case of a ball, which is easily deformed by external force (this will be referred to here as a dynamic object), it becomes necessary to set the impedance of the hand, joint, and muscle to appropriate levels corresponding to the impedance characteristics of the object.

To analyze the control characteristics of the coordinated actions of two hands, a dynamic object was made as shown in Fig. 5. The object is composed of a rigid body 0.25 m long ($m_c = 0.4$ kg) in the central section, two elements with the viscosity ($d = 6.82$ Ns/m) and stiffness ($k = 0.49$ N/m), and two endplates ($m_{cL} = m_{cR} = 1.125$ kg), and is deformed by the forces applied by two hands. The object is placed on a linear rail of negligible friction and can be easily moved by the forces from the two sides. Each end of the object was furnished with a distortion gauge (10 Hz in cutoff frequency), and the contact forces were measured. An encoder was installed in the center of the object to measure its displacement. In addition, electrodes were placed on the extensor and flexor muscles that drive the wrist joints of the subject and the surface electromyograph (EMG) was measured.

Each subject was asked to sit in front of the object and to move the center position of the object as quickly as possible by using only his wrist joints without oscillating the object. The displacement was set at 60 mm to the left and to the right. Three normal male students were selected as the subjects, and after 1000 rounds of practice, 10 trials were measured. No particular target value was set for the internal force.

4.2 Experimental Results

Figure 6 shows some representative EMG patterns for the case of a dynamic object. They are, from top to bottom, the EMG patterns of (a) the extensor

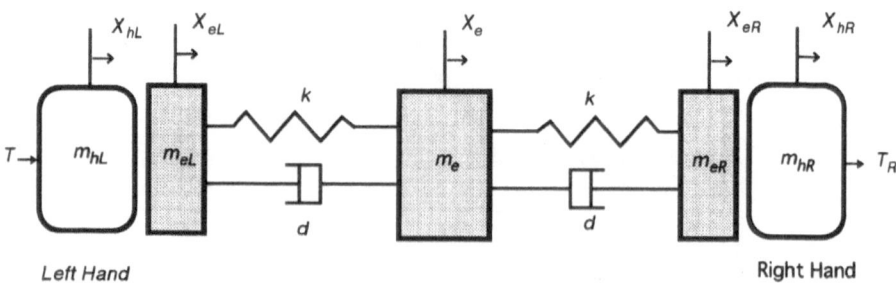

FIG. 5. Dynamic object for experiments on coordinated actions

FIG. 6a–d. Electromyograph
(EMG) patterns for a
dynamic object. **a** Extensor
muscle of right hand. **b**
Flexor muscle of right hand.
c Extensor muscle of left
hand. **d** Flexor muscle of
left hand

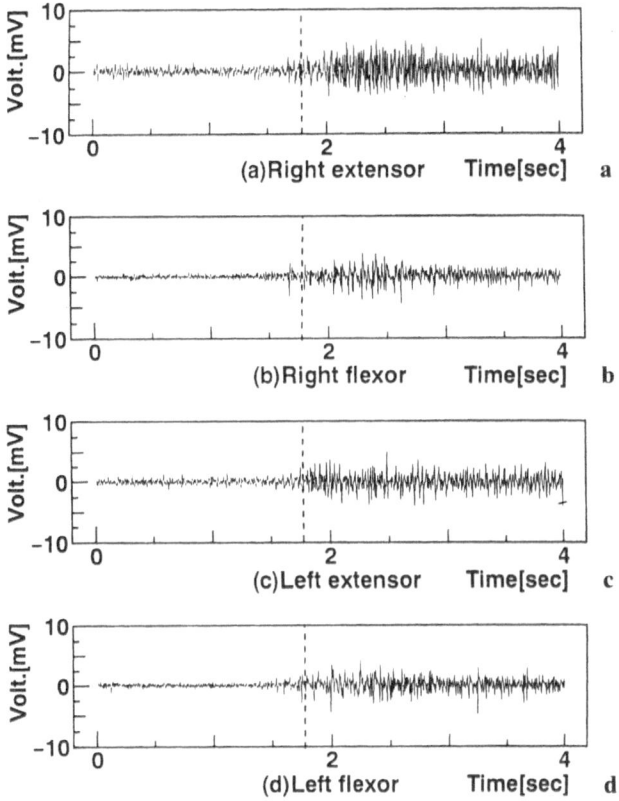

muscle of the right hand, (b) the flexor muscle of the right hand, (c) the extensor
muscle of the left hand, and (d) the flexor muscle of the left hand. In addition, Fig.
7 shows (a) the displacement of the object, (b) its velocity, and (c) the internal
force applied to the object under this condition. Figure 8 shows EMG patterns
obtained when the object was replaced with a rigid body. The broken lines in the
center show the time when the object began to move.

   In the case of a rigid object, it is seen from the EMG that the extensor muscle
of the right hand and the flexor muscle of the left hand are used to control the
object. By contrast, in the case of a dynamic object, the flexor and extensor
muscles of the left and right hands are coactivated. Why does the subject use such
a control strategy? Let us analyze this by using a bilinear control model.

4.3 Bilinear Control Model

The equations of motion involving two hands and an object after the Laplace
transformation are as follow:

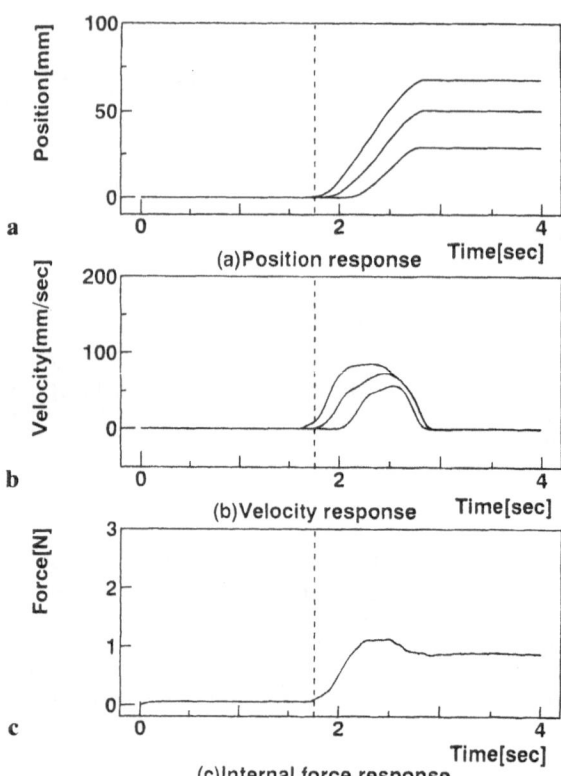

FIG. 7a–c. Coordinated actions for a dynamic object. **a** Displacement of object. **b** Velocity. **c** Internal force applied to object

(a)Position response

(b)Velocity response

(c)Internal force response

$$m_e s^2 X_e = Y(s)(X_{hL} + X_{hR} - 2X_e)$$
$$m_{hL} s^2 X_{hL} = T_L(s) - F_{intL}$$
$$m_{hR} s^2 X_{hR} = T_R(s) - F_{intR}$$
$$m_{eL} s^2 X_{hL} = F_{intL} - Y(s)(X_{hL} - X_e)$$
$$m_{eR} s^2 X_{hR} = -F_{intR} - Y(s)(X_{hR} - X_e)$$
$$Y(s) = k + ds \qquad (8)$$

Now, when the variable stiffness and viscosity of the muscle are approximated by a bilinear model of Eq. 7, then a block diagram as indicated in Fig. 9 is obtained. Here, the transfer function from the difference of contracting forces of the muscles $u_f - u_e$ (driving force) to a displacement X_e of the object is found to be

$$X_e = \left(D_L D_R - G_e Y(s)(D_L + D_R)\right)^{-1} \left(G_e D_R(u_{Lf} - u_{Le}) + G_e D_L(u_{Rf} - u_{Re})\right) \qquad (9)$$

FIG. 8a–d. EMG patterns for a rigid object. **a** Extensor muscle of right hand. **b** Flexor muscle of right hand. **c** Extensor muscle of left hand. **d** Flexor muscle of left hand

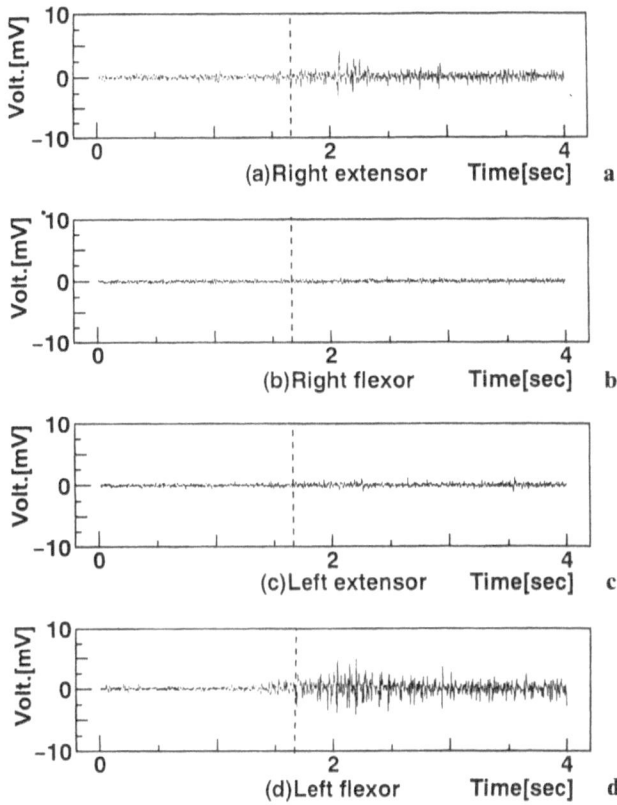

FIG. 9. Bilinear control model

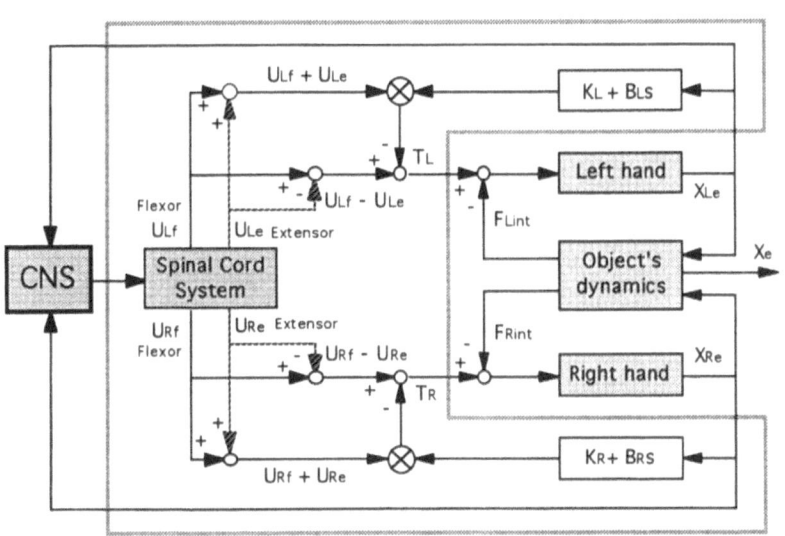

where

$$D_L = \left(m_{hL} + m_{eL}\right)s^2 + Y(s) + \left(k_L + B_L s\right)\left(u_{Lf} + u_{Le}\right) \tag{10}$$

$$D_R = \left(m_{hR} + m_{cR}\right)s^2 + Y(s) + \left(k_R + B_R s\right)\left(u_{Rf} + u_{Re}\right) \tag{11}$$

$$G_e = Y(s)\big/\left(m_e s^2 + Y(s)\right) \tag{12}$$

Note that the transfer function is a sixth-order system.

When the flexor and extensor muscles of the wrist joints of the left and right hands are coactivated and their activity levels are raised, $(u_{Lf} + u_{Le})$ and $(u_{Rf} + U_{Re})$ become bigger. When root loci are drawn with $(u_f + u_e)$ as a parameter, it is found that three poles are dominant. In other words, as the activity levels of the flexor and extensor muscles are raised and the joint impedance is made bigger, the complex sixth-order system can be approximated by a third-order system. From the relationship between the hands and the object, the impedance of the dynamic object itself cannot be modified. However, the transfer characteristics integrating the object and the musculoskeletal system can be reduced in dimension by adjusting the impedance of the joints. This example suggests that humans regulate the impedance of musculoskeletal systems skillfully according to the aim of motion.

5 Coordination Among Subsystems

Let us remember the very first time we rode a bicycle. We all made very awkward movements by stiffening the muscles of our legs and arms. Also, we all tried to adjust the center of gravity of our body to the left or right so as not to fall with the swaying of the bicycle. In many cases, however, we fell. As we practiced, the stiffness of the entire body disappeared, and we began to predict the movements of the bicycle and skillfully regulate the movements of each section of our body.

Thus, in the initial stage of motor learning, we coactivate the principal muscles and antagonist muscles and raise the impedance level. A high level of impedance results in making the movements of the arm and leg more robust against unexpected changes in the environment and, at the same time, results in lowering the degree of freedom of the entire body by making the joints stiff.

In movements after training, the complex impedance adjustment is carried out by skillfully controlling the variable elasticity and viscosity of the muscles, the reflection programs at the spinal cord level, and the posture adjustment of the skeletal system. In other words, it may be said that the purpose of training itself is to learn how to set up the impedance. This fact, however, does not necessarily mean the lowering of the impedance level; there are cases of raising the impedance of the wrist joints after training, as in the coordinated actions of two hands for a dynamic object. This suggests that the acquisition of a motor skill is not to learn the feedback parameter corresponding to a change in the environment but rather to create new relationships among lower subsystems (musculoskeletal system + reflection system). It is not that the degree of freedom is lowered dynamically simply by stiffening every joint, as in the initial stage of learning, but rather that the degree of freedom is reduced as a result of creating new relationships among various parts of the body via motor impedance. Such new dynamics created by the lower subsystems are here called "goal-directed motor dynamics" (see Fig. 10).

6 Functional Modules of Motor Control System

Let us now consider the reaching action when you move your hand to a cup in front of you. Figure 11 shows the information flow of the motor control system [5]. The visual information captured in the receptive field of the retina is sent to the primary and secondary visual areas. After processing, it is converted into the spatial position and velocity representation (parietal association area), which are not influenced by eye and head movements and pattern representation (temporal association area), such as shape and size. They are encoded on the visual space map.

At the same time, sensory information from the proprioceptive sensors at each part of the body is encoded on the proprioceptive map as the body coordinate representation (such as the joint angle). In addition, the hand positions on the visual space map and the body coordinates on the proprioceptive map are coupled through coordinate transformation. The relation between the hand and the other body parts, as well as the relation between the hand and the object, are represented thereon. It has been confirmed that the positioning accuracy of your hand depends greatly on whether or not you can see. This coordinate transformation corresponds to the forward and inverse kinematics.

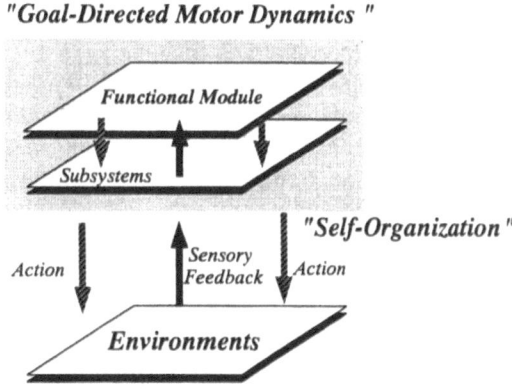

Fig. 10. Goal-directed motor dynamics

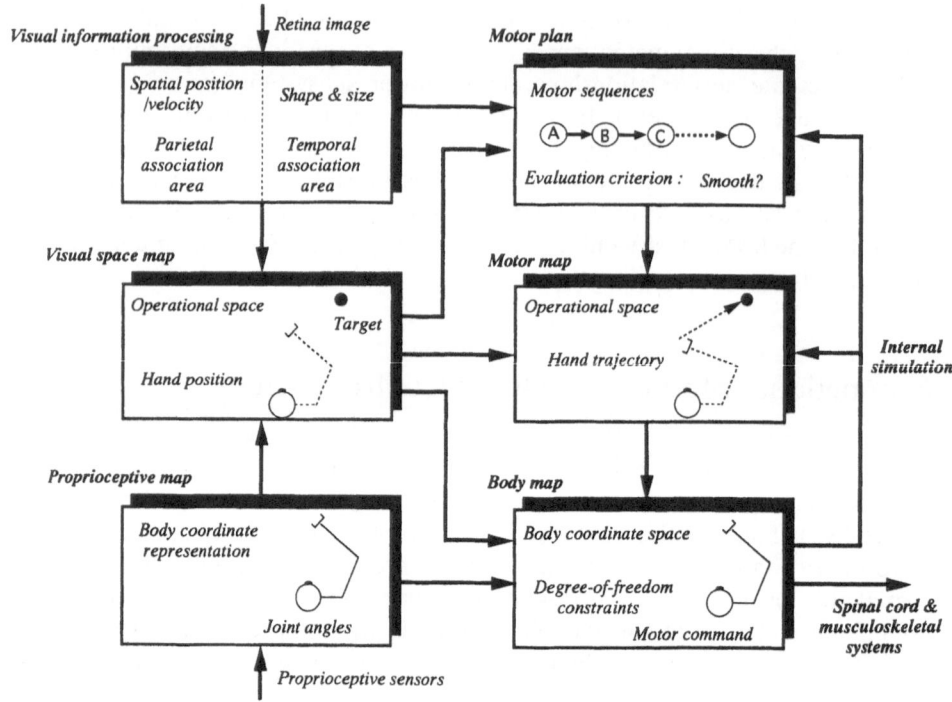

FIG. 11. Architecture of motor control system

In the motor planning module, not only are the motor sequences for achieving the intended motion generated but the evaluation criterion for realizing the individual motions is also set up on the basis of information from the visual space map and the proprioceptive map and other internal representations.

Next, in the motor map, the spatiotemporal motor pattern is produced from the motor sequences based on the given evaluation. It is hard to believe that this motor pattern is directly generated about the entire multiple-degrees-of-freedom dynamic system. It may be more reasonable to imagine, as mentioned earlier, that the motor pattern is produced in a certain low-dimensional operational space (the hand space in the case of the reaching action of the forearm, and the phase-difference space, in the case of locomotion). It is one of the important problems of motor control to define this abstract operational space and to analyze the mechanism for generating the motor pattern coupled with goal-directed motor dynamics.

The generated motor pattern is mapped into the body coordinate space (the joint–muscle space). A variety of degree-of-freedom constraints are necessary for defining this mapping. The motor impedance will be one of the constraint conditions. In addition, the motor pattern at the body coordinate is not only sent to the servomechanism at the spinal cord level as the motor command, but is also simulated internally using the forward kinematics and dynamics models and is fed back to the motor map or motor plan.

As described earlier, the spatiotemporal mapping of information is conducted in parallel among the modules. Information mapping among the different functions is made in the same way as fusing the information from different sensors or the formation of a motor map by converting the symbol processing information such as the motor plan into the spatial or temporal pattern. Furthermore, a group of homogeneous subsystems are activated cooperatively or competitively inside each module, e.g., in the body coordinate space, the dynamic subsystems such as the trunk, forearms, lower limbs, and hand coordinate with each other to generate a motor pattern.

Therefore, the problem is how to provide for the coordination and competition of the respective module outputs. For example, in the subsumption architecture of Brooks [6], each module autonomously takes in the information flowing from the sensor side or other module to execute its own information processing. Whether or not the action command of each module becomes available depends on the presence or absence of a suppression signal from the upper level. In the motor control system, various motor outputs from a simple motion like the bending reflex up to a high-degree voluntary movement are formed in parallel. This can be clearly seen from an athlete's skillful body actions. Our next step is to consider the frameworks of coordination and competition among the motion modules in addition to the suppression of the lower level by the upper level.

7 Conclusion

The phenomenal finger movements of a pianist, the dynamic carriage of a soccer player, and the dexterous hand movements of a potter are all worthy of the highest admiration, and the complexity and dexterity of their motion capabilities are of incalculable value. The motion/action of such a biological system is controlled on the basis of programmed motion patterns. In addition, a majority of those functions have been gained in a self-organizing manner through interactions with the environment.

In this vein, the recent study of complex adaptive systems by the Santa Fe Research Laboratory in the United States is attracting attention [7]. This study concerns the complexity generated by the competition and coordination of simple and local primitive elements, as represented by chaos, evolution, or artificial life, in other words, by the macrocosmic complexity caused by microcosmic behavior. It is important to clarify its principle and structure and to seek its applications to various fields, including the dynamic control of the musculoskeletal system.

Acknowledgments. This research was financed in part by the Scientific Research Foundation of the Ministry of Education, Japan (06452253 and 06213219), the

Research Foundation for the Electrotechnology of Chubu, and the Tokai Foundation for Technology. The author expresses his sincere appreciation to all concerned.

References

1. Ito K, Ito M (1991) Motion control in living bodies and robots. Society of Instrument and Control Engineers, Tokyo
2. Dowen RM (1980) Contractility. In: Mountcastle VB (ed) Medical physiology, 14th edn. Mosby, St Louis
3. Ito K, Tsuji T (1985) Bilinear characteristics of musculoskeletal motor systems and their application to prosthesis control. Trans Inst Elect Eng Jpn C-105(10):201–208
4. Hogan N (1984) Adaptive control of mechanical impedance by coactivation of antagonist muscles. IEEE Trans Auto Contr AC-29:681–690
5. Jeannerod M (1990) The representation of the goal of an action and its role in the control of goal-directed movements. In: Schwarts EL (ed) Computational neuroscience. MIT Press, Cambridge, pp 352–368
6. Brooks RA (1986) A robust layered control system for a mobile robot. IEEE J Robotics Automation RA-2:14–23
7. Langton CG (ed) (1991) Artificial life, vol II. Addison-Wesley, Reading, MA

Theoretical Analysis of Otoacoustic Emissions

HIROSHI WADA and SYU-ICHI NOGUCHI

Summary. The cochlea is the principal sensory organ of the mammalian auditory system. The high sensitivity and sharp tuning of the healthy cochlea have been realized. Moreover, an interesting phenomenon, that is, sound is emitted from the ears, was discovered by Kemp, and this phenomenon was named otoacoustic emissions (OAEs). OAEs are thought to be the products that the cochlea emits in the form of acoustic energy, and are considered to be transmitted to the external auditory meatus through the middle ear in a retrograde fashion. These findings suggest that the cochlea emits energy by itself and that the cochlea has the function of active processing as an amplifier. Concerning OAEs, various investigations have been carried out; however, the generation mechanism of OAEs is still unclear. Therefore, in this study the dynamic behavior of the cochlea was simulated by using a mathematical model of the cochlea. Then, an attempt was made to clarify the generation mechanism of transiently-evoked OAEs (TEOAEs) by comparing the numerical results with the experimental data.

Key words: Transiently evoked OAEs (TEOAEs)—Cochlear model—Outer hair cell (OHC)—Theoretical analysis—Active mechanism

1 Introduction

Sound—in other words, mechanical vibration of the air—is transmitted to the cochlea, which has the function of mechanical to electrical transduction through the middle ear, which consists of the tympanic membrane and three tiny bones called ossicles (ossicula). Many studies concerning auditory systems have been performed and have indicated that the cochlea works as not only a transducer but also as an amplifier.

Department of Mechanical Engineering, Tohoku University, Aoba, Aramaki, Aoba-ku, Sendai, Miyagi, 980-77 Japan

One of the phenomena that proves the cochlear amplifier function, is the amplification of basilar membrane motion [1–6]. Sharp frequency tuning of the basilar membrane has been measured in living animals [1–3]. Death or cochlear trauma causes a reducton of basilar membrane vibration and a disappearance of this sharp tuning [4–6]. The other phenomenon believed to be caused by cochlear amplification is otoacoustic emissions (OAEs), which were discovered by Kemp [7]. OAEs are thought to be the products that the cochlea emits in the form of acoustic energy, and are considered to be transmitted to the external auditory meatus through the middle ear in a retrograde fashion. OAEs can be detected in most humans and experimental animals with normal hearing [7,8]. In contrast, in hearing-impaired subjects that have a dysfunctional cochlea, OAEs either cannot be detected or the levels are significantly low [8,9]. These findings indicate that the cochlea emits energy by itself and has a function of active processing as an amplifier.

In recent measurements, the isolated outer hair cells (OHCs) removed the organ of Corti (composed of sensory and supporting cells) have been shown to be motile. The cells become shorter in response to depolarizing currents and longer in response to hyperpolarizing currents [10,11]. Brownell [12] demonstrated the relationship between the function of OHCs and OAEs by administering aspirin. These measurement results suggested that the OHCs generate force as an active source of mechanical energy by which basilar membrane motion is promoted and OAEs are generated.

Although many experiments that have been mentioned were carried out to clarify the mechanism of the cochlea, it is difficult to solve the question by experiment only. In measurement of basilar membrane motion, the sites that can be observed on the basilar membrane are limited to a narrow region [5,6]. Also, it is impossible to observe a human cochlea because the experiment is invasive. Insofar as OAEs are concerned, the measurements are noninvasive and clinical application using OAEs has been anticipated. However, because OAEs are detected by a probe microphone that is inserted into the external auditory meatus, cochlear function is demonstrated indirectly.

To compensate for the defects of such experiments and to clarify the mechanism of the cochlea, simulations with a mathematical or hardware cochlea model have been performed by many researchers [13–20]. A numerical simulation method for one-dimensional and two-dimensional cochlear models with nonlinear and active mechanical properties was presented by Diependaal et al. [13,14]. Zwicker [19,20] simulated the basilar membrane motion and OAEs using a hardware nonlinear model. Electrical models of the cochlea have been also used to describe the basilar membrane motion and the OAEs [21,22]. However, the OAE generation mechanism is still unclear. In this chapter, for the purpose of clarifying the generation mechanism of transiently evoked OAEs (TEOAEs), which are evoked by a transient acoustic stimulus such as a toneburst, the dynamic behavior of the cochlea is analyzed using a mathematical model of the cochlea.

2 Measurement

OAEs can be classified according to the type of stimulus. The classification is shown in Fig. 1. One major emissions class is spontaneously present without stimulation, and are called spontaneous OAEs (SOAEs). SOAEs are present in humans and several other species of mammal, but appear to be less prevalent in these other species than in humans [8,23]. The other principal class, evoked by different acoustic stimulation, are called evoked OAEs (EOAEs). EOAEs can be in general further divided into three classes. EOAEs evoked by a transient acoustic stimulus such as a click or a toneburst are called transiently evoked OAEs (TEOAEs). Stimulus-frequency OAEs (SFOAEs) are evoked by a single, continuous pure-tone stimulus. TEOAEs and SFOAEs are elicited in all normal-hearing humans [7,8]. However, the measurement of SFOAEs is more difficult than that of TEOAEs because SFOAEs are present at the same time and at the same frequency as the much larger stimulus. Further, it has been reported that TEOAEs and SFOAEs appear smaller in some experimental animals such as rabbits and rodents than in humans [8]. OAEs that occur at harmonic and intermodulation distortion products of frequencies present in the stimulus are distortion-product OAEs (DPOAEs). DPOAEs are evoked by two continuous pure tones and are generated by the nonlinear process of the cochlea. DPOAEs also are larger in rabbits and rodents than in human [8,24].

In this study, the measurement of TEOAEs was performed in normal-hearing humans using toneburst signals as the stimulus. In measuring TEOAEs, a commercially available OAE measuring apparatus, ILO88 (Otodynamics, Hatfield, UK) [25] was applied. A typical measurement result of TEOAE waveforms is shown in Fig. 2a. Two wave trains were clearly seen at about 10 ms and 15 ms after the onset of the stimulation, termed the fast and slow component of TEOAEs, respectively, by Tanaka et al. [26]. Input–output curves of the fast and slow components are displayed Fig. 2b. When the magnitude of the stimulation was small, only the slow component was measurable. The curve of the slow component was less steep than that of the fast component.

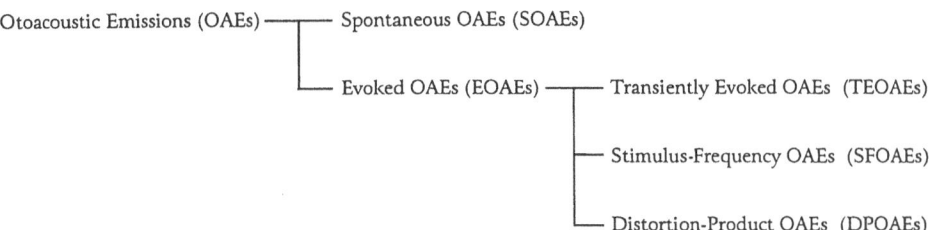

Fig. 1. Classification of otoacoustic emissions (*OAEs*)

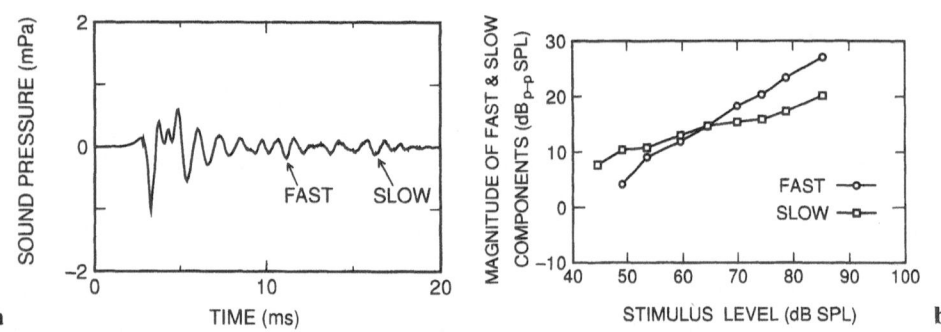

FIG. 2a,b. Measurement results when toneburst signals of 3 ms duration with 1 ms fall time, 1.0 kHz in frequency, were applied. **a** Typical transienthy evoked otoacoustic emissions (TEOAEs) waveforms. Tonebursts of 70 dB sound pressure level (*SPL*) were applied. The response window was set at 2.5–20.5 ms. **b** Input–output curves of the fast (*circles*) and slow (*squares*) components

3 Theoretical Analysis

As shown in Fig. 3, the cochlea is a long, spiral, fluid-filled structure that is divided into three chambers called the scala vestibuli, scala media, and scala tympani. At the apical end of the cochlea, the scala vestibuli and scala tympani are connected by the helicotrema. At the basal end, the scala vestibuli and scala tympani have the oval window and round window, respectively. The base of the stapes, called the foot plate, fits into the oval window and transmits the vibration of the middle ear to the fluid in the scala vestibuli.

The structure of the cochlea is very complicated. However, to avoid this complexity in the theoretical analysis in this study, the one-dimensional model of the cochlea obtained by Diependaal [13] is modified. The cochlea is assumed to be uncoiled and to be approximated by fluid-filled rigid-walled compartments separated by the basilar membrane; this is possible because Reissner's mem-

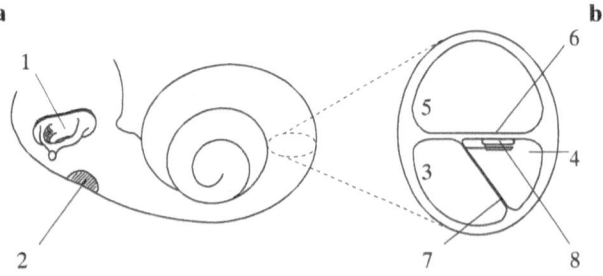

FIG. 3a,b. Cochlear configuration. **a** Outline of the cochlea. Three semicircular canals, which are connected to the basal end of the cochlea, have been omitted. **b** Cross section of the cochlea: *1*, stapes; *2*, round window; *3*, scala vestibuli; *4*, scala media; *5*, scala tympani; *6*, basilar membrane; *7*, Reissner's membrane; *8*, organ of Corti

brane, between the scala vestibuli and scala media, is acoustically transparent and does not influence the mechanical functions of the cochlea [27].

As shown in Fig. 4, the rest position of the basilar membrane (BM) is taken to be the x-axis; the height of each channel is H and its length is L. If p and u represent the difference in pressure between the scala vestibuli and scala tympani and the displacement of the BM, respectively, the corresponding equation of motion describing the response of the BM is given by

$$\partial^2 p(x, t)/\partial x^2 - (2\rho/H)\partial^2 u(x, t)/\partial t^2 = 0 \tag{1}$$

where ρ is the fluid density. The boundary conditions at the basal and apical ends are

$$\partial p(0, t)/\partial x = 2\rho\partial^2 a_s(t)/\partial t^2, \quad p(L, t) = 0 \tag{2}$$

where $a_s(t)$ is the displacement of the stapes. The initial conditions are

$$u(x,0) = \partial u(x,0)/\partial t = 0 \tag{3}$$

If a partition of the BM is assumed to be a vibration system with one degree of freedom, the equation of BM motion is given by

$$M(x)\partial^2 u(x, t)/\partial t^2 + R(x)\partial u(x, t)/\partial t + K(x)u(x, t) = p(x, t) + P_{OHC}(x, t) \tag{4}$$

where $M(x)$, $R(x)$, and $K(x)$ are the mass, damping, and stiffness of the BM per unit area, respectively. The characteristic frequency of each partition, which depends on the mass and stiffness, is shown in Fig. 5 as a function of the distance from the stapes.

As OHCs have been shown to contract and expand and generate force [10,11], it is believed that the cochlea's active mechanism is originated by the OHCs. Therefore, P_{OHC}, which is the force per unit area generated by the active behavior of the OHCs, is added to Eq. 4. Based on the report that input–output function for an OHC shows a compressive nonlinearity [28], the force of the OHCs is assumed to vary in conjunction with the velocity of the BM and the distance from the basal end, and is expressed by

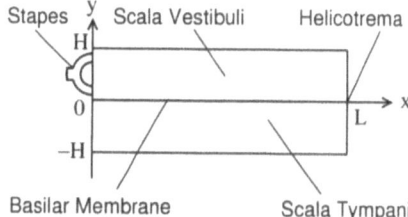

FIG. 4. One-dimensional model of the cochlea.
H, height; L, length

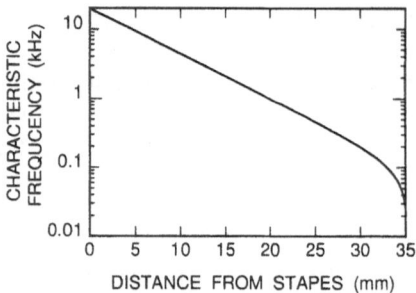

FIG. 5. Frequency map of the basilar membrane. The x-axis shows the distance from the stapes. Each cochlear partition has its own resonance frequency, $f = (K(x)/M(x))^{1/2}/2\pi$, where $K(x)$ and $M(x)$ are the stiffness and mass of the basilar membrane; their values are shown in Table 1. The resonance frequency is 19.4 kHz at the basal end ($x = 0$ mm), and 25 Hz at the apical end ($x = 35$ mm)

$$P_{OHC}(x,v) = \begin{cases} -a(x) \cdot b \cdot (c \cdot v_N + 1) \cdot v_N & (v \le -v_N) \\ a(x) \cdot b \cdot (c \cdot |v| + 1) \cdot v & (|v| \le v_N) \\ a(x) \cdot b \cdot (c \cdot v_N + 1) \cdot v_N & (v_N \le v) \end{cases} \tag{5}$$

$$a(x) = 2 \cdot (M \cdot K)^{1/2} \tag{6}$$

where v is the velocity of the BM and b, c, and v_N are constants. In Fig. 6, one example of the relationship between the pressure that acts on the BM and velocity of the BM is displayed. In this study, the middle ear is assumed to have one degree of freedom [29].

To solve the differential Eqs. 1 and 4 with the boundary and initial conditions (Eqs. 2 and 3), the finite-difference method and the fourth-order Runge–Kutta method are applied to discretize these equations in space and time. In this analysis, the cochlea is divided into 512 sections and the time step is taken to be 1/128 ms. Numerical values and parameters of the middle ear and cochlea used for the analysis are shown in Table 1.

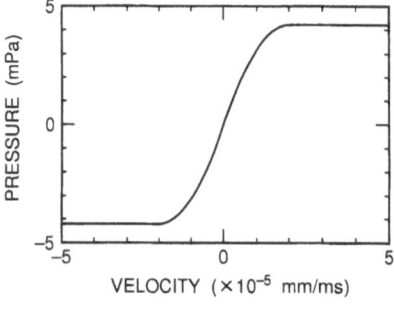

FIG. 6. Relationship between the force of the outer hair cells (OHCs) and the velocity of the basilar membrane (BM) at $x = 20$ mm. The force of OHCs is saturated when the velocity of the the BM is large

TABLE 1. Numerical values and parameters of the middle ear and cochlea.

Parameter	Value	Units
Length of BM	$l = 35.00$	mm
Height of cochlear scala	$h = 5.000$	mm
Density of cochlear fluids	$\rho = 1.034$	mg/mm^3
Mass of BM	$M(x) = 0.300$	mg/mm^2
Damping of BM	$R(x) = 0.24 \cdot (K(x) \cdot M(x))^{1/2}$	mg/(mm$^2 \cdot$ ms)
Stiffness of BM	$K(x) = 4.736 \times 10^3 e^{-0.3x} - 0.123$	mg/(mm$^2 \cdot$ ms^2)
Parameters of OHC	$a(x) = 2 \cdot (K(x) \cdot M(x))^{1/2}$	mg/(mm$^2 \cdot$ ms)
	$b = 0.112$	
	$c = -2.5 \times 10^4$	
	$v_N = 2.0 \times 10^{-5}$	mm/ms
Mass of middle ear	$M_{me} = 42.8$	mg
Damping of middle ear	$R_{me} = 63.5$	mg/ms
Stiffness of middle ear	$K_{me} = 1.47 \times 10^3$	mg/ms^2

BM, basilar membrane; OHC, outer hair cell.

4 Results

Figure 7a is a three-dimensional (3-D) expression of the force per unit area generated by the active behavior of OHCs when the behavior is assumed to be uniform. Figure 7a shows $|P_{OHC}(x, v)|$ calculated by Eqs. 5 and 6 when v is 2.0×10^{-3} mm/ms. In Eq. 6, $a(x)$ increases with an increase in x, because, as shown in Table 1, K in Eq. 6 increases as x increases. This is the reason why the pressure

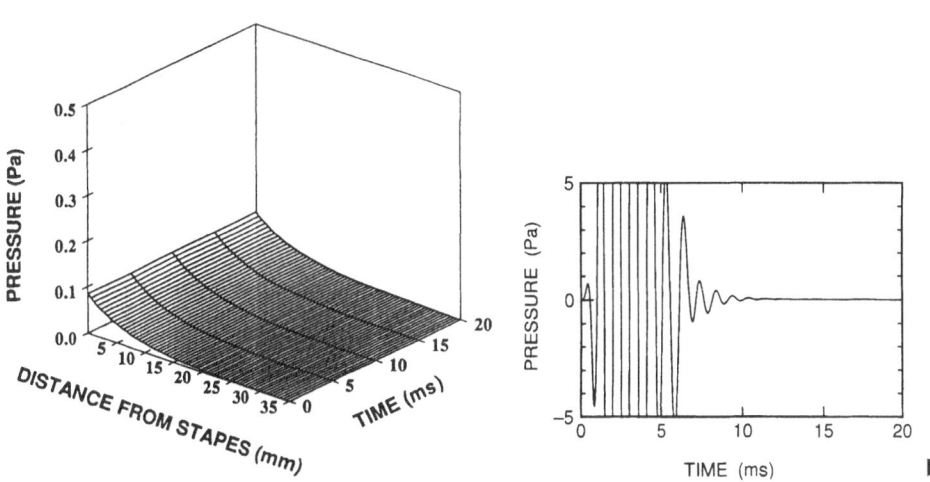

a

b

FIG. 7a,b. Numerical results. **a** Three-dimensional (3-D) expression of the force per unit area, that is, pressure versus BM position and time when the active behavior of the OHCs is assumed to be uniform. **b** Waveform when the the active behavior is expressed by **a**. TEOAE waveforms cannot be obtained

generated by the OHC in Fig. 7a is larger at the basal end than at the apical end of the cochlea. Fig. 7b is a numerical result of the waveforms when the toneburst signals at 1.0kHz and 70dB sound pressure level (SPL) are the stimulus. Such TEOAE waveforms as those displayed in Fig. 2a cannot be obtained.

This result suggests that the strength of the active behavior is not sufficient to generate TEOAEs and that stronger OHC behavior is necessary. Therefore, the active behavior of the OHCs at a region of the BM where the vibration amplitude evoked by the toneburst signal is large is assumed to be stronger than the active behavior of the OHCs at the other BM positions. The region of strong OHC activity is assumed to be between the position of the BM corresponding to a characteristic frequency (CF) equal to the stimulus frequency and the position corresponding to a CF a few hundred hertz higher than the stimulus frequency. Moreover, it is assumed that this strong active behavior begins at 7.5 ms after the onset of the stimulation and lasts for 3 ms. The active behavior of OHCs as a function of time and position on the BM and the corresponding waveforms are shown in Fig. 8a and 8b, respectively. At about 10 ms, one train can be seen clearly, and a comparison between this result and the measurement shown in Fig. 2a suggests that this train is the fast component.

To obtain the slow component, it is assumed that the active behavior of the OHCs becomes stronger for a second time between 12.5 ms and 15.5 ms after the onset of the stimulation (Fig. 9). In Fig. 9, the second period of active behavior of the OHCs is shown to be stronger than the first; however, it is assumed that this is not always the case. When the stimulus level is small, the second period of active OHC behavior is assumed to be stronger than the first.

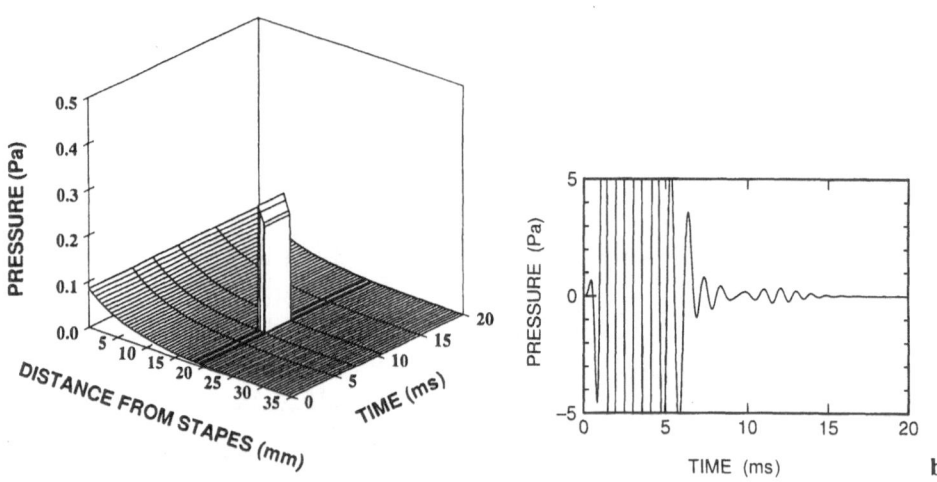

a   b

FIG. 8a,b. Numerical results. **a** 3-D expression of the pressure generated by OHCs. It is assumed that the active behavior of the OHCs becomes stronger between 7.5 ms and 10.5 ms after the onset of stimulation. **b** Numerical result of the waveforms shows the fast components

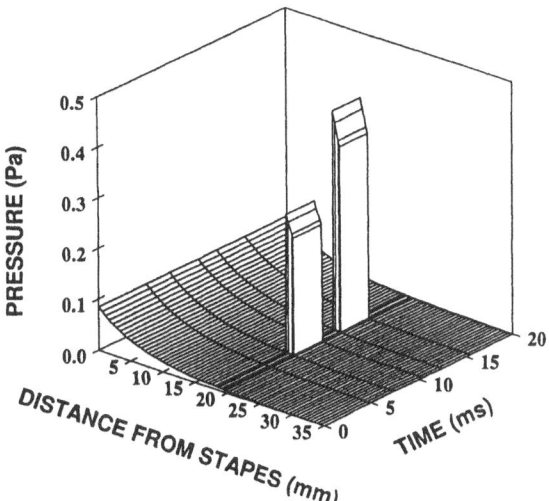

FIG. 9. A 3-D expression of the pressure generated by OHCs. It is assumed that the active behavior of the OHCs becomes stronger twice, between 7.5 ms and 10.5 ms and between 12.5 ms and 15.5 ms after the onset of stimulation

On the other hand, when the stimulus level is large, the first period is assumed to be stronger than the second. The numerical results of the waveforms and input–output curves of the fast and slow components are shown in Fig. 10a and 10b, respectively. These results are fairly consistent with the measured valves shown in Fig. 2.

5 Discussion

In the model shown in Fig. 4, the wave traveling along the BM cannot reflect at any point except at the apical end. When the model is stimulated by a click or toneburst signal, the frequency of the wave reflected from the apical end depends

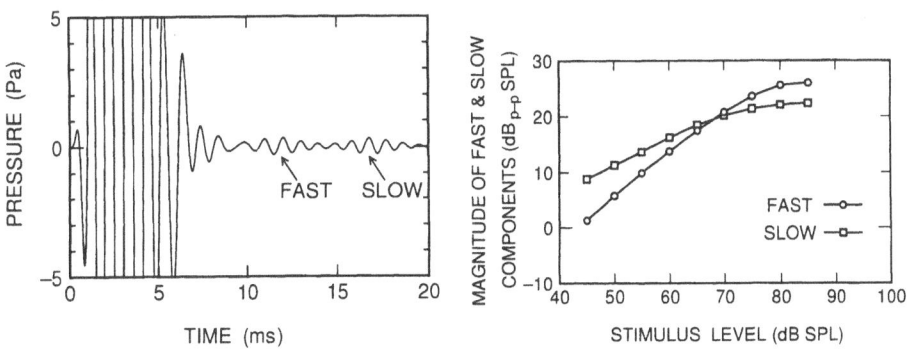

FIG. 10a,b. Numerical results when the active behavior of the OHCs is expressed by Fig. 9. **a** TEOAE waveforms. **b** Input–output curves of the fast and slow components

on its characteristic frequency, because natural vibration persists after transient vibration is diminished. Because the frequencies of TEOAEs are dependent on the spectrum of the stimulus [8], the reflected wave may not cause TEOAEs. In fact, the wave reflected from the apical end that influences the waveforms is too small to be seen in Fig. 7. Therefore, the generat or of TEOAEs may exist in another region of the BM.

Some researchers have introduced the irregularity of BM impedance in their cochlear model to explain the mechanism of TEOAE generation. Wit et al. [30] performed the simulation of TEOAEs stimulated by a click using a plain model assuming random irregularities in characteristic frequencies of the BM. Fukazawa [22] showed that a model with three discontinuities in BM damping can produce echoes similar to TEOAEs. It was explained that the fast and slow component were the beat of the waves reflected from the irregularities. In this study, the TEOAE waveforms are obtained when the active behavior of the OHCs is assumed to become strong twice.

The fast and slow components exhibit a different tendency in some experiments. The threshold of fast components is higher than that of slow components (see Fig. 2). Tanaka et al. [26] reported that the input–output function of fast components was more linear and less vulnerable to trauma than that of slow components. These findings may suggest that the fast and slow components are generated by a different mechanism.

Moreover, Whitehead et al. also suggested that DPOAEs consist of two components [24]. When the stimuli are low, the input–output function of one of the DPOAE components is nonlinear, and this component is not robust. The characteristics of this component are similar to those of the slow component of TEOAEs. In contrast, when the stimuli are high, the input–output function of the other DPOAE component is linear, and like the fast component of TEOAEs, this component is robust. Therefore, the active behavior of the cochlea may have two different mechanisms.

To obtain the latency between fast components and slow components, it is assumed that the strong active behavior of OHCs is inhibited between 10.5 ms and 12.5 ms after the onset of the stimulation. As far as the latency is concerned, it has been reported that OHC behavior is suppressed by medial olivocochlear efferents, which are activated by the ipsilateral tonal stimulation, and that the medial olivocochlear effect on suppression is a maximum at about 10 ms after stimulation in cats [31]. There is a possibility that interruption of OHC activity is caused by this suppression. Tavarkiladze et al. [32] investigated ipsilateral suppression effects on TEOAEs in normal-hearing human subjects, and showed that the most prominent suppression of TEOAEs under forward masking conditions was observed during the first 5–7 ms after masker click onset. Berlin et al. [33] reported that ipsilateral suppression effects on TEOAEs became maximum between 14 and 18 ms after white noise. The difference in suppression time between them may depend on the masker condition. These reports that OHC behavior is suppressed by ipsilateral stimulation for several milliseconds after the onset support our assumption that there are two periods of strong OHC activity.

6 Conclusions

An attempt was made to simulate the generation mechanism of TEOAEs by theoretical analysis. The following assumptions, when applied to our one-dimensional mathematical model of the cochlea, produced TEOAE waveforms fairly consistant with the measured values:

1. The active behavior of the OHCs becomes stronger twice after the onset of stimulation. The first period is from 7.5–10.5 ms and the second period is from 12.5–15.5 ms after the onset of stimulation. The strong active behavior is located between the parts of the BM where the CF corresponds to the stimulus frequency and a few hundred hertz above the stimulus frequency.

2. For weak stimulus signals the second period is stronger than the first. For more powerful stimulus signals the first period is stronger than the second.

Acknowledgment. This research is supported by the Ministry of Education of Japan under Scientific Research Grant No. 04237204, 05221207, and 06213207.

References

1. Patuzzi R, Johnstone BM, Sellick PM (1984) The alteration of the vibration of the basilar membrane produced by loud sound. Hear Res 13:99–100
2. Nuttall AL, Dolan DF, Avinash G (1991) Laser Doppler velocimetry of basilar membrane vibration. Hear Res 51:203–214
3. Johnstone BM, Patuzzi R, Yates GK (1986) Basilar membrane measurements and the travelling wave. Hear Res 22:147–153
4. Robles L, Ruggero MA, Rich NC (1986) Basilar membrane mechanics at the base of the chinchilla cochlea. I. Input–output functions, tuning curves, and response phases. J Acoust Soc Am 80:1364–1374
5. Sellick PM, Patuzzi R, Johnstone BM (1982) Measurement of basilar membrane motion in the guinea pig using the Mössbauer technique. J Acoust Soc Am 80:1375–1383
6. Ruggero MA, Rich NC (1991) Application of a commercially-manufactured Doppler-shift laser velocimeter to the measurement of basilar-membrane vibration. Hear Res 51:215–230
7. Kemp DT (1978) Stimulated acoustic emissions from within the human auditory system. J Acoust Soc Am 64:1386–1391
8. Probst R, Lonsbury-Martin BL, Martin GK (1991) A review of otoacoustic emissions. J Acoust Soc Am 89:2027–2067
9. Kemp DT, Bray P, Alexander L, Brown AM (1986) Acoustic emissions cochleography—practical aspects. Scand Audiol 25:71–95

10. Brownell WE, Bader CR, Bertrand D, Ribaupierre YE (1985) Evoked mechanical responses of isolated cochlear hair cells. Science 277:194–196
11. Ashmore JF (1987) A fast motile response in guinea-pig outer hair cells: the cellular basis of the cochlear amplifier. J Physiol (Camb) 388:323–347
12. Brownell WE (1990) Outer hair cell electromotility and otoacoustic emissions. Ear Hear 11:82–92
13. Diependaal RJ, Duifhuis H, Hoogstrten HW, Viergever MA (1987) Numerical methods for solving one-dimensional cochlear models in the time domain. J Acoust Soc Am 82:1655–1666
14. Diependaal RJ, Viergever MA (1989) Nonlinear and active two-dimensional cochlear models: time-domain solution. J Acoust Soc Am 85:803–812
15. Neely ST (1981) Finite difference solution of a two-dimensional mathematical model of the cochlea. J Acoust Soc Am 69:1386–1393
16. Neely ST (1985) Mathematical modeling of cochlear mechanics. J Acoust Soc Am 78:345–352
17. Viergever MA, Kalker JJ (1975) A two-dimensional model for the cochlea. I. The exact approach. J Eng Math 9:353–365
18. Viergever MA (1977) A two-dimensional model for the cochlea. II. The heuristic approach and numerical results. J Eng Math 11:11–28
19. Zwicker E (1986) Hardware cochlear nonlinear preprocessing model with active feedback. J Acoust Soc Am 80:146–153
20. Zwicker E (1986) Otoacoustic emissions in a nonlinear cochlear hardware model with feedback. J Acoust Soc Am 80:154–162
21. Furst M, Lapid M (1988) A cochlear model for acoustic emissions. J Acoust Soc Am 84:222–229
22. Fukazwa T (1992) Evoked otoacoustic emissions in a nonlinear model of the cochlea. Hear Res 59:17–24
23. Ohyama K, Wada H, Kobayashi T, Takasaka T (1991) Spontaneous otoacoustic emissions in guinea pig. Hear Res 56:111–121
24. Whitehead ML, Lonsbury-Martin BL, Martin GK (1992) Evidence for two discrete sources of $2f_1-f_2$ distortion-product otoacoustic emission in rabbit. I. Differential dependence on stimulus parameters. J Acoust Soc Am 91:1587–1607
25. Kemp DT, Ryan S, Bray P (1990) A guide to the effective use of otoacoustic emissions. Ear Hear 11:93–105
26. Tanaka Y, Suzuki M, Inoue T (1990) Evoked otoacoustic emissions in sensorineural hearing impairment: its clinical implications. Ear Hear 11:134–143
27. Dallos P (1992) The active cochlea. J Neurosci 12:4575–4585
28. Cody AR, Russell IJ (1987) The responses of hair cells in the basal turn of the guinea pig cochlea to tones. J Physiol (Camb) 383:551–569
29. Wada H, Ohyama K, Kobayashi T, Sunaga N, Koike T (1993) Relationship between evoked otoacoustic emissions and middle-ear dynamic characteristics. Audiology (Basel) 32:282–292
30. Wit HP, van Dijk P, Avan P (1994) Wavelet analysis of real ear and synthesized click evoked otoacoustic emissions. Hear Res 73:141–147
31. Gifford ML, Guinan JJ Jr (1987) Effects of electrical stimulation of medial olivocochlear neurons on ipsilateral and contralateral cochlear responses. Hear Res 29:179–194
32. Tavarkiladze GA, Frolenkov GI, Kruglov AV, Artamasov SV (1994) Ipsilateral suppression effects on transient evoked otoacoustic emission. Br J Audiol 28:1–12

33. Berlin CI, Hood LJ, Hurley A, Wen H, Kemp DT (1994) Bilateral and ipsilateral forward masking and TEOAE suppression. In: Popelka GR (ed) Abstracts of the seventeenth midwinter research meeting. Association for Research in Otolaryngology, Des Moines, p 52

Mechanical Model and Simulation of Respiratory System

SHIGEO WADA[1] and MASAO TANAKA[2]

Summary. A simulation approach based on the detailed mechanical model is applied to understand the complex system of lung respiration in terms of computational biomechanics. Mechanical models were established for the various elements of the respiratory processes such as air flow, tissue deformation, blood flow, and gas diffusion, and they are unified into a system model in a coupled manner. The simulation using the mechanical model represents the overall behavior of lung respiration as well as the behavior in detail of the elements. The mechanical model for each element is verified through system behavior, which is observed by experiments, and the respiratory system is analyzed by synthesis. Taking into account the hierarchical interaction of the mechanical phenomena in lung respiration, we attempted to seek an appropriate pressure condition in artificial ventilation.

Key words: Computational biomechanics—Simulation—Lung respiration—Mechanical model—Artificial ventilation

1 Introduction

The respiratory system consists of the mechanical processes of breathing, pulmonary circulation, and gas exchange, which include various mechanical phenomena such as gas flow, blood flow, tissue deformation, and gas diffusion. It is the primal function of lung respiration to exchange the carbon dioxide produced in the body with the oxygen in the external air, and respiration is a resultant of the interaction of these mechanical phenomena. Therefore, the lung respiratory system is large in scale and complex in mechanism because of geometrical nonlinearity, material nonlinearity, hierarchy in mechanism, and interactions among multiple fields [1].

[1]Research Institute for Electronic Science, Hokkaido University, N12 W6 Kita-ku, Sapporo, Hokkaido, 060 Japan
[2]Department of Mechanical Engineering, Faculty of Engineering Science, Osaka University, 1-3 Machikaneyama-cho, Toyonaka, Osaka, 560 Japan

The computational approach enables us to use detailed models of mathematical physics established in the theoretical approach and to cope with realistic model studies as in the experimental approach. That is, computaion is the third approach, complementing the theoretical and experimental approaches. The up-to-date simulation model is conceptually different from the traditional engineering model. Simplification is the fundamental principle of traditional modeling, and typical examples are the equivalent electric circuit and the bond graph model. This has been successfully applied to examine the overall behavior of the respiratory system [2,3]. The simulation model employs direct modeling element by element, and the mechanical phenomena have been described as mathematical models based on continuum mechanics as reported in the literature [e.g., 4–6]. The direct mechanical model has the potential to probe detailed mechanical behavior.

In the case of the lung respiratory system, interaction among the mechanical phenomena is an essential factor in the overall behavior of the system, and the isolated elements sometimes gives biased insights. The validity of the elements, or subsystems, should be examined under the environmental conditions expected in vivo, although in vivo observation is sometimes restricted by the disturbance caused by artificial treatment. This suggests that it is necessary to consider the behavior of the element in the context of the system behavior as a whole in the context of the practical simulation based on the detailed mechanical model. The current computer environment encourages us to proceed to computer simulation for the respiratory system [7,8].

The authors and co-workers have also been working on lung respiration using the simulation approach, that is, the approach of computational respiratory biomechanics [9–14]. The concept of analysis by synthesis is the key in both establishing the element and system models and understanding the element and system behaviors and functions, where the computational simulation is coupled with experimental observation. It is noted here that the current simulation is in a different category from numerical computation based on a theory established a priori. In this chapter, a system model is described for lung respiration based on the direct modeling principle, and model verification and system analysis are demonstrated by means of computer simulation. Some application studies are also included for artificial ventilation and its optimal operation design in the biomedical engineering field.

2 Respiratory Model

2.1 Breathing Model

Tissue deformation, including surface tension activity and gas flow in the branching airway, determines the breathing dynamics. These mechanical phenomena are coupled in the breathing model.

2.1.1 Lung Deformation

An inflation state of the lung in the thoracic cage is settled by the equilibrium relation

$$P_{al} = P_{pl} + \sigma \tag{1}$$

where P_{pl} is the pressure in pleural space, the alveolar pressure P_{al} represents the gas pressure in the lung, and the tension of the pleura is neglected [4]. Because the lung parenchyma is largely composed of microscale alveoli, the macroscopic stress σ can be defined as the sum of forces acting on the tissue including unit cross-sectional area [15]. Two stresses, the stress σ_e from tissue elasticity and the stress σ_s from surface tension, make the macroscopic stress σ,

$$\sigma = \sigma_e + \sigma_s \tag{2}$$

The elastic stress is derived from a pseudo-strain energy function W as

$$\sigma_{ei} = \frac{1}{\lambda_i^2} \frac{\partial(\rho_0 W)}{\partial \lambda_i} \quad (i = x, y, z) \tag{3}$$

where λ_i $(i = x, y, z)$ is the stretch ratio of lung tissue. For an idealized lung parenchyma composed of regular cubic alveoli, Fung [4] and Vawter et al. [16] have proposed an energy function:

$$\rho_0 W = \frac{1}{2} c \exp\left(a_1 E_x^2 + a_2 E_y^2 + 2a_4 E_x E_y\right)$$

+symmetrical terms by permutation $\tag{4}$

where ρ_0 is the density of parenchyma, c and a_j $(j = 1, 2, 4)$ are material constants, and E_i stands for Green's strain, defined as $E_i = (\lambda_i^2 - 1)/2$. For an uniform and isotropic inflation, the stresses for each principal direction become identical $\sigma_e = \sigma_{ei}$.

The stress σ_s due to the surface tension γ is represented as

$$\sigma_s = \frac{4\gamma}{\lambda \Delta} \tag{5}$$

where Δ is edge length of cubic alveolus [4]. It is known that in the lung, surfactants reduce the surface tension depending on the surface area change [17]. The hysteresis of the surface tension γ to the cyclic area change is expressed by the rate-type model [10]:

$$\frac{d\gamma}{dt} = \begin{cases} a(\gamma_u - \gamma)\dfrac{d\Lambda}{dt} & \text{for } \dfrac{d\Lambda}{dt} \geq 0 \\[2mm] a(\gamma - \gamma_l)\dfrac{d\Lambda}{dt} & \text{for } \dfrac{d\Lambda}{dt} < 0 \end{cases} \tag{6}$$

where γ_u and γ_l are the upper and lower bound of the surface tension, respectively, the coefficient a determines the degree of hysteresis, and Λ denotes the surface area ratio ($\Lambda = \lambda^2$). This surface tension model not only represents the essential features of the hysteresis observed in experiments [17,18] but also guarantees the convergence of the hysteresis loop for any range of surface area change. This adaptive feature is only expressed by using the rate-type model, not by a model fixed in the state space [19].

2.1.2 Gas Flow in the Airway

From the trachea, the airway bifurcates into two smaller branches 23 times on average until it reaches the alveoli of the human lung [20]. The gas flow model in the airway system is constructed by assembling the equation of motion

$$\frac{\partial u_i}{\partial t} + u_i \frac{\partial u_i}{\partial x_i} + \frac{1}{\rho_i}\frac{\partial P_i}{\partial x_i} + \lambda_f \frac{u_i^2}{4r_i} = 0 \tag{7}$$

and the equation of continuity

$$\frac{\partial \rho_i}{\partial t} + u_i \frac{\partial \rho_i}{\partial x_i} + \rho_i \frac{\partial u_i}{\partial x_i} + 2\rho_i \frac{\partial \varepsilon_\theta}{\partial t} = 0 \tag{8}$$

for each airway branch of generation i, which is assumed to be an elastic cylindrical tube. The equation of state under isothermal process, $\rho_i = k_p P_i$, relates the gas density ρ_i with the pressure P_i for compressive air flow. As the airway is embedded in the lung parenchyma, the circumferential strain ε_θ is determined by the transmural pressure $P_i - P_{al}$ through the finite deformation theory. The flow resistance is estimated as that at steady flow [21], and thus the coefficient of friction is $\lambda_f = 64/\mathrm{Re}$ for laminar flow and $\lambda_f = 0.3164/\sqrt[4]{\mathrm{Re}}$ for turbulent flow. The airway bifurcation is assumed to have a regular dichotomy [20], and the governing Eqs. 7 and 8 for each branch from the trachea ($i = 0$) to the alveoli ($i = N$) are assembled from gas continuity at the junction between generation i and $i + 1$

$$\rho_i A_i u_i \big|_{x_i = l_i} = 2\rho_{i+1} A_{i+1} u_{i+1} \big|_{x_{i+1} = 0} \tag{9}$$

and the energy conservation

$$k_p \log P_i + \frac{1}{2}u_i^2 \bigg|_{x_i = l_i} = k_p \log P_{i+1} + \frac{1}{2}(1+\zeta)u_{i+1}^2 \bigg|_{x_{i+1} = 0} \tag{10}$$

where A_i is the cross-sectional area of the airway and ζ denotes the energy loss coefficient.

The manner of coupling between lung deformation and gas flow is illustrated in Fig. 1. The alveolar pressure P_{al} in Eq. 1 provides one of the boundary

FIG. 1. Mechanical interaction in the breathing model (from [14] with permission)

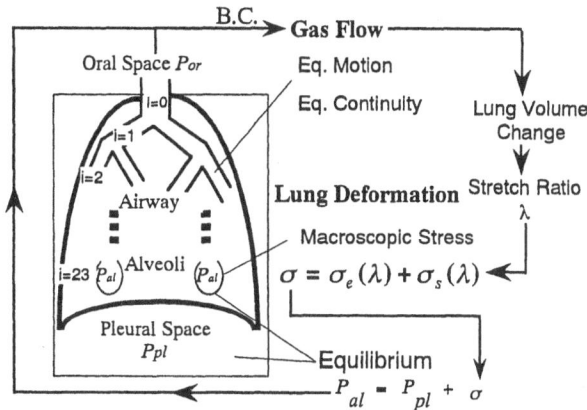

conditions for the gas flow model. The change of lung volume is calculated by integrating the gas flow at the trachea, and the inflation state then determines the stretch ratio of lung tissue, which is reflected in the macroscopic stress in the equilibrium relation.

2.2 Pulmonary Circulation Model

From the outlet of the right ventricle, the pulmonary artery bifurcates successively in the lung, arriving at the capillary network, while the venous vessels converge and terminate in the left atrium (Fig. 2). The blood flow model is constructed on the basis of the pulmonary circulation.

2.2.1 Blood Flow in the Arterial and Venous Tree

The blood flow in the arterial and venous tree is expressed by assembling the tube flow for each elastic vessel. The geometrical data of human vessels are provided by Singhal et al. [22] and Horsfield and Gordon [23]. The governing equations for incompressible blood flow with density ρ_b are written as

$$\frac{\partial u_{b(j)}}{\partial t} + u_{b(j)}\frac{\partial u_{b(j)}}{\partial x_{b(j)}} + \frac{1}{\rho_b}\frac{\partial P_{b(j)}}{\partial x_{b(j)}} + \lambda_{b(j)}\frac{u_{b(j)}^2}{4r_{b(j)}} = 0 \tag{11}$$

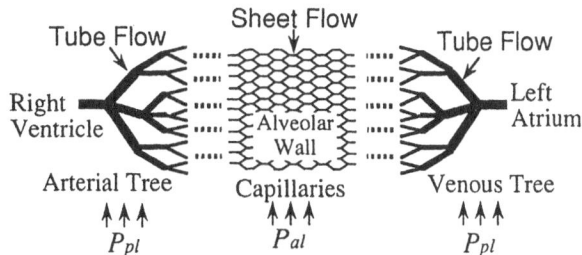

FIG. 2. Pulmonary circulation structure (from [14] with permission)

$$\frac{\partial r_{b(j)}}{\partial t} + u_{b(j)} \frac{\partial r_{b(j)}}{\partial x_{b(j)}} + \frac{r_{b(j)}}{2} \frac{\partial u_{b(j)}}{\partial x_{b(j)}} = 0 \tag{12}$$

where subscript $j (0 < |j| \le N_b)$ stands for the vessel order, $r_{b(j)}$ is radius of the vessel, and $P_{b(j)}$ and $u_{b(j)}$ are blood pressure and velocity, respectively. Negative vessel orders imply arterial vessels. The friction coefficient $\lambda_{b(j)}$ is modified from that of steady tube flow by the geometrical friction coefficient factor $f_{b(j)}$ [6]. The deformation of the vessel caused by the transmural pressure $\Delta P_{b(j)} = P_{b(j)} - P_{ex}$ is expressed by an equilibrium relation:

$$\alpha_j \beta_j \frac{\partial r_{b(j)}}{\partial t} + r_{b(j)} - r_{b0(j)} \left(1 + \alpha_j \Delta P_{b(j)}\right) = 0 \tag{13}$$

where $r_{b0(j)}$ is the radius in the natural state, and α_j and β_j are coefficients concerned with vessel compliance and viscosity, respectively [14]. The external pressure P_{ex} is the alveolar pressure P_{al} for the small vessels inside the lung, and the pleural pressure P_{pl} is for the large vessels outside the lung. For longitudinal deformation caused by the lung inflation, the stretch ratio of the vessel is assumed to be identical to that of the lung tissue λ.

2.2.2 Capillary Blood Flow

The concept of sheet flow proposed by Fung and Sobin [6] is employed in capillary blood flow. The one-dimensional blood flow between alveolar membranes supported by the elastic posts of connecting tissue is represented by

$$\frac{\partial u_{b(0)}}{\partial t} + u_{b(0)} \frac{\partial u_{b(0)}}{\partial x_{b(0)}} + \frac{1}{\rho_b} \frac{\partial P_{b(0)}}{\partial x_{b(0)}} + \lambda_{b(0)} \frac{3 u_{b(0)}^2}{8 h_b} = 0 \tag{14}$$

$$\frac{\partial h_b}{\partial t} + u_{b(0)} \frac{\partial h_b}{\partial x_{b(0)}} + h_b \frac{\partial u_{b(0)}}{\partial x_{b(0)}} = 0 \tag{15}$$

where subscript (0) indicates the capillary vessel. The alveolar gas pressure P_{al} applies to the alveolar membrane, and the height of the alveolar sheet h_b changes obeying the equilibrium relation

$$\Delta P_{b(0)} + R_b - \kappa T_b = 0 \tag{16}$$

where T_b is the membrane tension from lung inflation, that is, the sum of the elastic tension and the surface tension. The curvature κ of the alveolar membrane is written as

$$\kappa = \frac{-\partial^2 w_b / \partial x_{b(0)}^2}{\left\{1 + \left(\partial w_b / \partial x_{b(0)}\right)^2\right\}^{1.5}} \tag{17}$$

using the deflection $w_b = (h_b - h_{b0})/2$. The elastic posts are assumed to be distributed uniformly like a spring system, and the elastic resistance R_b is represented as

$$R_b = k_b w_b \quad (w_b \geq 0), \quad R_b = 0 \quad (w_b < 0) \tag{18}$$

The continuity relation at the junction between the j and $j+1$ vessels, including capillaries, is written as

$$N_{b(j)} A_{b(j)} u_{b(j)} \Big|_{x_{b(j)} = l_{b(j)}} = N_{b(j+1)} A_{b(j+1)} u_{b(j+1)} \Big|_{x_{b(j+1)} = 0} \tag{19}$$

$$P_{b(j)} + \frac{\rho_b}{2} u_{b(j)}^2 \Big|_{x_{b(j)} = l_{b(j)}} = P_{b(j+1)} + \frac{\rho_b}{2} u_{b(j+1)}^2 \Big|_{x_{b(j+1)} = 0} \tag{20}$$

where $N_{b(j)}$ is number of vessels at order j and $A_{b(j)}$ stands for the cross-sectional area of the vessel. These relations include the governing equations from the right ventricle to the left atrium.

2.3 Gas Exchange Model

The gas exchange model describes the transport phenomena of oxygen and carbon dioxide in the airway and the blood gas transport in the alveolar capillary in coupling. These phenomena are closely related to breathing and the pulmonary circulation.

2.3.1 Gas Transport in the Airway

The gas transport mechanism is governed by two fundamental processes: bulk convection and molecular diffusion. The combination of axial convection and lateral mixing by molecular diffusion results in an effective mechanism called augmented diffusion [24]. In the peripheral airway surrounded by the alveoli, oxygen diffuses into the capillary blood and carbon dioxide diffuses out. Taking into account both gas transport and gas exchange in the airway, the gas concentrations $C_{(g)i}(x_i, t)$ of oxygen ($g = O_2$) and carbon dioxide ($g = CO_2$) in each airway generation i are expressed by

$$\frac{\partial C_{(g)i}}{\partial t} + u_i \frac{\partial C_{(g)i}}{\partial x_i} - D_{eff} \frac{\partial^2 C_{(g)i}}{\partial x_i^2} + S_i D_{L(g)} \left(P_{(g)i} - \overline{P}_{b(g)} \right) = 0 \tag{21}$$

where S_i denotes the ratio of gas exchange area to volume [10] and $D_{L(g)}$ is the diffusing capacity in Fick's law [25]. Partial pressure $p_{(g)i}$ in the airway is converted from gas concentration $C_{(g)i}$. As the capillary position could not be specified at the interface with the airway space, the average partial pressure $\overline{p}_{b(g)}$ of the the blood gas is used. The gas velocity u_i in the convection term of Eq. 21 comes from the breathing model, and the effective diffusion coefficient D_{eff} involves the augmented diffusion. Among several expressions of the coefficient [26], we refer to the theoretical analysis by Watson [27]. The continuity that satisfies mass conservation at the branching point between generation i and $i+1$

$$C_{(g)i}\Big|_{x_i=l_i} = C_{(g)i+1}\Big|_{x_{i+1}=0} \tag{22}$$

$$D_{eff}A_i \frac{\partial C_{(g)i}}{\partial x_i}\Big|_{x_i=l_i} = 2D_{eff}A_{i+1}\frac{\partial C_{(g)i+1}}{\partial x_{i+1}}\Big|_{x_{i+1}=0} \tag{23}$$

assembles the model Eq. 21 for each generation ($i = 0\sim N$) to that for the whole airway system.

2.3.2 Gas Carriage by Blood Flow

The venous blood is arterialized during passage through the alveolar capillaries. Based on mass conservation of the blood gas in the capillary, the distributions of the oxygen and carbon dioxide concentrations $C_{b(g)}(x_{b(0)},t)$ along the capillary are expressed by

$$\frac{\partial C_{b(g)}}{\partial t} + u_{b(0)}\frac{\partial C_{b(g)}}{\partial x_{b(0)}} + S_b D_{L(g)}\left(p_{b(g)} - \overline{P}_{(g)}\right) = 0 \tag{24}$$

where S_b is the ratio of the gas exchange area to the capillary volume and $\overline{p}_{(g)}$ denotes the average partial gas pressure over the peripheral airway with the alveoli. The pulmonary circulation model provides the distribution of blood velocity $u_{b(0)}$ in the capillary. The gas concentration $C_{b(g)}$ is converted to the partial pressure $p_{b(g)}$ by the dissociation curves, including Bohr and Haldane effects [28].

The total amount of the gas exchange calculated from the airway side is

$$F_{a(g)} = \sum_{i=20}^{N} 2^i \int_0^{l_i} A_i S_i D_{L(g)}\left(P_{i(g)} - \overline{P}_{b(g)}\right)dx_i \tag{25}$$

and that from the capillary side is

$$F_{b(g)} = \int_0^{l_{b(0)}} A_{b(0)} S_b D_{L(g)}\left(\overline{P}_{(g)} - P_{b(g)}\right)dx_{b(0)} \tag{26}$$

where $l_{b(0)}$ is the capillary length. These values must be identical to the average flux

$$\overline{F}_{(g)} = A_s D_{L(g)}\left(\overline{P}_{(g)} - \overline{P}_{b(g)}\right) \tag{27}$$

where A_s stands for the total surface area for the gas exchange, and the average partial pressures $\bar{P}_{(g)}$ and $\bar{P}_{b(g)}$ are determined so as to satisfy $F_{a(g)} = F_{b(g)} = \bar{F}$.

3 Discretization of the Model and Simulation Procedure

To solve the respiratory model numerically, the model written in partial differential equations is discretized by the finite-element method based on the adjoint variational principle. As this method has been concretely explained in the literature [8,14,29], only the general outline is described here.

3.1 Adjoint Variational Principle

In the gas flow model of the airway and the blood flow model of the vessel tree, the governing equations are $\mathbf{f}_i(\mathbf{w}_i(x_i,t)) = 0$ $(N_1 \leq i \leq N_2)$ along with the continuity $\mathbf{g}_i(\mathbf{w}_i(0,t),\mathbf{w}_{i+1}(l_i,t)) = 0$ $(N_1 \leq i \leq N_2-1)$ at the branching points where vector $\mathbf{w}_i$ represents the physical variables as the pressure and velocity. According to the Lagrangian multiplier method, a functional is formulated as

$$\mathbf{J} = \sum_{i=N_1}^{N_2} \int_0^T \int_0^{x_i} \boldsymbol{\phi}_i^T \mathbf{f}_i dx_i dt + \sum_{i=N_1}^{N_1-1} \int_0^T \boldsymbol{\eta}_i^T \mathbf{g}_i dt \qquad (28)$$

using Lagrangian multipliers $\boldsymbol{\phi}_i(x_i,t)$ and $\boldsymbol{\eta}_i(x_i,t)$. The first variation of the functional $\mathbf{J}$ after successive integration by parts leads to the original governing equations $\mathbf{f}_i = 0$ as the primal part and that for the Lagrangian multipliers as the adjoint part. In this case the physical meaning of the multipliers is not straightforward because the variational problem is nonself-adjoint. However, the connecting compatibility of the Lagrangian multipliers $\boldsymbol{\phi}_i$ corresponding to $\mathbf{g}_i = 0$ for the primal part is obtained by eliminating $\boldsymbol{\eta}_i$ [14]. These connecting relations are used in the finite-element discretization.

3.2 Finite-Element Discretization

The space variables in the functional $\mathbf{J}$ are discretized by the finite-element method. In the finite element i, the space variables $\mathbf{w}_i(x_i,t)$ $\boldsymbol{\phi}(x_i,t)$ are interpolated by the element vectors $\mathbf{w}_i^e = [\mathbf{w}_i(0,t)^T, \mathbf{w}_i(l_i,t)^T]$ and $\boldsymbol{\phi}_i^e = [\boldsymbol{\phi}_i(0,t)^T, \boldsymbol{\phi}_i(l_i,t)^T]$ using the polynomial shape functions $\mathbf{N}^w$ and $\mathbf{N}^\phi$, respectively. Furthermore, the element vectors are represented by the global vector $\mathbf{w}^s$ and $\boldsymbol{\phi}^s$, which consist of the independent variables at the nodal points. As a result, the space variables are discretized as

$$\mathbf{w}_i(x_i,t) = \mathbf{N}^{w^T}\mathbf{w}_i^{e^T} = \mathbf{N}^{w^T}\mathbf{B}_i^{w^T}\mathbf{w}^{s^T}, \quad \boldsymbol{\phi}_i(x_i,t) = \boldsymbol{\phi}_i^e\mathbf{N}^\phi = \boldsymbol{\phi}^s\mathbf{B}_i^\phi\mathbf{N}^\phi \qquad (29)$$

where the matrices $\mathbf{B}_i^w$ and $\mathbf{B}_i^\phi$ consist of the continuity derived from the variational principle. It is noted that the matrices $\mathbf{B}_i^w$ and $\mathbf{B}_i^\phi$ correspond to the Boolean in the standard finite-element method, but their components are not always zero and unity. By substituting Eq. 29 into Eq. 28, the stationary condition of the discretized functional gives the ordinary differential equations

$$\sum_{i=N_1}^{N_2}\left[\mathbf{B}_i^\phi\mathbf{K}_i^1\mathbf{B}_i^{w^T}\frac{d\mathbf{w}^{s^T}}{dt}+\mathbf{B}_i^\phi\mathbf{K}_i^2\left(\mathbf{w}^s\right)\mathbf{B}_i^{w^T}\mathbf{w}^{s^T}\right]=\sum_{i=N_1}^{N_2}\mathbf{B}_i^\phi\mathbf{q}_i \qquad (30)$$

where $\mathbf{K}_i^1$ and $\mathbf{K}_i^2$ are the elemental coefficient matrices and $\mathbf{q}_i$ denotes the elemental free term vector. The obtained ordinary differential equations are solved under an appropriate boundary and initial conditions. The time derivative is handled by the numerical integration combined with the conventional iterative technique resulting from the quasi-linearization for the nonlinear terms.

3.3 Simulation Procedure

The simulation procedure is briefly illustrated in Fig. 3. The pleural pressure P_{pl} and the oral pressure P_{or} are given as the driving force for normal respiration and artificial ventilation, respectively. The gas pressure P_{al} and P_{pl} in the lung and the stretch ratio λ of the tissue obtained from the breathing model are used in the pulmonary circulation model. The blood pressure or the velocity at the inlet of the artery and at the outlet of the vein are prescribed as the boundary condition. The gas velocity in the airway from breathing and the blood flow in the capillary from the pulmonary circulation are incorporated into the gas exchange model. For the boundary condition of gas exchange, the inhaled gas concentration is given and the partial pressure is set at that of venous blood returning to the lung.

4 Verification of the Model Through System Behavior

4.1 Breathing Dynamics Considering Surface Tension Activity

The relationship between pleural pressure P_{pl} and the lung volume change ΔV was examined by using a closed chamber imitating the thoracic cage. Five lung specimens were excised from white rabbits weighing about 3 kg for the measurement. This system behavior is compared with the simulation of breathing to verify the breathing model. The tissue elasticity of each lung specimen was also measured by the biaxial tension test [14], and the material constants were used in the simulation (Table 1). In the simulation, the airway size of the human lung [20] is scaled down to one-third (for the rabbit lung) and the alveolar size is assumed to be $\Delta = 100\,\mu m$. The unknown model parameters, that is, the lung volume in the natural state V_0, the hysteresis coefficient a of the surface tension, and the pressure loss coefficient ζ in the airway, are identified from the P_{pl}–ΔV relation

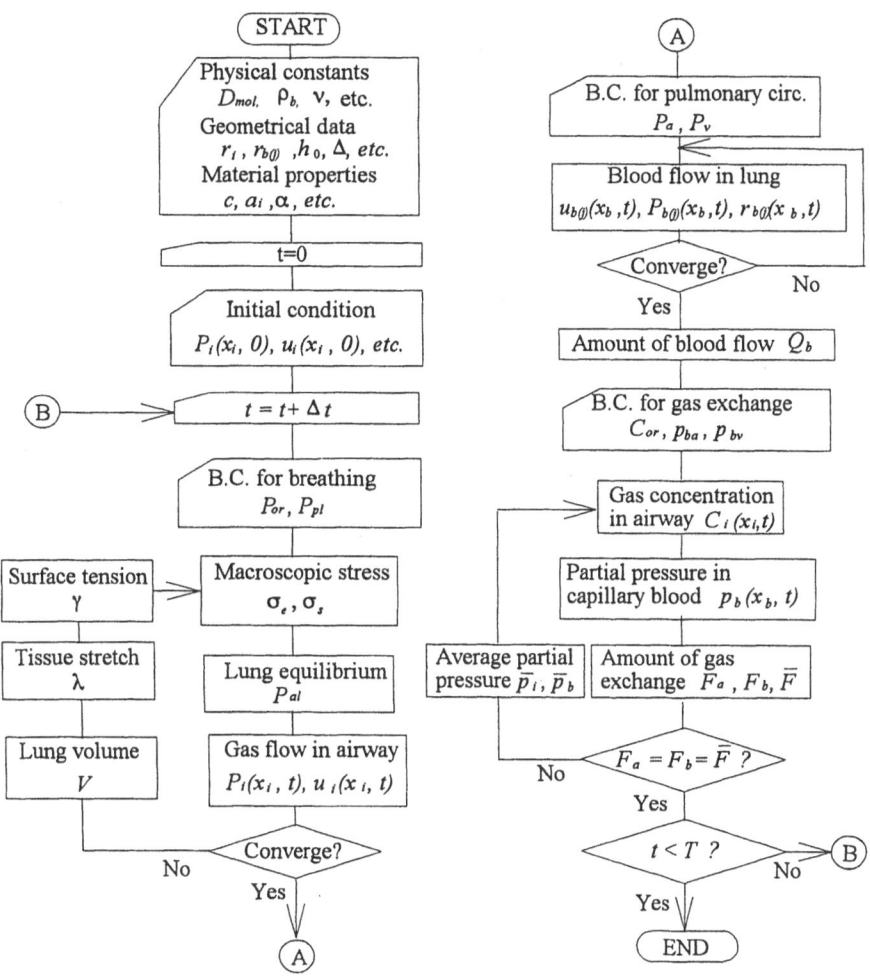

FIG. 3. Flowchart of simulation procedure (from [14] with permission)

TABLE 1. Material constants and identified model parameters.

Specimen	Material constants			Identified parameters			Resultant error R_{VH} (%)	
	c (Pa)	$a_1 = a_2$	a_3	V_0 (cm³)	a	ξ	$f = 0.2$ Hz	$f = 5$ Hz
I	19.1	1.48	0.117	21	2.9	1.5	8.9	11.9
II	22.1	1.75	0.411	22	3.1	3.0	12.0	19.6
III	39.7	1.90	0.509	26	2.7	2.0	9.8	14.1
IV	106	0.824	0.152	18	1.7	1.5	4.7	10.8
V	62.5	1.35	0.316	37	3.9	1.5	7.9	25.1

with the pressure amplitude of 0.25 kPa (case A), 0.49 kPa (case B), and 0.74 kPa (case C) at the frequencies 0.2 Hz and 0.5 Hz. The relative errors $R_{v(k)}$ and $R_{H(k)}$ between the simulation and experiment are defined for the tidal volume and for the hysteresis area, respectively. The model parameters are then identified so as to minimize the resultant error:

$$R_{VH} = \sqrt{\frac{1}{6}\sum_k \left(R_{V(k)}^2 + R_{H(k)}^2 \right)} \tag{31}$$

where subscript k distinguishes the pressure amplitude condition.

The identified model parameters are listed in Table 1 along with the resultant error in the P_{pl}–ΔV relation. It was confirmed that the identification gives a meaningful value for every specimen by evaluating the sensitivity of the model parameters to the error [13]. Examples of simulated P_{pl}–ΔV relations compared with experimental results are shown in Fig. 4a–c, where the pleural pressure P_{pl} oscillates in the sinusoidal waveform with the frequencies of 1 Hz and 5 Hz, and in trapezoid waveform with 0.5 Hz, respectively. It is found that the simulation using a single set of model parameters for each lung specimen represents the breathing dynamics observed by the experiments for various pressure conditions and specimens. This agreement supports the validity of the prediction by the simulation for inside phenomena of the lung such as the surface tension behavior as shown in Fig. 5.

4.2 Pulmonary Blood Flow Affected by the Gas Pressure in the Lung

Four Japanese white rabbits weighing about 3 kg were killed by an anesthetic following heparin treatment. A constant gas pressure P_L was applied to the trachea and the chest was opened. Keeping the hydrostatic pressure P_t constant at the reservoir tank connected to the pulmonary artery, the blood flow out of the vein was measured. The blood as the working fluid was diluted with saline to 20%. The relationship between the volumetric blood flow Q_b and the lung gas pressure P_L is shown by the solid symbols in Fig. 6. The experiment is also simulated using the pulmonary circulation model. The geometry and elasticity of the vessel are borrowed from those of the cat lung [30]. By using a suitable geometric friction coefficient $f_{b(j)} = 2.2$, the blood flow Q_b and its dependency on static gas pressure P_L show a good agreement with the experimental result, as shown by the open symbols in Fig. 6.

The simulation enables us to interpret the experimental result through the inner mechanical phenomena of the lung.

Figure 7a shows the distribution of alveolar sheet thickness, that is, the height of the capillary network from the entrance to the exit of the alveolar sheet. The gas pressure P_L in the lung compresses the alveolar sheet, and the collapse of the alveolar capillaries appears downstream in the sheet flow when the gas pressure becomes $P_L = 1.96$ kPa. This phenomenon corresponds to the decrease of blood

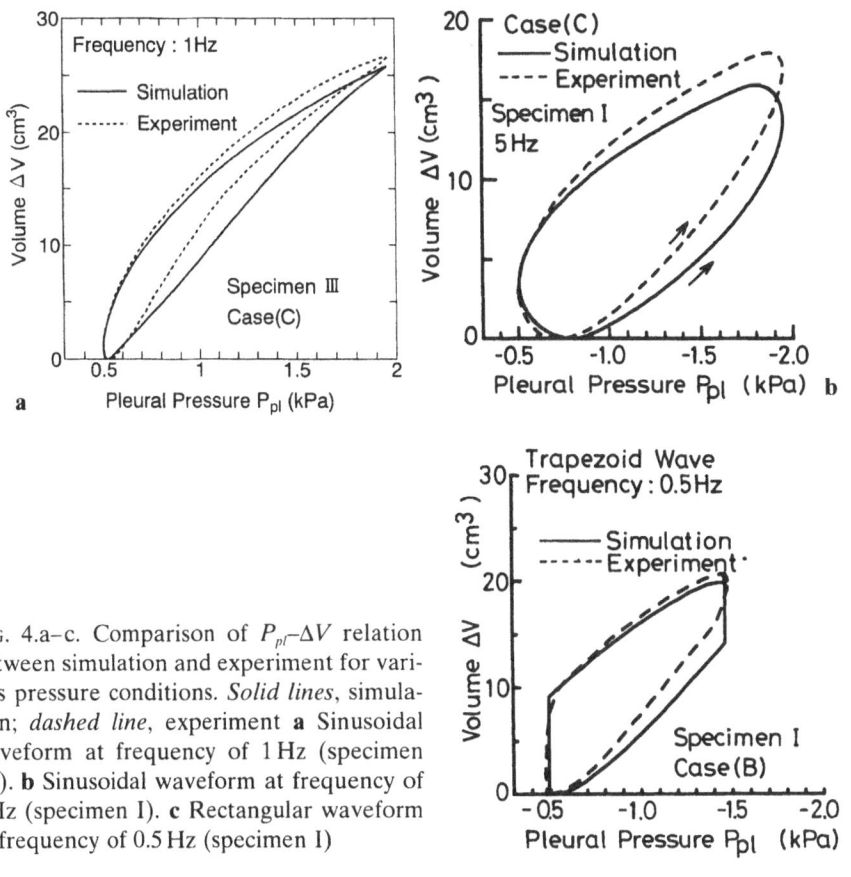

FIG. 4.a–c. Comparison of P_{pl}–ΔV relation between simulation and experiment for various pressure conditions. *Solid lines*, simulation; *dashed line*, experiment **a** Sinusoidal waveform at frequency of 1 Hz (specimen III). **b** Sinusoidal waveform at frequency of 5 Hz (specimen I). **c** Rectangular waveform at frequency of 0.5 Hz (specimen I)

FIG. 5. Surface tension behavior predicted by simulation (specimen III). *Solid line*, case A; *dashed line*, case B; *broken line*, case C

flow observed by both simulation and experiment. The volumetric blood flow Q_b decreases almost linearly below gas pressure up to $P_L = 1.47$ kPa (dotted line, Fig. 6), and the decrease of Q_b is accelerated at a gas pressure about $P_L = 1.96$ kPa.

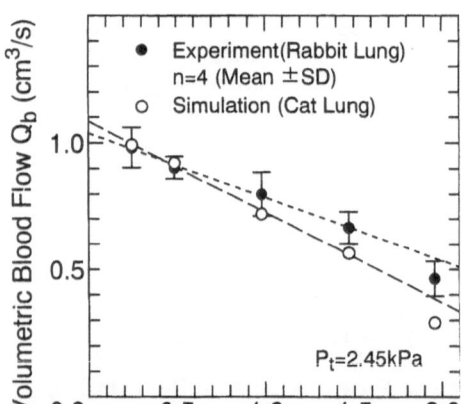

FIG. 6. Volumetric blood flow affected by gas pressure in the lung. *Solid circles*, experiment; *open circles*, simulation

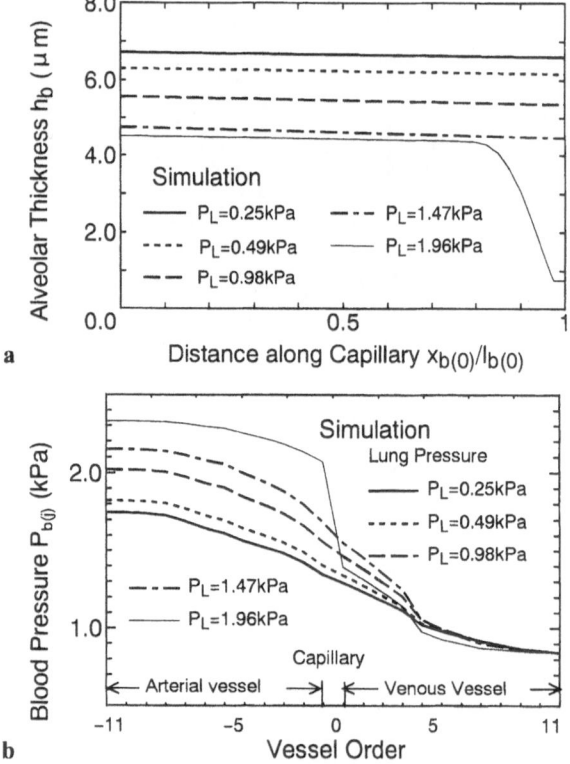

a

b

FIG. 7.a,b. Inside phenomena in the pulmonary circulation (from [14] with permission) **a** Alveolar sheet thickness h_b along capillary. **b** Blood pressure distribution over pulmonary circulation

Figure 7b shows the distribution of blood pressure along the pulmonary vessels. The abscissa indicates vessel order. Compression of the capillary by gas pressure increases the flow resistance significantly, resulting in high blood pressure in the arterial vessels, and the raise of blood pressure supports the alveolar sheet to free it from complete collapse. This mechanism of regulation by blood pressure is only explained by taking into account the correlation between the element phenomena and system behavior.

4.3 *Normal Respiration of the Human Lung*

To evaluate the total respiratory model including breathing, circulation, and gas exchange, normal respiration is simulated under physiological conditions. The pleural pressure P_{pl} is oscillated between $-0.49\,\mathrm{kPa}$ and $-0.88\,\mathrm{kPa}$ with a frequency of $0.2\,\mathrm{Hz}$, keeping the oral pressure P_{or} equal to atmospheric pressure. Because the pulmonary valve prevents the blood from returning to the right ventricle, the boundary condition at the inlet of the pulmonary is set as $P_{b(-Nb)}(0,t)$ $= P_c(t)$ for the open valve and $u_{b(-Nb)}(0,t) = 0$ for the closed valve. The cardiac output pressure P_c is given by an intermittent wave pattern between $0.54\,\mathrm{kPa}$ and $3.81\,\mathrm{kPa}$ with a frequency of $1\,\mathrm{Hz}$. Blood pressure at the output of the pulmonary vein is assumed to be constant, $P_{b(Nb)}(l_b,0) = 0.54\,\mathrm{kPa}$. For ventilation, air is inhaled and the gas tension in the venous blood is set to $p_{v(O_2)} = 40\,\mathrm{mmHg}$ for oxygen and $p_{v(CO_2)} = 46\,\mathrm{mmHg}$ for carbon dioxide. Other model parameters such as geometry and material properties are based on the normal human lung (see Table 2).

Corresponding to the oscillation of pleural pressure and cardiac output pressure, the lung volume changes between $3018\,\mathrm{cm}^3$ and $3441\,\mathrm{cm}^3$ (Table 3) and pulsatile blood flow is observed at the pulmonary artery (Fig. 8). According to the analysis of blood pressure and flow by discrete Fourier transforms, the frequency of the first impedance minimum appears at $3\,\mathrm{Hz}$ and the average impedance modulus is $17\,\mathrm{dyn \cdot s/cm^5}$. These characteristics are identical with the experimental results [31]. As the result of combining breathing and circulation, the respiratory functions listed in Table 3 fall within the physiological state of normal lung respiration.

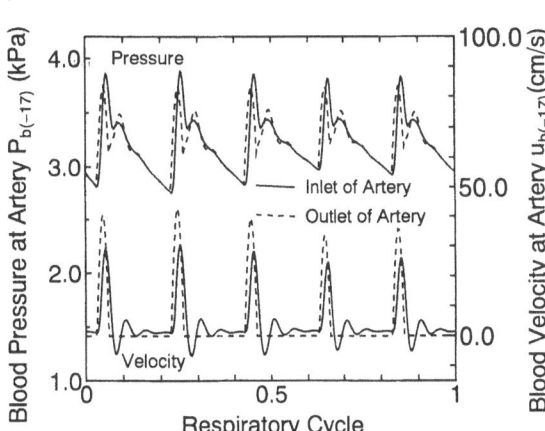

FIG. 8. Pulsatile blood pressure and velocity at pulmonary artery

TABLE 2. Representative model parameters for human lung.

Parameter		Reference
Breathing Model		
Material constants of lung tissue	$c = 10.1\,N/m$	33
	$a_1 = a_2 = 0.565$	
	$a_3 = 0.355$	
Edge length of alveoli	$\Delta = 149\,\mu m$	20
Surface tension	$a = 3.0$	13, 34, 35
	$\gamma_a = 30\,dyn/cm$	
	$\gamma_l = 2\,dyn/cm$	
Airway geometry	See reference	20
Gas constant	$k_p = 8.69 \times 10^4\,J/kg$	
Gas viscosity	$\mu = 18.69\,\mu Pa\cdot s$	
Lung volume at natural state	$V_0 = 1000\,cm^3$	10
Pulmonary Circulation Model		
Vessel geometry	See reference	22, 23
Capillary length	$l_{b(0)} = 600\,\mu m$	29, 30
Blood density	$\varrho_b = 1.05\,g/cm^3$	1
Vessel compliance	$\alpha = 1.4 \times 10^{-4}\,Pa^{-1}$	14
Blood viscosity	$\mu_b = 2.0\text{--}3.0\,mPa\cdot s$	6,30
Sheet thickness	$h_{b0} = 3.5\,\mu m$	29
Spring coefficient of connecting post	$k_b = 1.54 \times 10^5\,N/m^3$	14,29
Gas Exchange Model		
Capillary blood volume	$V_c = 70\,cm^3$	20
Alveolar–capillary interface	$A_s = 80\,m^2$	20
Hemoglobin content in blood	$0.147\,g/cm^3$	
Hemoglobin O_2 capacity	$1.34\,cm^3/g$	
O_2 molecular diffusion coefficient	$D_{mol.O_2} = 0.206\,cm^2/s$	
CO_2 molecular diffusion coefficient	$D_{mol.CO_2} = 0.164\,cm^2/s$	
Diffusing capacity	See reference	25, 36
O_2 reaction rate	See reference	37

TABLE 3. Boundary conditions for normal respiration and simulated results.

Boundary condition	
Pleural pressure P_{pl}	$-0.49 \sim -0.88\,kPa$, $0.2\,Hz$
Oral pressure P_{or}	$0\,kPa$ (atmospheric pressure)
Blood pressure at left atrium P_v	$0.54\,kPa$ ($4\,mmHg$)
Cardiac output pressure P_c	$0.54 \sim 3.81\,kPa$ ($4 \sim 28\,mmHg$), $1\,Hz$
Inhaled gas	Air
O_2 tension at inlet of capillary $P_{v(O_2)}$	$40\,mmHg$
CO_2 tension at inlet of capillary $P_{v(CO_2)}$	$46\,mmHg$
Results	
Lung volume V	$3018 \sim 3441\,cm^3$
Tidal volume V_T	$423\,cm^3$
Blood flow Q_b	$5027\,cm^3/min$
O_2 tension at outlet of capillary $p_{a(O_2)}$	$97.2 \sim 102\,mmHg$
CO_2 tension at outlet of capillary $p_{a(CO_2)}$	$39.6 \sim 41.6\,mmHg$
O_2 intake	$255\,cm^3/min$
CO_2 exhaust	$178\,cm^3/min$

5 Model-Based Approach to Optimal Artificial Ventilation

In spite of much improvement in respirators, because of a lack of information about the lung misoperation sometimes occurs, resulting in mechanical damage to the lung [32], especially in newborn infants. The simulation approach based on the theoretical model gives a fundamental assessment to the conventional technique for optimal ventilation.

5.1 Determination of Pressure Condition by Simulation

Simulation of artificial ventilation is carried out by oscillating the oral pressure P_{or} as the inhaled gas pressure. The change of pleural pressure P_{pl} following the lung volume change is approximated as a quadratic function of the volume ratio to the functional residual capacity [14]. Two typical wave patterns, shark-fin plateau (SFP) and sharp shark-fin (SSF), having a period between the inspiration and expiration phase, are prepared for inhaled gas pressure (Fig. 9). The former is recognized from clinical experience as the best pattern in conventional mechanical ventilation. The pressure amplitude is determined at several frequencies by the simulation (Fig. 10). The exhaust of carbon dioxide is considered when the air is inhaled because the oxygen supply can be adjusted over a wide range by raising the oxygen concentration of inhaled gas. The end-expiratory pressure is atmospheric pressure, and the pressure amplitude is adjusted so that the average carbon dioxide tension of the arterialized blood becomes a normal value ($p_{a(co_2)} =$ 40 mmHg) at the steady state. The metabolic rates of oxygen and carbon dioxide in the body are assumed to be 250 cm³/min and 200 cm³/min, respectively, and the gas tensions of blood returning to the lung are calculated from those of blood flowing out of the lung depending on the amount of blood flow affected by the applied gas pressure.

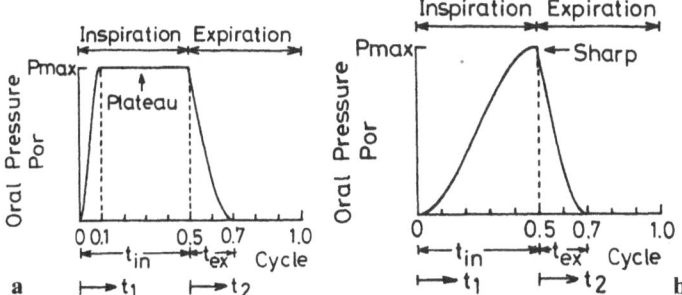

FIG. 9.a,b. Applied gas pressure pattern. **a** Shark-fin plateau (SFP). **b** Sharp shark-fin (SSF)

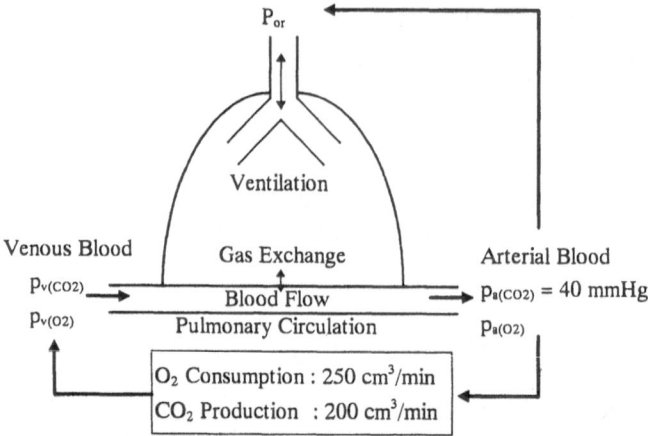

FIG. 10. Determination problem of inhaled gas pressure amplitude

5.2 Influence of Frequency

Figure 11 contrasts the oxygen distribution along the airway during inspiration by the SSF pressure pattern at the low-frequency oscillation (0.1 Hz) with that at a relatively high frequency (5 Hz). Both ventilation conditions maintain the normal CO_2 exhaust, and the resultant tidal volumes are 776 cm³ and 193 m³, respectively. The gradient of gas concentration indicates that the bulk flow dominates gas transport in the conduction airway and that diffusion takes over in the peripheral airway at the frequency of 0.1 Hz, while diffusion also contributes in the conduc-

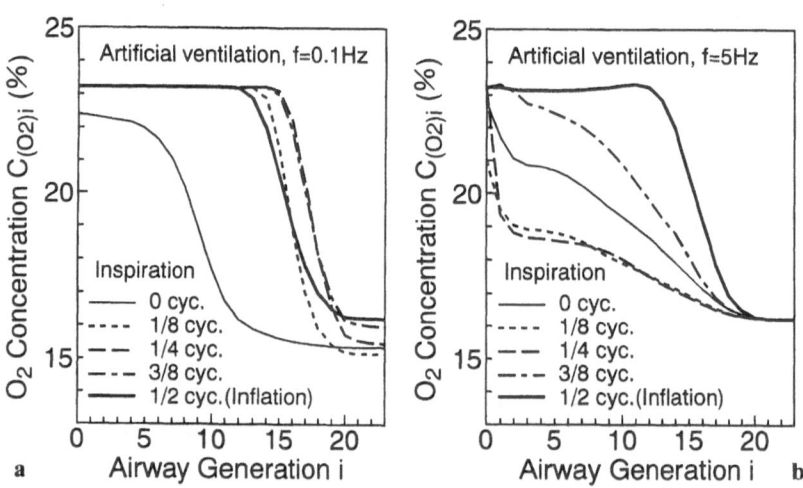

FIG. 11a,b. Distribution of oxygen concentration along airway during inspiration. **a** At frequency of 0.1 Hz. **b** At frequency of 5 Hz

FIG. 12a–c. Peak-to-peak pressure amplitude to maintain normal CO_2 exhaust at various frequencies of oscillation and resultant tidal volume and volumetric blood flow. **a** Peak-to-peak amplitude of applied gas pressure P_{or}. **b** Tidal volume V_T. **c** Blood flow ratio Q_b/Q_{bNorm} to that normal respiration

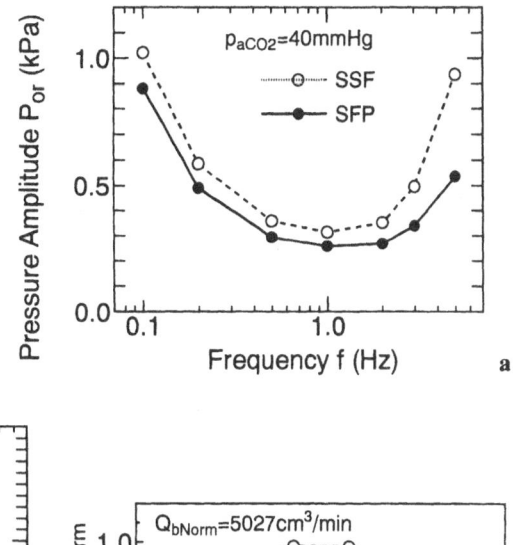

a

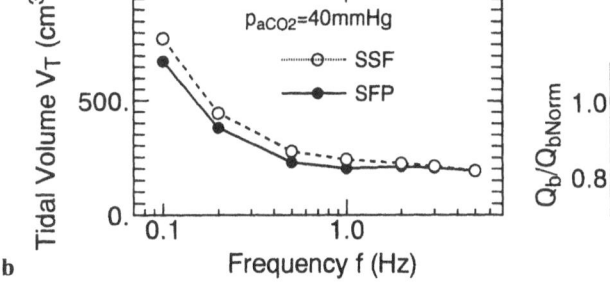

b

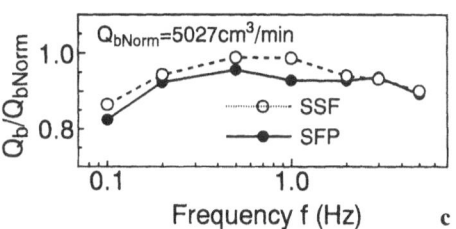

c

tion airway at 5 Hz. That is, the augmented diffusion described in Section 2.3.1 is effective for the high-frequency oscillation, which makes it possible to ventilate with a small tidal volume.

Figure 12a,b shows the peak-to-peak amplitude of inhaled gas pressure and the resultant tidal volume to maintain normal CO_2 exhaust by artificial ventilation at several frequencies. A higher frequency of oscillation promotes gas transport in the airway and decreases the necessary tidal volume, as mentioned earlier. However, the pressure amplitude to ensure the same tidal volume increases as frequency increases because of the gas flow dynamics in the airway. As the result of the interaction between the ventilation effect and breathing dynamics the pressure amplitude to maintain the normal CO_2 exhaust level becomes a minimum at a frequency of 1 Hz for both pressure patterns. In terms of preventing mechanical damage of the lung, minimization of the gas pressure is a criterion for determining optimal ventilation parameters.

5.3 Effect of Pressure Pattern

The pressure pattern also affects the ventilation status, and the SFP oscillation pattern lowers the pressure amplitude to maintain the CO_2 exhaust level over the frequency range (Fig. 12). The reason why the SFP pressure pattern rather than the SSP pattern is effective in reducing the pressure amplitude is interpreted from

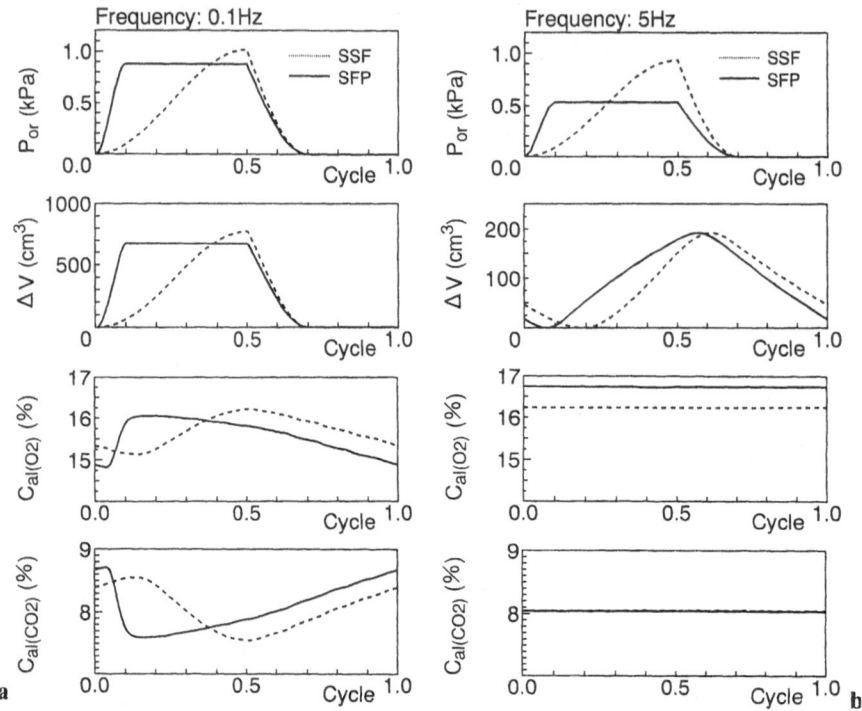

FIG. 13.a,b. Change of lung volume ΔV, alveolar oxygen concentration $C_{al(O_2)}$ and carbon dioxide concentration $C_{al(CO_2)}$ depending on the pressure pattern. **a** At low frequency of 0.1 Hz. **b** At high frequency of 5 Hz

the simulation results as follows. Figure 13 shows the lung volume change and gas concentration in the alveolar space succeeding the pressure oscillation at 0.1 Hz and 5 Hz. The change of lung volume follows the applied gas pressure in an oscillation pattern similar to that at the low frequency, 0.1 Hz. The rapid inspiration and subsequent holding period in the case of the SFP pressure pattern make gas diffusion in the peripheral airway sufficient, which reduces the necessary tidal volume resulting in lower pressure amplitude. On the other hand, the phase lag between the pressure and volume change invalidates the advantage of gas transport in the SFP pressure pattern at the high frequency of 5 Hz. However, the holding period of SFP pressure pattern moderates the phase lag of the gas flow dynamics as compared with the case of SSP pattern, lowering the pressure amplitude.

It should be recognized that gas pressure applied to the lung affects the blood flow in the lung and reduces the ability of gas carriage by the blood circulation. The decrease of blood flow depends not only on the magnitude of the applied gas pressure but also on its wave pattern, and the blood flow of the SFP pressure pattern is less than that of the SSF pattern (Fig. 12c). In this simulation, the normal healthy lung is ventilated with a relatively low pressure amplitude, and therefore the decrease of blood flow does not significantly disturb the gas exchange. In the case of a diseased lung that needs a high gas pressure to ventilate, it is necessary to pay attention to the circulation blockage effect of the SFP pressure pattern.

6 Conclusion

In this chapter, a mechanical model of lung respiration consisting of the breathing process, the pulmonary circulation process, and the gas exchange process was established by assembling the mathematical model for each mechanical phenomenon in the processes, and the capability of the simulation approach using the respiratory model was discussed in terms of computational biomechanics.

Simulation using the respiratory model represents not only the element phenomena but also the overall behavior of lung respiration. The mathematical model for each element was verified through the system behavior, which was observed by experiment. Through case studies compared with experimental observations, it was demonstrated that the simulation based on the mechanical model enables us to express the system behavior from the element details and to identify the internal phenomena of the lung respiration that could not be directly observed by experiment. This is an analysis by synthesis in terms of computational biomechanics, and it allows investigation of the complex respiratory system.

As an application of the simulation approach for the clinical field, artificial ventilation was simulated and the applied pressure condition to retain normal ventilation was investigated, taking into account both the ventilation function by breathing and the circulation function by blood flow. The model-based approach of the simulation gave a fundamental assessment for the conventional technique, and it was demonstrated that a holding period after inspiration was effective to reduce the pressure amplitude, although the mechanism differs according to the frequency of oscillation.

Because the repiratory model was built up from fundamental mechanical phenomena, it is possible to incorporate different values of geometry and different material properties into the model. The simulation based on personal properties allows us to compare experimental data of different species and to handle differences due to individuality. Such a personalized insight into the simulation is a key to evolve the computational biomechanical findings toward agreement with those in the clinical field.

Acknowledgment. The authors wish to thank Dr. H. Togari of Nagoya City University, Prof. T. Karino of Hokkaido University, and Profs T. Horikawa and H. Nakamura of Ryukoku University for their encouragement. This work was supported in part by Grant-in-aid for Scientific Research on Priority Areas (No. 05221237 and No. 06213235) and Grant-in-aid for Encouragement of Young

Scientists (No. 06780738) from the Ministry of Education, Science & Culture of Japan.

References

1. Fung YC (1981) Biomechanics. Springer-Verlag, New York
2. Fredberg JJ, Horning A (1978) Mechanical response of the lungs at high frequencies. Trans ASME J Biomech Eng 100:57–65
3. Shore DL, Tabrizi M (1983) Acoustic modeling of lung dynamics using bond graphs. Trans ASME J Biomech Eng 105:84–91
4. Fung YC (1975) Stress, deformation, and atelectasis of the lung. Circ Res 37:481–496
5. Hoshimiya N, Tanaka M, Matsuo T (1974) Finite-length collapsible-tube of the check-valve in expiration. Jpn J Med Electron Biol Eng 12(6):41–48
6. Fung YC, Sobin SS (1969) Theory of sheet flow in lung alveoli. J Appl Physiol 26(4):427–488
7. Seguchi Y, Fung YC, Maki H (1984) Computer simulation of dynamics of fluid-gas-tissue systems with a discretization procedure and its application to respiration dynamics. In: Fung YC, Fukada E, Wang JJ (eds) Biomechanics in China, Japan, and USA. Chinese Science Press, Beijing, pp 224–239
8. Seguchi Y, Fung YC, Ishida T (1986) Respiratory dynamics-computer simulation. In: Schmid-Schonbein GW, Woo SLY, Zweifach BM (eds) Frontiers in biomechanics. Springer-Verlag, New York, pp 377–391
9. Wada S, Seguchi Y, Tanaka M, Fung YC (1988) Simulation of respiratory dynamics considering breathing and ventilation. In: Miller GR (ed) Advances in bioengineering, BED-8. American Society of Mechanical Engineers, New York, pp 135–138
10. Seguchi Y, Wada S, Fung YC, Tanaka M (1989) Simulation of combined breathing and ventilation of a lung. In: Fung YC, Hayashi K, Seguchi Y (eds) Progress and new direction of biomechanics. Mita Press, Tokyo, pp 171–181
11. Wada S, Seguchi Y, Tanaka M (1990) Simulation of breathing and ventilation combined with body circulation. In: Goldstein SA (ed) 1990 Advances in bioengineering, BED-17. American Society of Mechanical Engineers, New York, pp 67–70
12. Wada S, Seguchi Y, Tanaka M (1991) Breathing-ventilation model, and simulation of high-frequency ventilation. Jpn Soc Mech Eng Int J I-34(1):98–105
13. Wada S, Seguchi Y, Tanaka M, Matsuda M, Adachi T, Fujigaki M (1991) Parameter identification for respiratory dynamics by personalized simulation and experiment. Jpn Soc Mech Eng Int J I-35(2):170–178
14. Wada S, Tanaka M (1995) Coupled behavior of lung respiration: computational respiratory mechanics approach. In: Power H (ed) Bio-fluid mechanics. Computational Mechanics, Southampton, pp 219–264
15. Fung YC (1974) A theory of elasticity of the lung. Trans ASME J Biomech Eng 41:8–14
16. Vawter DL, Fung YC, West JB (1979) Constitutive equation of lung tissue elasticity. Trans ASME J Biomech Eng 101:38–45
17. Clements JA, Tierney DF (1965) Alveolar instability associated with altered surface tension. In: Fenn WO, Rahn H (eds) Handbook of physiology, vol 3. American Physiology Society, Washington, DC, pp 1565–1583
18. Bachofen H, Hildebrandt J, Bachofen M (1970) Pressure-volume curves of air- and liquid-filled excised lung: surface tension in situ. J Appl Physiol 29(4):422–431

19. Vawter DL, Shields WH (1982) Deformation of the lung: the role of interfacial forces. In: Gallagher RH, Simon BR, Johnson PC, Gross JF (eds) Finite elements in biomechanics. Wiley, New York, pp 84–110
20. Weibel ER (1963) Morphometry of the human lung. Springer-Verlag, New York
21. Streeter VL, Wylie EB (1967) Hydraulic transients. McGraw-Hill, New York
22. Singhal S, Henderson R, Horsfield K, Harding K, Cumming G (1973) Morphometry of the human pulmonary arterial tree. Circ Res 33:190–197
23. Horsfield K, Gordon WI (1981) Morphometry of pulmonary veins in man. Lung 159:211–218
24. Fredberg JJ (1980) Augmented diffusion in the airways can support pulmonary gas exchange. J Appl Physiol Respir Environ Exercise Physiol 48(3):710–716
25. Forster RE (1957) Exchange of gases between alveolar air and pulmonary capillary blood: pulmonary diffusing capacity. Physiol Rev 37(4):391–542
26. Drazen JM, Kamm RD, Slutsky AS (1984) High-frequency ventilation. Physiol Rev 64(2):505–543
27. Watson EJ (1983) Diffusion in oscillatory pipe flow. J Fluid Mech 133:233–244
28. Gomez DM (1961) Considerations of oxygen-hemoglobin equilibrium in the physiological state. Am J Physiol 200(1):135–142
29. Fung YC (1990) Biomechanics: motion, flow, stress, and growth. Springer-Verlag, New York
30. Zhuang FY, Fung YC, Yen RT (1983) Analysis of blood flow in cat's lung with detailed anatomical and elasticity data. J Appl Physiol Respir Environ Exercise Physiol 55(4):1341–1348
31. Piene H (1986) Pulmonary arterial impedance and right ventricular function. Physiol Rev 66(3):606–652
32. Pinsky MR (1990) The effects of mechanical ventilation on the cardiovascular system. Crit Care Clin 6(3):663–678
33. Zeng YJ, Yager D, Fung YC (1987) Measurement of the mechanical properties of the human lung tissue. Trans ASME J Biomech Eng 109:169–174
34. Schurch S (1982) Surface tension at low lung volumes: dependence on time and alveolar size. Respir Physiol 48:339–355
35. Smith JC, Stamenovic D (1986) Surface forces in lung: I Alveolar surface tension-lung volume relationships. J Appl Physiol 60(4):1341–1350
36. Wagner PD (1977) Diffusion and chemical reaction in pulmonary gas exchange. Physiol Rev 57(2):257–312
37. Staub NC, Bishop JM, Forster RE (1962) Importance of diffusion and chemical reactions in O_2 uptake in the lung. J Appl Physiol 17:21–27

Subject Index